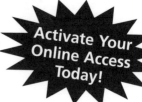

theclinics.com

# PHYSICAL MEDICINE AND REHABILITATION CLINICS OF NORTH AMERICA

## Multiple Sclerosis: A Paradigm Shift

GUEST EDITORS
Theodore R. Brown, MD, MPH,
George H. Kraft, MD, MS

CONSULTING EDITOR
George H. Kraft, MD, MS

May 2005 • Volume 16 • Number 2

**SAUNDERS**

An Imprint of Elsevier, Inc.
PHILADELPHIA   LONDON   TORONTO   MONTREAL   SYDNEY   TOKYO

W.B. SAUNDERS COMPANY
A Division of Elsevier Inc.

1600 John F. Kennedy Blvd. • Suite 1800 • Philadelphia, Pennsylvania 19103

http://www.theclinics.com

PHYSICAL MEDICINE AND REHABILITATION     Volume 16, Number 2
CLINICS OF NORTH AMERICA     ISSN 1047-9651
May 2005     ISBN 1-4160-2867-6
Editor: Molly Jay

Physical Medicine and Rehabilitation Clinics of North America (ISSN 1047-9651) is published quarterly by W.B. Saunders Company, Corporate and Editorial Offices: 1600 John F. Kennedy Blvd., Suite 1800, Philadelphia, PA 19103-2899. Accounting and Circulation Offices: 6277 Sea Harbor Drive, Orlando, FL 32887-4800. Periodicals postage paid at Orlando, FL 32862, and additional mailing offices. Subscription price per year is $155.00 (US individuals), $238.00 (US institutions), $78.00 (US students), $188.00 (Canadian individuals), $305.00 (Canadian institutions), $108.00 (Canadian students), $215.00 (foreign individuals), $305.00 (foreign institutions), and $108.00 (foreign students). Foreign air speed delivery is included in all Clinics subscription prices. All prices are subject to change without notice. POSTMASTER: Send address changes to Physical Medicine and Rehabilitation Clinics of North America, W.B. Saunders Company, Periodicals Fulfillment, Orlando, FL 32887-4800. Customer Service: 1-800-654-2452 (US). From outside of the US, call 1-407-345-4000.

Physical Medicine and Rehabilitation Clinics of North America is indexed in Excerpta Medica, Index Medicus, Cinahl, and Cumulative Index to Nursing and Allied Health Literature.

Printed in the United States of America.

# CONSULTING EDITOR

**GEORGE H. KRAFT, MD, MS,** Professor, Department of Rehabilitation Medicine; Adjunct Professor of Neurology; Director, Electrodiagnostic Medicine, Multiple Sclerosis Clinical Center; and Co-Director, Muscular Dystrophy Clinic, The University of Washington, Seattle, Washington

# GUEST EDITORS

**THEODORE R. BROWN, MD, MPH,** Clinical Assistant Professor, Department of Rehabilitation Medicine, University of Washington School of Medicine; MS Hub Medical Group, Seattle, Washington

**GEORGE H. KRAFT, MD, MS,** Professor, Department of Rehabilitation Medicine; Adjunct Professor of Neurology; Director, Electrodiagnostic Medicine, Multiple Sclerosis Clinical Center; and Co-Director, Muscular Dystrophy Clinic, The University of Washington, Seattle, Washington

# CONTRIBUTORS

**CHARLES H. BOMBARDIER, PhD,** Associate Professor, Multiple Sclerosis Rehabilitation Research and Training Center, Department of Rehabilitation Medicine, University of Washington School of Medicine, Harborview Medical Center, Seattle, Washington

**JAMES BOWEN, MD,** Associate Professor, Department of Neurology, University of Washington, Seattle, Washington

**THEODORE R. BROWN, MD, MPH,** Clinical Assistant Professor, Department of Rehabilitation Medicine, University of Washington School of Medicine; MS Hub Medical Group, Seattle, Washington

**JACK S. BURKS, MD,** Clinical Professor of Medicine (Neurology), University of Nevada School of Medicine, Reno, Nevada; Vice President and Chief Medical Officer, Multiple Sclerosis Association of America, Cherry Hill, New Jersey; President, Multiple Sclerosis Alliance, Englewood, Colorado; President, Burks & Associates, Reno, Nevada

**JIMMY Y. CUI, MD, PhD,** Clinical Assistant Professor, Department of Rehabilitation Medicine, University of Washington, Seattle, Washngton

**DAWN M. EHDE, PhD,** Associate Professor, Department of Rehabilitation Medicine, University of Washington School of Medicine, Harborview Medical Center, Seattle, Washington

ROBERT T. FRASER, PhD, Professor, Departments of Neurology and Rehabilitation Medicine, University of Washington School of Medicine, Seattle, Washington

JODIE K. HASELKORN, MD, MPH, Director, MS Center of Excellence West, Veterans Health Administration, VA Puget Sound Health Care System; Associate Professor, Department of Rehabilitation Medicine; Adjunct Associate Professor, Department of Epidemiology, University of Washington, Seattle, Washington

MARK P. JENSEN, PhD, Professor, Department of Rehabilitation Medicine, University of Washington School of Medicine, Harborview Medical Center; and Multidisciplinary Pain Center, University of Washington Medical Center–Roosevelt, Seattle, Washington

KURT L. JOHNSON, PhD, CRC, Associate Professor and Head, Division of Rehabilitation Counseling, Department of Rehabilitation Medicine, University of Washington, Seattle, Washington

ESTELLE R. KLASNER, PhD, Instructor, Rehabilitation Medicine, University of Washington, Seattle, Washington

GEORGE H. KRAFT, MD, MS, Professor, Department of Rehabilitation Medicine; Adjunct Professor of Neurology; Director, Electrodiagnostic Medicine, Multiple Sclerosis Clinical Center; and Co-Director, Muscular Dystrophy Clinic, The University of Washington, Seattle, Washington

LAUREN B. KRUPP, MD, Professor of Neurology, Director, National Pediatric Multiple Sclerosis Center, State University of New York at Stony Brook, Stony Brook, New York

JOHN F. KURTZKE, MD, Consultant in Neurology and Neuroepidemiology, Neurology Service, Veterans Affairs Medical Center; Professor Emeritus, Department of Neurology, Georgetown University School of Medicine, Washington, DC

CHIARA LAROTONDA, MSW, Research Coordinator, Multiple Sclerosis Rehabilitation Research and Training Center, Department of Rehabilitation Medicine, University of Washington School of Medicine, Harborview Medical Center, Seattle, Washington

SHARON LOOMIS, MD, Director, Inpatient Rehabilitation, VA Puget Sound Health Care System; Clinical Associate Professor, Department of Rehabilitation Medicine, University of Washington, Seattle, Washington

WILLIAM S. MacALLISTER, PhD, Assistant Professor of Research/Neurology; Director of Pediatric MS Research, National Pediatric Multiple Sclerosis Center, State University of New York at Stony Brook, Stony Brook, New York

TRAVIS L. OSBORNE, PhD, Postdoctoral Fellow, Department of Rehabilitation Medicine, University of Washington School of Medicine, Harborview Medical Center, Seattle, Washington

MARY PEPPING, PhD, Associate Professor, Department of Rehabilitation Medicine, University of Washington School of Medicine, Seattle, Washington

JACK H. SIMON, MD, PhD, Professor of Radiology, Neurology, Neurosurgery, Psychiatry; Vice Chairman-Radiology, University of Colorado Health Sciences Center, Denver, Colorado

**KATHRYN M. YORKSTON, PhD, BC-NCD,** Professor and Head, Division of Speech Pathology, Rehabilitation Medicine, University of Washington, Seattle, Washington

**ROHINI WADHWANI, BS,** Research Care Manager, Multiple Sclerosis Rehabilitation Research and Training Center, Department of Rehabilitation Medicine, University of Washington School of Medicine, Harborview Medical Center, Seattle, Washington

# CONTENTS

> The geographic distribution of multiple sclerosis (MS) has changed markedly in the last 50 years. Migrants from high MS areas to low MS areas keep the risk of their birthplace, only if they move after age 15; those who move from low to high MS areas increase their risk of MS even beyond that of their new homeland for moves between birth and age 40 or so. MS occurred in the Faroe Islands as successive epidemics following the occupation by British troops in World War II. All of these findings are compatible with the view that clinical MS is the rare result of a unique, but unknown, widespread persistent infection that is acquired most often between age 11 and 45 or so, and has a prolonged latent or incubation period between acquisition and clinical disease.

> The precise cause of multiple sclerosis (MS) remains unknown, although immunopathologic studies provide solid evidence of participation of activated immune cells in the formation of MS lesions. Cell-mediated and antibody-mediated (humoral) immune responses are involved in the immunopathogenesis of MS. The Th1 and Th2 cells, by releasing a variety of pro- or anti-inflammatory cytokines, work in opposition to balance the immune response and

determine the net effect of the inflammation. Current understanding of immunopathogenesis shapes the contemporary approach as to the treatment of MS. The article also reviews the mechanisms of action of commonly used immunotherapy agents and their impact on the immune response of patients who have MS.

Resources and recommendations for health care providers to assist their patients in maintaining, securing, or leaving employment are presented.

Multiple sclerosis (MS) is a multifaceted condition that can be viewed from many perspectives. It is clear that the individual living with MS, the insider, has a somewhat different perspective than that of a physician or a physical or occupational therapist. The purpose of this article is to (1) review the literature related to the insider's experience of MS, focusing especially on taking part in valued activities; (2) suggest a model for understanding/measuring the adequacy of participation, including factors that may influence it and domains such as employment that are key to the construct; and (3) suggest strategies that health care providers can employ as mentors or partners in achieving the goal of full participation.

# FORTHCOMING ISSUES

# RECENT ISSUES

---

## VISIT OUR WEB SITE

The Clinics are now available online!
Access your subscription at **www.theclinics.com**

---

ELSEVIER
SAUNDERS

Phys Med Rehabil Clin N Am
16 (2005) xiii–xv

PHYSICAL MEDICINE
AND REHABILITATION
CLINICS OF
NORTH AMERICA

Foreword

# Multiple Sclerosis: A Paradigm Shift

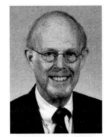

George H. Kraft, MD, MS
*Consulting Editor*

Several decades ago, physiatrists—trained in the comprehensive re-habilitation of patients with spinal cord injury, stroke, and other neurologic diseases—were not rehabilitating patients with multiple sclerosis (MS). One of the major reasons was that one of the pioneers in the field of rehabilitation medicine was reputed to have taught that rehabilitating patients with MS was essentially a waste of time and money—they would merely progress in their disability, and all of the effort would be for naught.

MS patients were generally diagnosed by neurologists, and because no medicines were available to control the disease, the prevailing philosophy of care was—as so pithily stated by one of the early MS specialists, Dr. Labe Scheinberg—"diagnose and adios." Consequently, neither physiatry nor neurology paid much attention to the rehabilitation of patients with this disease. Although rudimentary care was provided, care was mainly—as it was so euphemistically described—"supportive."

The situation is quite different now, and this is the theme of this issue of the *Physical Medicine and Rehabilitation Clinics of North America*. At the time of this writing, there are six FDA-approved medications available in the United States to modify the disease course, a host of agents effective in managing its multiple symptoms, and rehabilitation is recommended by the National MS Society (http://www.nmss.org).

This work was supported by the National Institute on Disability and Rehabilitation Research grant H133B031129-04.

MS care may be looked at as having three stages. Several decades ago, MS was considered to be a disease of ambulation. That was it. Indeed, the widely used Expanded Disability Status Scale (EDSS), developed by Dr. John Kurtzke, is mainly an ambulation measure at higher disability levels. Dr. Labe Scheinberg thought that because MS was a disease of ambulation, physiatrists should be involved in its management, and he recruited me. This might be considered Phase I: MS was a disease of ambulation.

The next phase—Phase II, occurring throughout the 1980s and early 1990s—came about through the work of investigators at the Albert Einstein School of Medicine MS Rehabilitation Research and Training Center (MSRRTC), under the leadership of the aforementioned Dr. Scheinberg. These investigators, along with others, identified many abnormalities other than the obvious ambulation impairment in patients with MS. Affected systems included cognition, memory, and emotional control, among others. The field of MS management was advanced as studies were performed of these and other symptomatic systems.

The University of Washington MSRRTC started in 1998, and is now at the beginning of its second 5-year term. Work done at this center suggests that the total disability of MS is more than the sum of each affected system. Evaluating the impairment in each system and adding them together often does not begin to describe the severity of the disability. Patients tend to do better on evaluation of individual systems than they do when all systems are forced to perform simultaneously—the multitasking of life, as it were. The gestalt is what is important.

An example of this is an MS patient with an EDSS of 6.5 who might ambulate safely with a cane when focusing on ambulation. However, when s/he is walking along and talking with a friend, s/he might trip and fall. As another example, a patient might perform very well as a schoolteacher but would need to spend an excessive amount of time preparing lessons and grading papers. Although the teacher was doing well in her/his vocation, s/he might have little energy left over for maintaining the home and caring for the family. If each of life's requirements were evaluated in isolation, s/he could do it well. But s/he could not sustain quality function in all areas over an extended period. It is as if such enormous energy must be expended on one aspect of life, that there is little left over for other areas. This may result in a paradigm shift in our understanding of this disease and help us understand why some patients who we think should do well just don't.

This first became apparent to us at the University of Washington MSRRTC when we looked at patients from the "insider's perspective"—a structured but open-ended interview process allowing subjects to describe how the disease affects them. We think that this may account for the surprising observation that well-educated and highly motivated persons with MS are employed at a much lower rate than would be expected.

These findings surprise some people, especially because verbal communication is preserved in most patients well into the advanced stages of the disease. Consequently, when such a patient is seen in a health professional's office, s/he may appear to be far better than s/he is ("But she talks so well...").

This awareness—that the sum of impairments leads to a greater disability gestalt than adding the impairments together—might be termed Phase III in our understanding of persons with MS. This may alter how we look at MS and how we care for patients who have this disease. Research from our MSRRTC discussing this explains the title of this issue.

I would like to thank my Co-Guest Editor, Ted Brown, MD, for his enormous help in editing this issue. Truly, without his able assistance, this issue would not have come about. I have had the highest regard for Dr. Brown for over a decade, beginning with his service as Chief Resident in our program. Subsequently, I followed his career during the time he spent in northern Thailand, where he assisted in the conversion of a leprisorium into a rehabilitation hospital, and later through his M.P.H studies at Berkley. I was pleased when he became the 2003–2004 multiple sclerosis Fellow at the University of Washington, and have been gratified that he has decided to devote his talents to the full-time care of MS patients.

In addition, I would like to thank all of the authors who have contributed to this issue of the *Physical Medicine and Rehabilitation Clinics of North America*; they have preformed a tremendous service in caring for persons who have MS. I hope that readers find this issue to be a valuable resource in the management of this disability.

George H. Kraft, MD, MS
*Department of Rehabilitation Medicine*
*University of Washington School of Medicine*
*1959 NE Pacific Ave, Box 356490*
*Seattle, WA 98195-6490, USA*

*E-mail address:* ghkraft@u.washington.edu

ELSEVIER
SAUNDERS

Phys Med Rehabil Clin N Am
16 (2005) xvii–xx

PHYSICAL MEDICINE
AND REHABILITATION
CLINICS OF
NORTH AMERICA

Preface

# Multiple Sclerosis: A Paradigm Shift

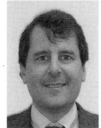 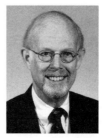

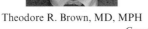

Theodore R. Brown, MD, MPH     George H. Kraft, MD, MS
*Guest Editors*

We are pleased to present this issue of the *Physical Medicine Rehabilitation clinics of North America* on multiple sclerosis (MS), and want to thank the distinguished authors, both from without and from within the University of Washington, who have contributed to this issue.

MS is a rapidly changing field. Only a little over 10 years ago, no FDA-approved immunomodifying agents were available for treating this disease. Research looked promising, but nothing was available.

Then, an explosion!

So much has happened in this field over the last 10 years. We now have six disease-modifying agents available, with much exciting research in progress. Furthermore, as readers of this issue will see, there are now new concepts in the understanding of the disease. This issue documents the current state of the science of MS care—and the thrust of research of the University of Washington MS Research and Training Center (MSRRTC).

This issue begins with an article by Dr. John Kurtzke, outlining some of his new concepts regarding the etiology of this disease. Dr. Kurtzke is the most distinguished of MS researchers—having both studied the patterns of the development of MS as well as developing the most widely used scale of MS severity, the Expanded Disability Status Scale. His epidemiologic

This work was supported in part by the United States Association project #659 and the Department of Education, National Institute on Disability and Rehabilitation Research grant #H133B031129-04.

studies of MS in the islands of the North Atlantic are legendary, and the first article of this issue contains an exciting and very convincing argument of his latest thoughts about the cause of this disease.

Following this, Jimmy Cui, MD, PhD, our first MS Fellow at the University of Washington, provides a very readable description of current concepts of the immunology and pathology of MS. James Bowen, MD, our esteemed colleague, MSRRTC researcher, and friend, then describes how to distinguish MS from those diseases often confused with it. Next, Dr. Jack Simon provides a salient description of radiologic imaging in the various stages of MS and how it can assist in the diagnosis and management of this disease.

One of the major developments of the past two decades is the awareness that MS is more than just a disease of ambulation—it affects cognition and emotion as well. Drs. Mary Pepping and Dawn Ehde of the MSRRTC provide an outstanding discussion on cognitive impairment, while Dr. Charles Bombardier and Dr. Ehde discuss depression, including many practical suggestions regarding diagnosis and management.

We are pleased that our good friend Dr. Jack Burks helped us address the practical application of the many disease-modifying agents for MS. It is somewhat ironic that just over 10 years ago no medications were FDA-approved for modifying the course of MS; now there are six, and physicians and patients need assistance in determining which ones to use.

Of all of the disabling symptoms of MS—and among the most refractory to treatment—are tremor and spasticity. We are indebted to the Director of the Department of Veterans Affairs MS Center of Excellence West, Jodie Haselkorn, MD, MPH, for her description of the management of these symptoms. Fatigue is another important MS symptom—not mentioned until our studies of the 1980s—that is discussed in this issue by two leaders in the field: Drs. Lauren Krupp and William MacAllister. Dr. Krupp has done more than anyone else in taking the study of fatigue to the next level of understanding.

Pain is a huge problem in some patients with MS. Although it has come under scrutiny only recently, pain can be the most devastating of MS symptoms. We need new methods of managing it, and Dr. Mark Jensen and Dr. Ehde from our research group offer us new insights on management techniques. The comprehensive article on exercise and rehabilitation gives details of these management techniques.

The last three articles expand on the work of the University of Washington MSRRTC, which is discussed in the Foreword for this issue. These articles discuss Phase III: the new paradigm in the understanding of MS. Drawing from our interest in nonpharmacologic treatment of the symptoms and complications of MS, Dr. Bombardier and colleagues from our research group present our approach to wellness promotion. Drs. Kathryn Yorkston, Kurt Johnson, and Estelle Klasner eloquently present the concept of participation in MS as the ultimate assessment of function (see the discussion of Phase III in the Foreword). Drs. Johnson and Fraser then discuss the issues of employment and MS.

MS is a complex disease, and the patient-centered, Phase III management-oriented approach of this issue is beholden to the basic research preceeding it. It seems fitting to pay credit to the creatures who have allowed us to learn so much about it. Much of what is known about the immune process of MS has been acquired through experimentation and inference using an animal model of the disease. In experimental autoimmune encephalomyelitis (EAE), rodents are injected with murine spinal cord homogenate in complete Freund's adjuvant which contains killed *Mycobacterium tuberculosis*. The inflammatory response in the host central nervous system may cause acute monophasic illness with paralysis or a chronic progressive form of paralysis. We have learned that this disease is T cell–mediated, because the brains of mice with EAE become infiltrated with T cells and because cloned T helper cell ($T_H1$) lines from an EAE mouse can produce the same response when transferred to an unexposed syngeneic mouse. Feeding myelin basic protein to mice before the inflammatory exposure causes a shift toward anti-inflammatory T cell lines ($T_H2$ bias) that inhibits development of the disease [1]. EAE research has already yielded two FDA-approved disease-modifying drugs for MS. First was glatiramer acetate (Copaxone), which has molecular homology with myelin basic protein, a key constituent of central nervous system myelin. Recently, the cell adhesion molecule inhibitor natalizumab (Tysabri®) has also sprung from the EAE model into the repertoire of disease-modifying MS therapies.

EAE is not a perfect model for MS, however, as several drug trials have shown. For example, tissue necrosis factor alpha (TNF-α) triggers signals for cell proliferation and apoptosis in the induction of an immune response. TNF-α inhibitors showed a distinctly ameliatory effect on pathogenesis and demyelination in EAE and in the treatment of at least one autoimmune disease (rheumatoid arthritis). In contrast, human MS trials of TNF-α inhibitors demonstrated a paradoxical increase in inflammatory markers as measured by MRI and cerebrospinal fluid pleocytosis and increase in number of clinical exacerbations. [2] Recently, examination of the initial stages of the destructive disease process in MS has been achieved in a small number of patients with relapsing remitting MS. Apoptotic oligodendrocyte death in a circumscribed and relatively small area was discovered preceding leukocyte infiltration and demyelination in 7 of 12 cases [3]. This novel finding questions basic concepts of the pathogenesis of MS. In the words of Bruce Trapp, "It is time to ask ourselves if modeling all aspects of MS after experimental allergic encephalomyelitis is justified or prudent... there is a true missing link in our understanding of MS and we must be open to surprises" [4]. Although mechanisms of T cell–mediated demyelination have been described in detail in EAE, the corresponding mechanism by which the immune system is tricked into seeing myelin as foreign in MS patients has been elusive. The investigators who quarry this prey will be deserving of the Nobel Prize.

The relationship between EAE and MS may be akin to that between mouse and man. We can learn something about the one from the other, but never approach a full understanding in this manner. The words of Francis Peabody come to mind: "Disease in man is never exactly the same disease in an experimental animal, for in man the disease at once affects and is affected by what we call the emotional life" (ie, the human experience) [5].

This issue of the *Physical Medicine and Rehabilitation Clinics of North America* contains an up-to-date discussion of MS and its immunologic, radiologic, physical, psychologic, and social ramifications. We hope that it will help you to treat people with MS and that it will encourage you toward further discovery—for there are many more mysteries waiting to be unraveled before we find the cure.

Theodore R. Brown, MD, MPH
*MS Hub Medical Group*
*1100 Olive Way, Suite 150*
*Seattle, WA 98101 USA*

*E-mail address:* berktocm@yahoo.com

George H. Kraft, MD, MS
*Department of Rehabilitation Medicine*
*University of Washington School of Medicine*
*1959 NE Pacific Ave, Box 356490*
*Seattle, WA 98195-6490, USA*

*E-mail address:* ghkraft@u.washington.edu

## References

[1] Janeway CA, Travers P, Walport M, editors. Immunobiology. 50th edition. New York: Garland Publishing; 2001.
[2] Wiendl H, Hohlfeld R. Therapeutic approaches in multiple sclerosis: lessons from failed and interrupted treatment trials. BioDrugs 2002;16:183–200.
[3] Barnett MH, Prineas JW. Relapsing and remitting multiple sclerosis: pathology of the newly forming lesion. Ann Neurol 2004;55:458–68.
[4] Trapp BD. Pathogenesis of multiple sclerosis: the eyes only see what the mind is prepared to comprehend. Ann Neurol 2004;55:455–7.
[5] Peabody FW. The care of the patient. Oxford (UK): Oxford University Press; 2004 [quoted in *The Oxford Dictionary of Medical Quotations* by Peter McDonald].

ELSEVIER
SAUNDERS

Phys Med Rehabil Clin N Am
16 (2005) 327–349

PHYSICAL MEDICINE
AND REHABILITATION
CLINICS OF
NORTH AMERICA

# Epidemiology and Etiology of Multiple Sclerosis

## John F. Kurtzke, MD*

*Neurology Service, Veterans Affairs Medical Center, Washington, DC*

The generally accepted view is that multiple sclerosis (MS) primarily is an autoimmune disease that is precipitated by undefined environmental factors in a genetically predisposed host. The author's interpretation of the epidemiologic information, however, is that the "environmental factors" include the principal cause of this illness. Epidemiologic works are concerned with the frequency of diseases, and their characteristics by race, sex, geography, and other risk factors, as well as with the severity and course of the illness. Such information is needed and should be used by all aspects of the health care system, from government to clinician. The epidemiologic unit is a person who has a given disorder. After diagnosis, the basic question is "How common is the disease?" This frequency should be described by the best count of the number of cases as the numerator within the specific populations at risk as the denominator. These ratios, with the addition of the time period to which they pertain, are referred to as rates.

The population-based rates that are in common use are the incidence rate, the mortality rate, and the prevalence "rate." The incidence or attack rate is defined as the number of new cases of the disease beginning clinically in a unit of time within the specified population. Usually, this is given as an annual incidence rate in cases per 100,000 population per year. The mortality or death rate refers to the number of deaths with the disease as the (underlying) cause of death that occur within a unit of time and population, and thus, an annual death rate per 100,000 population. The point prevalence "rate" more properly is called a prevalence ratio, and it refers to the number of the affected within the community at one point in time, again expressed per unit of population.

The Association for Research in Nervous and Mental Disease meets annually in New York to present a symposium on one specific topic. Their

---

* 7509 Salem Road, Falls Church, VA 22043-3240.
*E-mail address:* kurtzke2@aol.com

1047-9651/05/$ - see front matter © 2005 Elsevier Inc. All rights reserved.
doi:10.1016/j.pmr.2005.01.013
*pmr.theclinics.com*

first session in 1920 dealt with von Economo's encephalitis. The second was
on MS; this was the first comprehensive assessment of MS in the United
States (references to this and other uncited works are in [1]). The
Commission concluded that MS affected chiefly young adults and men
more than women. Duration averaged 8 years, and it seemed to affect skilled
manual workers more often. Geographically, in the United States it was
most common near the Great Lakes, whereas in Europe is was more
common in the north than in the south. The male excess was found for most
of the European studies and all those from the United States, with an overall
average of 3:2 (male:female).

Male preponderance also was seen for MS death rates near 1960 in the
United States, but only among those of older age. White women were clearly
in excess at younger ages (Fig. 1) [2]. Incidence and prevalence rates in
Denmark near 1950 had a similar pattern, with higher rates for women
among the younger patients and equal rates by sex in the older ones. An
increasing excess of women in Denmark has characterized the incidence
rates for more than 50 years, however. Two regions of Norway also
demonstrated a growing female excess over time. Sweden also has shown an
increasingly higher majority among women [3]. By 1980, white women had
the highest death rates in the United States at all ages (Fig. 2). Young black
women seemed then to have rates similar to the whites.

We studied MS in the United States among some 5300 veterans of World
War II or the Korean Conflict, who were service connected by the
Department of Veterans Affairs (VA) for MS. They were matched with
preillness peers from the military. White women had nearly twice the risk of
MS as the white men, with a relative risk ratio of 1.79. There seems to have
been a change from a disorder that affected men more often to one that

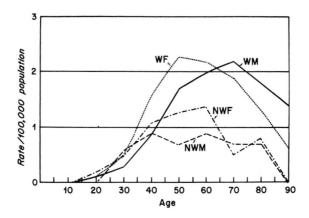

Fig. 1. Average annual age specific death rates per 100,000 population for multiple sclerosis by
sex and color, United States 1959–1961. F, female; M, male; NW, nonwhite; W, white.
(*Modified from* Kurland LT, Kurtzke JF, Goldberg ID. Epidemiology of neurologic and sense
organ disorders. Cambridge (MA): Harvard University Press; 1973. p. 70; with permission.)

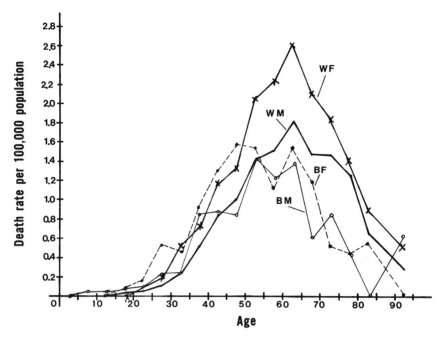

Fig. 2. Average annual age specific death rates per 100,000 population for MS by sex and race, United States 1979–1981. B, black; F, female; M, male; W, white. (*From* Kurtzke JF. Epidemiology of multiple sclerosis. Does this really point toward an etiology? Neurol Sci 2000;21:386; with permission.)

shows an increasing preponderance among women. The excess among whites versus those of other races persisted, however. Relative risk ratios were 0.44 for black males and 0.22 for other men (nonwhite, nonblack).

A more recent series is under study. This includes more than 5000 U.S. veterans with military service in the Vietnam War, or later, up to 1994, who also were service connected for MS by the VA, and who were matched on a 1:2 basis with military peers [4]. Women of all races, whether white, black, or other, now have a greater risk of MS than white men, with relative risk ratios of nearly 3 to 1. Black men have a significantly greater risk ratio of 0.67 than they showed in the World War II series, although their risk is still less than that of white men. Men of other races had little change, with a relative risk of 0.30. There has to be an environmental reason for the growing predominance of women who have MS. The changing ratios by race also suggest that these differences also are based more on environment than genes.

Geographic distributions are defined best by prevalence studies, of which there are now more than 300 for MS. Prevalence surveys from the 1960s to 1980 indicated that most of northern Europe was of high frequency, with rates of 30 or more per 100,000 population (Fig. 3) [5]. Southern Europe had a distinctly lower frequency, with rates reflecting medium frequency

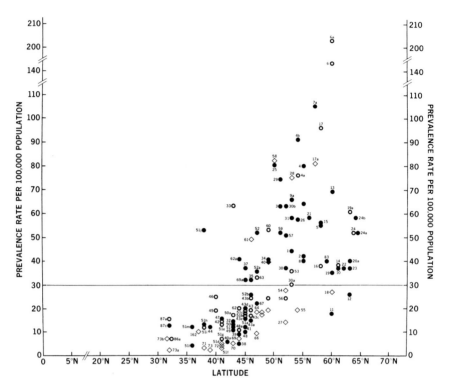

Fig. 3. Prevalence rates per 100,000 population for probable MS in Europe and the Mediterranean area as of 1980, correlated with geographic latitude. Solid circles represent class A (best) studies, open circles represent class B (good) studies, open diamonds represent class C (poor, cited only when there is no better survey for the site). Numbers identify specific surveys in the references below. (*From* Kurtzke JF. Geographic distribution of multiple sclerosis: an update with special reference to Europe and the Mediterranean region. Acta Neurol Scand 1980;62:70; and Kurtzke JF. A reassessment of the distribution of multiple sclerosis. Part One, Part Two. Acta Neurol Scand 1975;51:110–57; with permission.)

(5 to 29 per 100,000). The pattern was similar in North America, with high rates in Canada and the northern United States, whereas the southern United States had a medium frequency. Southeastern Australia had a high frequency whereas the rest of the country had a medium frequency. New Zealand also was in the high range, whereas Asia had a low frequency (prevalence less than 5 per 100,000 population).

Prevalence studies, however, are mostly "spot surveys" of small areas, and may tell little about areas that are not examined. Nationwide surveys by one team at one time permit complete geographic coverage. When such studies are repeated at a later time, we also can see if distributions have changed. The country of Denmark was surveyed twice, the old series for 1921 to 1933 disability cases, the new for 1949 prevalence. Rates were maximal across the north-central part of the Jutland peninsula on to the island of Funen, just to the east. Switzerland also had two national estimates, the old one for 1918 to 1922, the new for 1956; both showed a strong northwestern geographic concentration. Norway also had two surveys over time; highest rates were noted in the southeast. When percentages by county of each national mean are compared between the old and the new series in each of these three countries, each are correlated highly (old versus new), but with the same regression line that shows a clear diffusion over time, with an intercept far off the 0 point on the X-axis (Fig. 4) [6].

Spread of MS may be from within this Fennoscandian focus of high frequency of MS, and from a source within the southern inland lake region of Sweden (Fig. 5). Spread from this region eastward to Finland, southward to the continent, and westward to Norway and then Denmark would provide the diffusion. Currently under investigation is whether the European spread outside of the Baltic region may have had its first dissemination with the movements of the army of King Gustav Adolf of Sweden into Germany from 1630 to 1632 during the Thirty Years War of 1618 to 1648 [7].

The long held view of a north-south gradient for MS may be little more than a reflection of this spread from Sweden—a different type of big bang theory. Compatible with this view is the finding that the high-frequency regions of France are mostly in the northeast and those of Switzerland are in the northwest. But this spread takes years. The prevalence rates (see Fig. 3) for Europe in 1980 were similar to those that were seen earlier. By 1994, however, there were major differences. Fig. 6 shows that the entire northern Mediterranean basin is now an area of high frequency; Portugal and Greece also now exhibit high frequency of MS, with prevalence rates per 100,000 population in the 40s. Diffusion is a hallmark of this disease.

The spread is not limited to Europe. In the United States, the World War II series showed a marked excess for residents in the north (Fig. 7). This was seen for both sexes among whites and for black men, with a north to south difference of almost 3 to 1. The Vietnam War and later service veterans still showed a gradient, but it was much less. All southern states were calculated to lie within the high-frequency zone, with prevalence rates that were estimated at well more than 30 per 100,000 population. For all races and sexes, the north to south difference was only 2 to 1.

In Asia and Africa, earlier assessments provided low prevalence rates—less than 5 per 100,000—except for English-speaking whites of South Africa, who had a medium prevalence. This distribution is now more complex. Rates are still low in the few surveys from Korea, China, and southeast Asia, but not in the former Soviet Union or in Japan. For the latter, two recent studies reported rates of 9 [8] and 10 [9] per 100,000, respectively. Boiko [10] of Moscow summarized prevalence studies from Russia and other parts of the former Soviet Union. In the southern region of the Ukraine, the Volga area, the Caucasus, and into Novosibirsk and

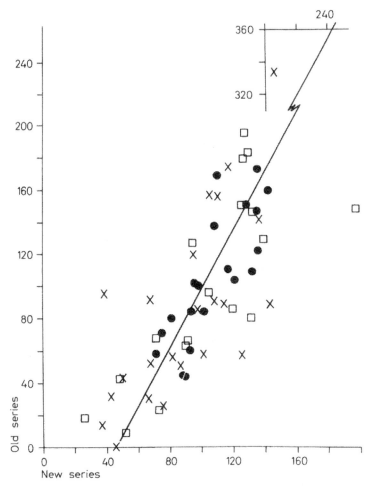

Fig. 4. Correlation of the distributions of MS by county between old series and new series of nationwide prevalence studies of three countries, each covering different generations of patients. Each county rate is expressed as the percentage of its respective national (mean) rates. ●, Denmark; □, Norway; X, Switzerland. (*From* Kurtzke JF. Further features of the Fennoscandian focus of multiple sclerosis. Acta Neurol Scand 1974;50:490; with permission.)

Kazakhstan, rates generally were in the medium prevalence range, whereas more easterly lands had a low prevalence. In easternmost Russia, medium rates reappeared, with high rates in parts of the Amur region near the Pacific Ocean north of China.

Now the southern littoral region of the Mediterranean has a medium prevalence, and the Canary Islands, Cyprus, and Israel have a high prevalence. In Latin America, the Caribbean region, including Mexico, also may have a medium frequency now, as well as Argentina, Brazil, Chile, Uruguay, and Peru, whereas Venezuela and Colombia may have a low

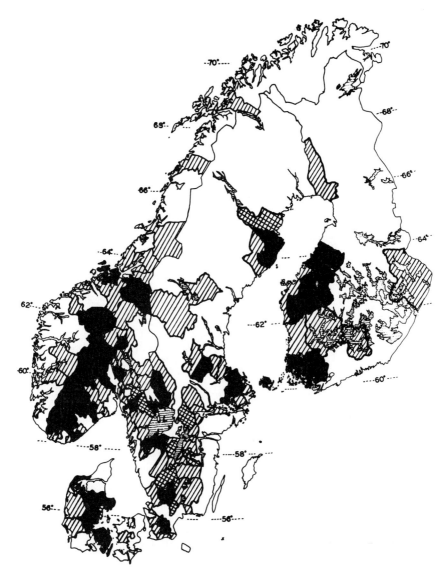

Fig. 5. Distribution of MS in Fennoscandia from nationwide surveys. Areas whose frequency of MS is significantly greater than their respective national means are in solid black; areas whose frequency of MS is increased, but of dubious statistical significance are cross-hatched; areas whose frequency of MS is insignificantly increased are diagonal-lined; and areas whose frequency of MS is less than the national mean are unshaded. Unit boundaries are omitted. Fine horizontal shading represents lakes in Sweden and Finland. (*From* Kurtzke JF. Further features of the Fennoscandian focus of multiple sclerosis. Acta Neurol Scand 1974;50:491; with permission.)

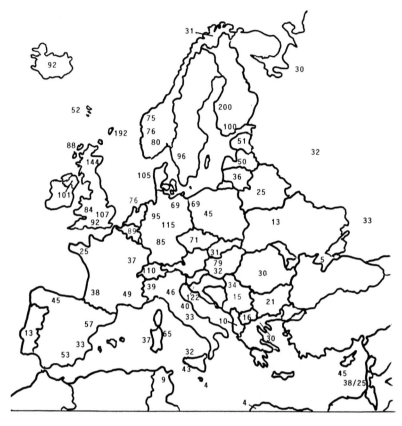

Fig. 6. Prevalence rates per 100,000 population for MS in Europe and the Mediterranean basin from publications 1980–1994. (*Modified from* Lauer K. Multiple sclerosis in the old world: the new map. In: Firnhaber W, Lauer K, editors. Multiple sclerosis in Europe. An epidemiological update. Darmstadt (Germany): LTV Press; 1994. p. 18.)

frequency. Even Cuba may have a high prevalence. Many of the Latin American studies, although well-done, have not appeared in the peer-reviewed literature.

The general worldwide distribution of MS still seems to be well-described by a division into three regions: high prevalence (30+ per 100,000 population), medium prevalence (5 to 29 per 100,000 population), and low prevalence (<5 per 100,000 population) (Fig. 8). With each iteration of this map in the last quarter century, the areas in white (unstudied) have shrunk appreciably, as expected; however, progressively more of the world has been marked in black (high prevalence).

The fate of migrants who move into regions of differing risk of MS is critical to our understanding of this disease. If migrants retain the risk of their birthplace, then either the disease is innate or it is acquired early in life.

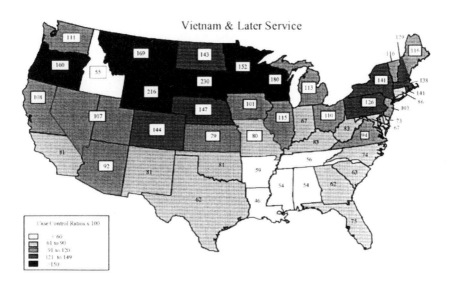

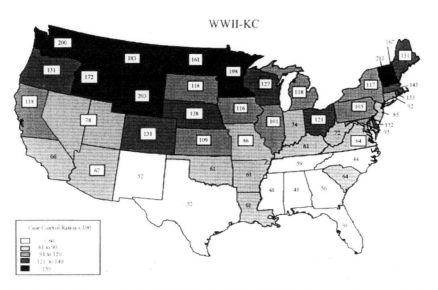

Fig. 7. Adjusted case control ratios (×100) for white male U.S. veterans service connected for MS by state of residence at entry into service. KC, Korean Conflict; WW II, World War II. (*From* Wallin MT, Page WF, Kurtzke JF. Multiple sclerosis in United States veterans of Vietnam era and later military service. 1. Race, sex and geography. Ann Neurol 2004;55:68; with permission.)

If they do change their risk upon moving, a major environmental cause or precipitant is active in their disorder well after birth.

MS-control ratios for birthplace and for preillness residence at service entry were compared for the white male veterans of World War II or

Korean service to assess migration. Ratios where these are the same locations (north-north, middle-middle, south-south tiers of residence) give MS:control ratios for nonmigrants; cells off this diagonal define the ratios for migrants. These nonmigrant ratios are 1.48 (north), 1.03 (middle), and 0.56 (south). For migrants, those who were born in the north and entered service from the middle tier have a ratio of 1.27. If they entered from the south, their ratio is 0.74, only half that of the nonmigrants. Birth in the middle tier is marked by an increase in the MS:control ratio for northern entrants to 1.40, and a decrease to 0.73 for the southern ones. Migration after birth in the south seems to increase the ratios to 0.65 (middle) and 0.70 (north). All of these changes except the last are statistically significant. The southern-born migrants were really too few to calculate valid ratios.

In a study of European immigrants to South Africa, the MS prevalence rate, adjusted to a population of all ages, was 13 per 100,000 for immigration under age 15; this was the same medium prevalence rate as native-born, English-speaking, white South Africans. For age groups that were older at immigration, the prevalence was 30 to 80 per 100,000, the same as expected from their high-risk homelands. This change was sharp and occurred at age 15 (Fig. 9). Each patient is represented by a bar, whose location on the Y-axis denotes age at immigration, and whose length on the X-axis shows the number of years between immigration and clinical onset. This also indicates that natives of high-risk areas are not susceptible to MS acquisition much before age 15, and that there is a long incubation period between acquisition and onset of symptoms.

Inferences as to the opposite migration (low-frequency areas to high-frequency areas), were afforded by the mostly white northern African migrants to France who came from Morocco, Tunisia, and especially Algeria. The migrants who had an onset of MS more than 1 year after immigration provided an age-adjusted MS prevalence rate that was 1.5 times greater than for all of France. If the rate for France is taken at 50 per 100,000 population, their adjusted rate is 77. The others who had presumed acquisition in northern Africa gave the same rate of 17 per 100,000 as expected for residents of those lands. For migrants who acquired MS in France, at each single year of age at migration there was a mean interval of 13 years between immigration or age 11 and clinical onset, with a minimum of 3 years. Only one of the four patients who had migrated after age 40 had had onset (at age 48) in France (Fig. 10). Note the solitary patient who migrated at 1 year of age and had the onset of symptoms at age 9; this supports the rarity of childhood MS.

The migrant series provide further support for the theses that MS primarily is an environmental disease that is acquired after childhood, and that acquisition requires prolonged or repeated exposure, followed by a prolonged latent or incubation period between acquisition and symptom onset.

The simplest explanation is that MS is the result of a geographically-delimited persistent infectious agent with a long latency and an age-limited

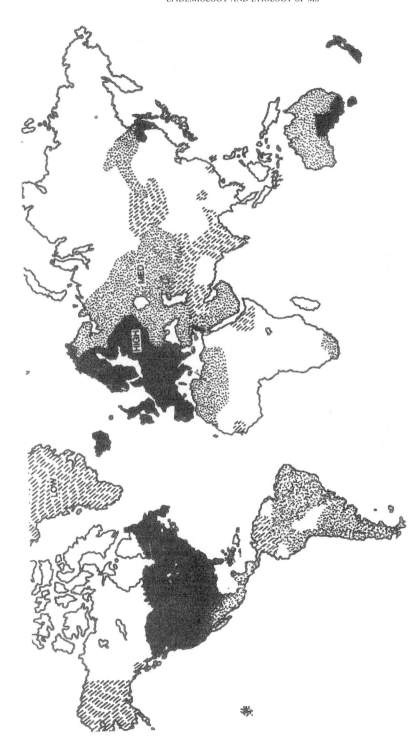

Fig. 8. Worldwide distribution of MS as of 2003 with high (prevalence 30+ per 100,000; solid), medium (prevalence 5–29; dotted), and low (prevalence 0–4; dashed) regions defined. Blank areas are regions without data, or people. (*From* Kurtzke JF. Epidemiología y esclerosis múltiple una revisión personal. Cuadernos de Esclerosis múltiple. [Epidemiology and multiple sclerosis: a personal review. Notebooks on Multiple Sclerosis.] Quarterly Journal 2003;16:17;l [in Spanish]; with permission.)

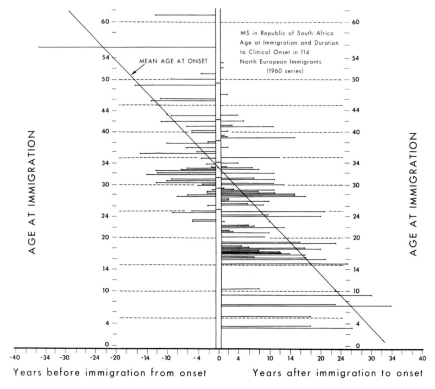

Fig. 9. MS in migrants from northern Europe to South Africa by age at immigration and years between immigration and clinical onset who were ascertained in 1960 MS prevalence survey of South Africa. (*Modified from* Kurtzke JF, Dean G, Botha DPJ. A method of estimating the age at immigration of White immigrants to South Africa, with an example of its importance. S Afr Med J 1970;44:668; with permission.)

host susceptibility. If this is true, what we call "MS" must be much more widespread than clinical cases indicate, or there must be a nonhuman reservoir. This hypothesis would have much stronger support if it could be shown that there epidemics of MS have occurred. An epidemic has been defined as disease occurrence that clearly is in excess of normal expectancy and is derived from a common or propagated source. Epidemics are divisible into two types; type 1 epidemics occur in susceptible populations who are exposed for the first time to a virulent infectious agent. Type 2 epidemics occur in populations within which the organism already is established. If the entire populace is exposed to a type 1 epidemic, the ages of those who are affected clinically will define the age range of susceptibility to the infection. Type 2 epidemics tend to have a young age at onset, because the effective exposure of the patients will be greatest for those who first reach the age of susceptibility.

Epidemics of MS seem to have occurred in the ethnically similar populations of several groups of islands in the North Atlantic Ocean: Iceland, the Shetland-Orkneys, and the Faroe Islands.

Data about all known patients in Iceland who had an onset of MS between 1900 and 1975 were collected in 1980. Annual incidence rates reveal that there seems to have been at least one definite type 2 epidemic of MS in Iceland which began in 1945. The average annual incidence rate from 1923 to 1944 was 1.6 per 100,000. For 1945 to 1954, it was significantly greater (3.2 per 100,000), and then it declined significantly to 1.9 per 100,000 for 1955 to 1974. Age at clinical onset in the 1945 to 1949 interval (23 years) was significantly younger than for any other 5-year period from 1935 to 1969.

For Shetland and the Orkneys for 1911 to 1985, the average annual incidence rates indicated that the occurrence after 1970 was significantly less than for the previous 30 or 35 years. With the small populations of these islands, the incidence rates showed considerable fluctuations and apparently differed in peaks and valleys between the islands. The overall impression of at least one epidemic between 1941 and 1970 seems to be valid, as does the clear decline after 1970.

The Faroe Islands are a semi-independent part of the Kingdom of Denmark that lies in the North Atlantic at 62°N latitude and 7°W longitude. Population numbered more than 44,000 in 1998. The Faroe Islands include 17 major volcanic islands that are made of basaltic rock, all with steep hills that reach the shore or bays and fjords. Almost all of the villages are in such inlets. Travel between many islands and even between a few villages on the same island is by boat.

The author has worked with the late Kay Hyllested and Anne Heltberg—both neurologists of Denmark—to investigate MS on the Faroe Islands since the early 1970s. At least one of the investigators examined every person on the Faroe Islands in whom MS was suspected between 1960 and June 1999. To find all possible cases of MS from 1900 on, every conceivable resource of medical information was used. Denmark, including the Faroe Islands, has had state-provided health care since the 1920s; Danish medical and health records are unsurpassed. All medical records for each suspected case was obtained and independently reviewed by each investigator.

There is no evidence that MS occurred in this century, before 1943, among native-born resident Faroese who had not lived off the islands for 3 or more years before clinical onset. July 1943 is the earliest date when symptom-onset was discovered to have taken place in such residents. There were 21 patients among the 26,000 Faroese who constituted a point source type 1 epidemic of MS on the Faroe Islands, beginning in 1943.

Inclusion of patients for this epidemic—and later ones—was dependent on two criteria: age of at least 11 years at "exposure" and "exposure" for 2 years. Thus, the "exposure" period here was 1941 to 1942 (2 years before

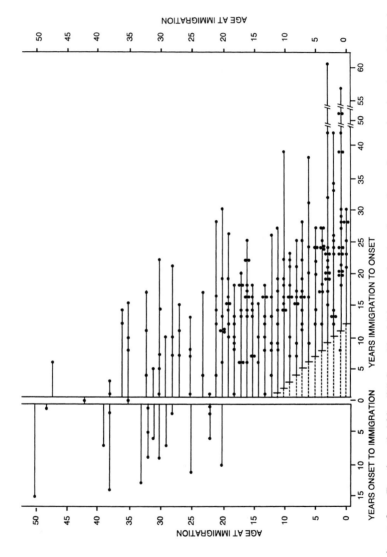

Fig. 10. MS in migrants from French north Africa (2/3 from Algeria) by age at immigration and years between immigration and clinical onset of MS. (*From* Kurtzke JF, Delasnerie-Lauprêtre N, Wallin MT. Multiple sclerosis in North African migrants to France. Acta Neurol Scand 1998;98:306; with permission.)

earliest onset) for 20 patients, and 1943 to 1944 for the last patient. What the Faroese must have been "exposed" to had to be an exogenous agent that was brought into the Faroe Islands in 1941 to 1944. We believe that this agent is a specific infection that we call the primary MS affection (PMSA). Age at first exposure to PMSA extended from 11 to 45 years. Thus, susceptibility to PMSA in this populace is limited to Faroese who were aged 11 to 45. Older and younger Faroese were not susceptible. Annual incidence rates show the striking appearance—and disappearance—of this epidemic, which peaked at annual incidence rates of 10 per 100,000 population for 1945 and 1946 (Fig. 11). Residence at the time of exposure indicates the wide scattering of these cases throughout the islands (see later discussion).

The Faroe Islands were occupied by British military forces for 5 years during World War II, from April 1940 to September 1945. Army troops were the main force, although Navy and Air Force units were present as well. The War Diaries identified the units by type, time, manning, and location. Local sources were used to confirm or deny the recorded British occupation sites.

By 1941, 1500 troops were stationed in the Faroe Islands. In 1942, the numbers increased to 7000, exceeded 4000 between June 1942 and August 1943, and were still near 1000 or so through 1944 (Fig. 12). It is clear that troop locations match the residences of the patients who had MS (Fig. 13). We concluded that the British troops brought MS to the Faroese in the Faroe Islands in 1941 to 1944.

Therefore, the troops brought something to the Faroe Islands that later resulted in an epidemic of clinical MS. This had to be an infection or a toxin, with either one geographically widespread on the islands from 1941. A toxin could not be responsible for later epidemics. Therefore, if there are later ones (and there are), then there must have been an infection that was carried by a large proportion of British troops (because of its wide distribution) in an asymptomatic fashion (because they were healthy troops). This must be a persistent infection that takes time (here 2 years) to be transmitted to a naïve populace, the Faroese. We call this agent the PMSA, which we have defined as a specific, but unknown, widespread, persistent infection that only rarely leads to clinical neurologic MS years after its acquisition.

Fig. 14 provides a model of transmission of PMSA from the British troops to that population cohort of Faroese of all ages which was first exposed geographically to this agent in 1941. Proportions of exposed persons who actually were affected are unknown, but must have been high.

After the British left, any further disease would have to be the result of transmission from F1 A to the next cohort of Faroese. If all of the F1 A persons were able to transmit PMSA lifelong, there would have been a steady input for new cases into the twenty-first century, and no further epidemics. Now, clinical MS patients do not transmit any disease. Thus, if this concept is valid, if there were later epidemics, transmissibility should have ended by the usual age of clinical onset—which we have taken as age

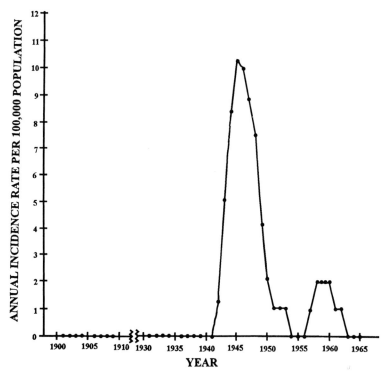

Fig. 11. MS in native resident Faroese. Annual incidence rates per 100,000 population calculated as 3-year centered moving averages for the 21 subjects of epidemic I. (*From* Kurtzke JF, Heltberg A. Multiple sclerosis in the Faroe Islands: an epitome. J Clin Epidemiol 2001; 54:7; with permission.)

27. This F1 affected and transmissible (A + T) cohort would contain three times as many Faroese in the first 7 years (1945–51) as in the next 6 years (1952–57). On the basis that the number of persons that is available to transmit determines the frequency of acquisition for the newly exposed next cohort of exposed and susceptible Faroese (F2 E + S) as they reach age 11 each year in essentially equal numbers, this would provide three times as many PMSA-affected persons in the first 7 years as in the next 6 years; this high-low pattern would repeat itself over time. If, in turn, there is a fixed ratio between PMSA and clinical neurologic MS (CNMS), such a model could explain the later occurrence of consecutive type 2 epidemics with peaks at 13-year intervals, as illustrated in the upper part of Fig. 15.

After epidemic I there were three later epidemics of clinical disease. The occurrence of epidemic IV was predicted by this transmission model. Membership in the epidemics has been defined by the time of exposure to PMSA for each patient (see lower part of Fig. 15). The 10 patients in epidemic II were exposed in 1945 to 1957; the 10 patients of epidemic III

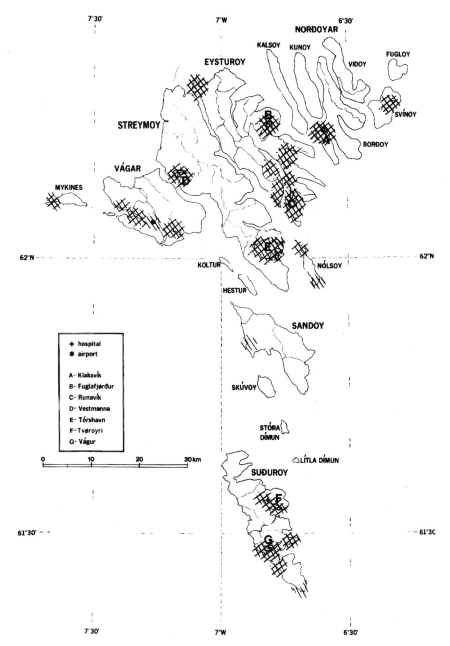

Fig. 12. British troop encampments on the Faroe Islands in World War II. Camps within Faroese villages are cross-hatched, those where no Faroese lived are diagonal-lined. (*From* Kurtzke JF, Heltberg A. Multiple sclerosis in the Faroe Islands: an epitome. J Clin Epidemiol 2001;54:10; with permission.)

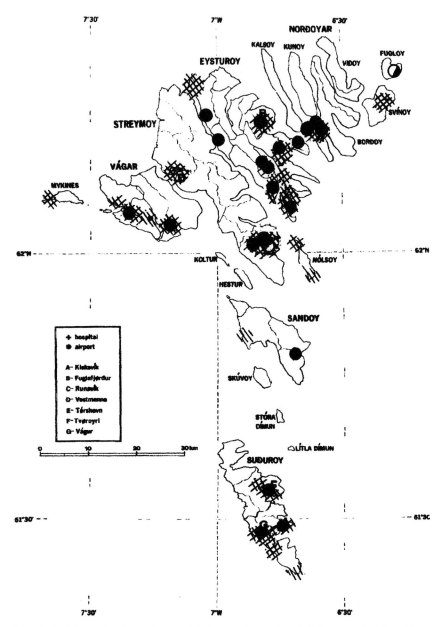

Fig. 13. Residence of patients of epidemic I (●) superimposed on British occupation sites. (*From* Kurtzke JF, Heltberg A. Multiple sclerosis in the Faroe Islands: an epitome. J Clin Epidemiol 2001;54:16; with permission.)

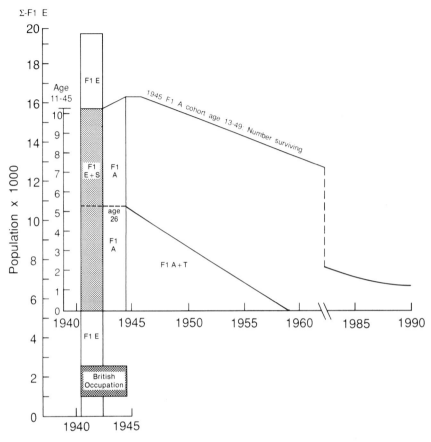

Fig. 14. Transmission model for the first population cohort of Faroese (F1) who were exposed to PMSA. Rectangle at lower left represents British occupation 1941–1944 when at least 1500 troops were stationed on the Faroe Islands. Long vertical bar represents the entire 1941 Faroese population, all ages, who were geographically at risk of PMSA (the F1 E [exposed] cohort). Only those who were 11 to 45 years of age in 1941 were susceptible to PMSA (F1 E + S) based upon the ages of the patients who had MS in epidemic I (shaded part of bar). After 2 years, the F1 E + S cohort became the F1 A (affected) cohort. If transmissibility ceases by age 27, then only that part of the F1 A cohort that was aged 13 to 26 would make up the F1 A + T cohort (affected and transmissible), which would decline to 0 in 1958 as its members attain age 27. (*From* Kurtzke JF, Hyllested K, Heltberg A. Multiple sclerosis in the Faroes: transmission across four epidemics. Acta Neurol Scand 1995;91:321–5; with permission.)

were exposed in 1958 to 1970. Open boxes indicate first exposure beyond age 11 (because of residence), as found for 4 of the 13 patients of epidemic IV whose exposure period was 1971 to 1983. Annual incidence rates per 100,000 population do show four epidemic peaks (Fig. 16). Furthermore, the male excess of epidemic I has changed to an increasing female preponderance for each later epidemic.

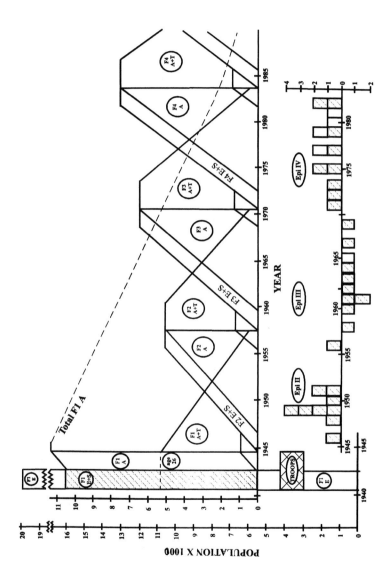

Fig. 15.  Summation of PMSA transmission with actual population numbers for British, and for Faroese geographically at risk, F1 through F4 cohorts, with time of exposure of patients of epidemics II through IV (lower portion); each rectangle represents one patient at age 11 (dotted) or at older age of first exposure (open), by calendar time. (From Kurtzke JF, Heltberg A. Multiple sclerosis in the Faroe Islands: an epitome. J Clin Epidemiol 2001;54:15; with permission.)

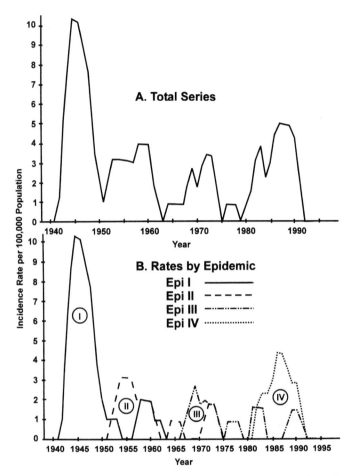

Fig. 16. Annual incidence rates per 100,000 population for clinical MS in native resident Faroese, calculated as 3-year centered moving averages, 1998. (*From* Kurtzke JF, Heltberg A. Multiple sclerosis in the Faroe Islands: an epitome. J Clin Epidemiol 2001;54:17; with permission.)

Most of the patients who had MS in epidemics II through IV lived in the same villages, which also were much the same as for patients in epidemic I and for the locations of British troops in World War II (Fig. 17). All patients of epidemics II though IV lived during the time of PMSA exposure in a location in which patients from epidemic I or occupying troops had lived. The disease has remained geographically stable for more than half a century on the Faroe Islands which makes it the ideal location to search for this agent. We must leave this task for other investigators. Because we could not receive permission from the Faroese authorities to draw the necessary samples, our work on the Faroe Islands has come to an end.

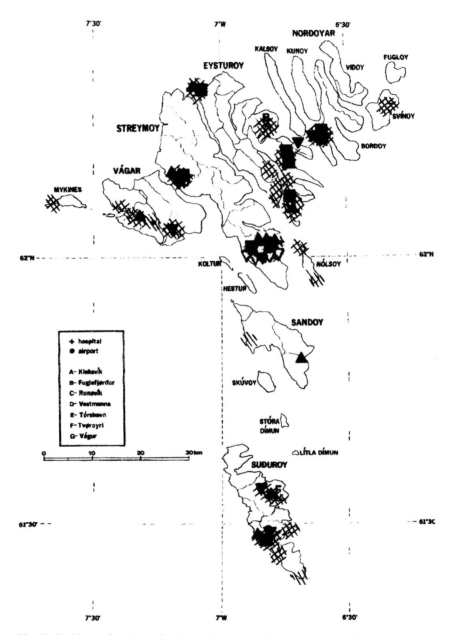

Fig. 17. Residence of patients of epidemics II through IV superimposed on British occupation sites of World War II. ▲, epidemic II; ■, epidemic III; ▼, epidemic IV. (*From* Kurtzke JF, Heltberg A. Multiple sclerosis in the Faroe Islands: an epitome. J Clin Epidemiol 2001;54:20; with permission.)

## Summary

The author believes that the Faroese saga provides major insight into what seems to him to be the essential nature of MS:

- There is a specific, widespread, but unidentified, infection that we call the primary multiple sclerosis affection (PMSA).
- PMSA is a persistent infection that is transmitted from person to person.
- A small proportion of persons who has PMSA will develop clinical neurologic multiple sclerosis (CNMS) years later.
- Prolonged exposure is needed to acquire PMSA. Acquisition follows first adequate exposure.
- Susceptibility to PMSA is limited to approximately age 11 to age 45 at start of exposure.
- CNMS is not transmissible.
- PMSA transmissibility is limited to a period that is less than the usual age of onset of CNMS. On the Faroe Islands, this period is approximately from age 13 to age 26.
- The existence of PMSA now must be inferred from the presence of CNMS.

## References

[1] Kurtzke JF. Epidemiology of multiple sclerosis. Does this really point toward an etiology? Neurol Sci 2000;21:383–403.

[2] Kurland LT, Kurtzke JF, Goldberg ID. Epidemiology of neurologic and sense organ disorders. Cambridge (MA): Harvard University Press; 1973.

[3] Landtblom A-M, Riise T, Boiko A, et al. Distribution of multiple sclerosis in Sweden based on mortality and disability compensation statistics. Neuroepidemiology 2002;21:167–79.

[4] Wallin MT, Page WF, Kurtzke JF. Multiple sclerosis in United States veterans of Vietnam era and later military service. 1. Race, sex and geography. Ann Neurol 2004;55:65–71.

[5] Kurtzke JF. Geographic distribution of multiple sclerosis: an update with special reference to Europe and the Mediterranean region. Acta Neurol Scand 1980;62:65–80.

[6] Kurtzke JF. Further features of the Fennoscandian focus of multiple sclerosis. Acta Neurol Scand 1974;50:478–502.

[7] Kurtzke JF. Epidemiología y esclerosís múltiple una revisión personal. Cuadernos de Esclerosis múltiple. [Epidemiology and multiple sclerosis: a personal review. Notebooks on Multiple Sclerosis.] Quarterly Journal 2003;16:6–31 [in Spanish].

[8] Houzen H, Niino M, Kikuchi S, et al. The prevalence and clinical characteristics of MS in northern Japan. J Neurol Sci 2003;211:49–53.

[9] Itoh T, Aizawa H, Hashimoto K, et al. Prevalence of multiple sclerosis in Asahikawa, a city in northern Japan. J Neurol Sci 2003;214:7–9.

[10] Boiko AN. Multiple sclerosis prevalence in Russia and other countries of the former USSR. In: Firnhaber W, Lauer K, editors. Multiple sclerosis in Europe. An epidemiological update. Darmstadt (Germany): LTV Press; 1994. p. 219–30.

ELSEVIER
SAUNDERS

Phys Med Rehabil Clin N Am
16 (2005) 351–358

PHYSICAL MEDICINE
AND REHABILITATION
CLINICS OF
NORTH AMERICA

# Multiple Sclerosis: An Immunologic Perspective

Jimmy Y. Cui, MD, PhD

*Department of Rehabilitation Medicine, University of Washington,
1959 NE Pacific Street, Seattle, WA 98195, USA*

Multiple sclerosis (MS) is a chronic recurrent inflammatory disorder of the central nervous system (CNS). The precise cause of MS remains unknown, although immune dysregulation or immune-mediated mechanisms almost certainly are involved. Advances in the field of basic and clinical immunology strongly influenced the concepts of the immunopathogenesis of MS and the contemporary approach in treating patients who have MS.

## Immunopathology of MS

Increasing evidence indicates that a complex immunologic cascade leads to the formation of the characteristic MS lesion. The hallmark of neuropathology in MS is the presence of multifocal plaques (lesions). Histologically, the MS lesion has a demarcated area of demyelination with inflammatory infiltrates. In addition, the presence of axonal degeneration is evident and recently was emphasized for its association with irreversible neurologic impairment and long-term disability in MS [1]. The inflammatory response is dominated by lymphocytes and macrophages. In acute MS lesions, B cells and plasma cells also are found. Other evidence for immune system involvement in MS includes class II major histocompatibility complex (MHC) antigen expression in lesions, up-regulation of cellular adhesion molecules, blood–brain barrier (BBB) disruption that allows autoreactive T cells to enter the CNS, and elevated levels of cytokines released from T cells [2]. The entire cascade of immune system events eventually causes CNS tissue damage. In chronic MS lesions, active inflammation is less conspicuous. It is characterized by hypocellularity with gliosis and axonal loss to a variable degree.

*E-mail address:* jcui66@hotmail.com or jcui@u.washington.edu

1047-9651/05/$ - see front matter © 2005 Elsevier Inc. All rights reserved.
doi:10.1016/j.pmr.2005.01.008                                       *pmr.theclinics.com*

*T cells*

T cells are dominant immunologic players in MS. With involvement of T cells, the cellular immunity is remarkably active and highly specific. Normally, these cells are not able to pass through the BBB or traffic through the CNS. When activated, they can gain entry into the CNS by up-regulation of their cell-surface receptors in conjunction with up-regulation of adhesion molecules on endothelial cells that maintain the BBB. Activated T cells, thereby, are able to adhere to endothelial cells and pass through the tight junctions of the BBB. Initial attachment of T cells involves interactions between members of the selectin family of adhesion molecules. Subsequent binding involves integrins. The prime autoantigen that elicits the autoimmune response in MS is unclear; however, researchers have suggested several possible candidates, such as myelin basic protein, myelin oligodendrocyte glycoprotein, and myelin-associated proteolipid protein. [3,4]. Once within the CNS, activated T cells release inflammatory cytokines. They recruit other immune cells to the region and increase the local permeability of the BBB. Meanwhile, microglial cells and astrocytes in the CNS also can secrete proinflammatory cytokines upon activation by T-cell released cytokines. This attracts more inflammatory cells to the lesion.

T cells have two major subtypes ($CD4^+$ and $CD8^+$ cells). $CD4^+$ cells, in turn, can be divided further into T helper cells type I (Th1) and T helper cells type II (Th2). Typically, $CD4^+$ cells are responsible for delayed type hypersensitivity, cell-mediated immune responses, and provide help to B cells that are necessary for antibody responses.

$CD8^+$ cells can be divided into cytotoxic T cells that are capable of lysing cells that are infected with virus, and suppressor T cells that are capable of inhibiting Th1 cells. The immune function of $CD4^+$ and $CD8^+$ cells is linked directly to a variety of cytokines that is generated in these cells.

In the presence of antigens, the $CD4^+$ T cells complete the antigen-recognition process by interacting with MHC class II molecules on the surface of antigen-presenting cells (APC). MHC class II molecules are commonly expressed in macrophages, microglia, endothelial cells, and astrocytes. These cells represent potential APCs for $CD4^+$ T-cell reactions in the human CNS. Inflammatory reactions in the CNS can result in tremendous increased expression of MHC class II molecules that further promote the $CD4^+$ T-cell reactions. The $CD8^+$ T cells usually recognize antigens when complexed with MHC class I molecules. MHC class I molecules are expressed on the surface of all nucleated cells. Upon antigen recognition, $CD4^+$ and $CD8^+$ T cells generate a variety of cytokines that is released subsequently. Essentially, they determine the nature of the immune response and the extent of the immune reaction.

*Cytokines*

Cytokines are soluble proteins that are a functionally diverse set of signaling molecules that are produced and released by T cells and macrophages. They play a pivotal role in the immunopathogenesis of MS. Cytotoxic $CD8^+$ cells may generate perforin, which is capable of inducing lysis of oligodendrocytes. Suppressor $CD8^+$ cells may release transforming growth factor (TGF)-$\beta$, which can inhibit Th1 cells. Studies found that most cytokines that are generated in Th1 cells are proinflammatory, whereas those in Th2 cells are anti-inflammatory. Interferon (IFN)-$\gamma$, tumor necrosis factor–$\alpha$, and lymphotoxin are cytokines that are produced in Th1 cells, whereas interleukin (IL)-4 and IL-10 are generated in Th2 cells.

Th1 and Th2 cells work in opposition to balance the immune response; the balance of these two types of cells determines the net effect of the inflammatory reaction and may influence the course of disease. Th1 cells secrete IL-2 and IFN-$\gamma$ that recruit and activate macrophages. Th2 cells may help myelin-specific B cells activate and, importantly, release IL-4 and IL-10 to down-regulate Th1 cells.

Recent studies indicate that immune cells also are capable of producing several potentially neuroprotective factors and neurotrophic mediators, such as neurotrophin-3, nerve growth factor, TGF-$\beta$, and platelet-derived growth factor. It was reported that brain-derived neurotrophic factor (BDNF), which can prevent neuronal damage, is expressed in immune cells, including T cells, macrophages, and microglia in MS lesions. New therapeutic targets could be developed in the future, based on enhancing neuroprotective effects to preserve axons [5,6].

*B cells*

There is accumulating evidence that B cells participate in the immuno-pathology in at least some types of MS [7]. B cells have been identified in acute MS lesions and antibodies that were detected in cerebrospinal fluid. Humoral immunity normally relies on circulating antibodies that are produced by B cells. Binding the correct antigen with B-cell receptors activates the B cell. B cells could be activated by certain cytokines that are released from autoreactive T cells, and subsequently, secrete antibodies that could cause demyelination in CNS.

The humoral immune response is triggered by interaction of B cells with antigen and leads to a clonally expanded population of plasma cells. Antigen-specific antibody is then produced by plasma cells. The antibodies are able to bind to target cells and certain components of the CNS, including myelin, and consequently, inflammatory attack occurs. Antibodies can activate the complement system, and cause membrane damage of myelin, and enhance phagocytosis, which further destroys myelin.

*Macrophages*

All cells in the immune system, including monocytes and lymphocytes, are derived from hematopoietic stem cells in bone marrow and certain lymphatic tissues. Macrophages probably originate from monocytes that are recruited from the blood to sites of inflammation. Macrophages, together with microglial cells and astrocytes, are considered APCs. These cells have a unique function that is known as antigen processing. Following this process, APCs take a specific portion of "processed" antigen to present on their cell surfaces. T cells then become activated by interaction of the T-cell receptor and MHC/antigen peptide complex and undergo proliferation. This is a critical step in the immunopathogenesis in patients who have MS, and could be a potential target of future treatment. Furthermore, microphages release cytokines, oxygen free radicals, and nitric oxide at the site of inflammation and involve antibody-mediated phagocytosis.

*Other cells in the central nervous system*

The CNS traditionally is believed to be exempt from active immune reactivity, but now it is clear that it is subject to immune surveillance and can be the site of immune responses [8]. In addition to the immune cells that were discussed above, some potential players in the CNS involve the immunologic reaction and inflammatory process in MS. They include microglia, endothelial cells, astrocytes, and oligodendrocytes. The exact roles of these cells remain uncertain, but studies implicate their participation in different stages of immune response, such as antigen presentation, signal transduction, BBB breakdown, cytokine production, and neuroprotection [8–10]. Future study on these cells and their interactions may shed additional light on the immunopathology of MS.

## Immunotherapy in MS

Multiple agents are used for treating MS; however, the precise mechanism of action for most of these agents has not been well-established. Almost all therapeutic agents that are available for treating MS are related to their immunomodulating or immunosuppressive properties.

Although mounting evidence has led to the recommendation of early implementation of immunomodulating therapy, initial decision-making by physicians who care for patients who have MS can be difficult under some circumstances, even after a careful risk-benefit analysis of each individual drug and cost-benefit assessment. How to make the best treatment recommendation for patients who have MS is beyond the scope of this article; however, physician knowledge of the mechanisms of action of these drugs will contribute to patient education and facilitate the shared decision-making process. Common agents that are used in treating patients who have MS and their influence on the immune response in MS are reviewed briefly below.

*Immunosuppressive agents*

Mitoxantrone (Novantrone) is a potent immunosuppressive drug that is used for relapsing-remitting (RR) and secondary progressive MS. It is a cytotoxic agent that is related to antineoplastic agents, such as doxorubicin. The exact mechanism of action is not well-elucidated. The agent seems to have a dual effect on nucleic acids. It participates in intercalation with DNA and induces DNA cross-links and DNA strand breakage. Furthermore, the drug interferes with RNA and inhibits topoisomerase II, a special enzyme that is responsible for repairing DNA damage. Thus, the drug suppresses the activity of T cells, B cells, and macrophages [11].

Other immunosuppressive drugs, such as methotrexate, azathioprine, and cyclophosphamide have been tried in MS to suppress the proliferation of active immune cells and cell products (eg, cytokines and immunoglobulins). More aggressive immune suppressive treatment has been tried in the forms of high-dose cyclophosphamide in combination with total body irradiation and antithymocytic globulin, followed by autologous peripheral stem cell (CD34$^+$ cell) transplantation. The preliminary result is encouraging. This study was based on the hypothesis that more complete immunosuppression might be more effective or even curative in autoimmune diseases [12].

Glucocorticoids primarily have been prescribed for patients who have MS and who have acute exacerbations. The detailed mechanism of action is not well-established. It seems that steroids are able to restore the BBB integrity, and suppress the release of cytokines from immune active cells, and thereby, dampen the inflammatory response in MS lesions.

*Immunomodulatory therapy*

Three interferons have been used as immunomodulating agents in treating MS, including interferon-β–1b (Betaseron), interferon-β–1a (Avonex) and another interferon-β–1a (Rebif). The mechanism of action is not clear, but studies suggest that INF-β inhibits antigen presentation and T-cell activation and prevents clonal expansion of activated Th1 cells. The migration of activated T cells from the periphery into the CNS also is prevented by IFN-β, and thereby, the proinflammatory cytokines are reduced and inflammatory reaction is diminished [13].

Glatiramer acetate (GA; Copaxone) is synthetic polypeptide that is composed of a randomized mixture of four amino acids: L-alanine, L-lysine, L-glutamatic acid, and L-tyrosine in a set molar ratio that resembles that of myelin-basic protein. GA seems to exert its immunomodulating effect by way of at least two modes of action at various stages of the immune response. First, able to cross the BBB, activated GA-specific Th2 cells release anti-inflammatory cytokines, such as IL-4, IL-6 and IL-10 [14]. Second, GA-specific T cells may mediate neuroprotection through the secretion of specific neurotrophic factors, including BDNF [15].

*Neutralizing antibodies*

High titers of IFN neutralizing antibodies (NABs), which develop in the course of INF treatment of cancer and hepatitis, can reverse some measures of efficacy or even result in treatment failure. Hence, NABs have become an important issue in treating patients who have MS with interferon-β, because NAB was detected in approximately one third of patients who received interferon-β-1b. It also was noted that NABs are cross-reactive against all three interferon-β preparations. Data suggest that the frequency of NABs ranges from 5% to 42% [16].

The presence of NABs could demolish or abrogate these drugs' efficacy. Physicians could be encountered with questions as to whether immunomodulating agents need to be altered in dosage or changed to another preparation when NABs are positive. It is clear that therapeutic regimen change is a clinical judgment; however, our knowledge about the immunologic reaction in the formation of NABs in the patient who has MS can help us to understand its possible clinical significance.

Tremendous controversy has been raised when treating patients who have RR MS with interferon-β in the presence of NABs. It generally is believed that interferon-β–1b is more immunogenic than an interferon-β-1a preparation because interferon-β–1b is manufactured from purified *Escherichia coli* through genetic engineering technology. Furthermore, interferon-β–1b is nonglycosylated, has a deletion of the N-terminal methionine residue, and has an amino acid substitution of cysteine for serine. Interferon-β–1a is glycosylated and is generated by recombinant DNA technology with use of mammalian cells, and therefore, is less immunogenic.

The NAB may block a surface molecule that is required for antigen activation. When NABs interfere with the binding of the IFN molecule to T-cell receptors, IFN-β's influence on the transmembrane signal transduction cascade and subsequent immunologic response is hampered. In the study of IFN-β–1b, the development of NAB appeared to be associated with loss of efficacy. Since then, several investigations have been conducted. Not all investigators have been convinced of a NAB effect.

It has been observed that small proportions of patients who have untreated MS have IFN-specific NABs [17]. Moreover, it apparently is difficult to compare the data of these three major IFNs. The result of positive titers could be significantly different, depending on how they were measured. No clear consensus exist about what constitutes a positive titer, or a standardized method to compute the result.

Studies revealed the disappearance of NABs in some patients who had MS who continued to use interferon-β. Rice et al [18] reported that the mean time for NABs to disappear was approximately 20 months in the patient who had MS and was treated with interferon-β–1b. Sixty percent of patients who had MS in a trial of interferon-β–1b and had positive NAB titer, became NAB negative [19]. There is no clear reason for the late disappearance of NAB. It could be explained by B-cell tolerance. Further immunologic study is warranted to elucidate this phenomenon further and its true influence on the efficacy of these immunomodulating agents.

GA, another important immunomodulating drug, also is known to have immunogenicity. The anti-GA antibodies, predominantly of the IgG class, were found in patients who had MS and were treated with GA [20]. It is not clear whether anti-GA antibodies have a neutralizing property or have any potential negative consequence on the drug's bioactivity and immunomodulating effect, although some studies showed that the antibody has no interference with GA's biologic function. Further research is needed to clarify the clinical significance of anti-GA antibodies.

## Summary

The precise cause of MS remains unknown, although immunopathologic studies provide solid evidence of participation of activated immune cells in the formation of MS lesions. Cell-mediated and antibody-mediated (humoral) immune responses are involved in the immunopathogenesis of MS. The Th1 and Th2 cells, by releasing a variety of pro- or anti-inflammatory cytokines, work in opposition to balance the immune response and to determine the net effect of the inflammation. The current understanding of immunopathogenesis shapes the contemporary approach to the treatment of MS. The article also reviewed the mechanisms of action of commonly used immunotherapy agents and their impact on the immune response of patients who have MS.

## Acknowledgments

The author is grateful to Dr. Ning Yu from Western Washington University at Bellingham, Washington for his critical review of the manuscript and invaluable suggestions.

## References

[1] Trapp BD, Peterson J, Ransohoff RM, et al. Axonal transection in the lesions of multiple sclerosis. New Engl J Med 1998;338:278–85.
[2] Al-Omaishi J, Bashir R, Gendelman HE. The cellular immunology of multiple sclerosis. J Leukoc Biol 1999;65:444–52.
[3] Allegretta M, Nicklas JA, Sriram S, et al. T cells responsive to myelin basic protein in patient with multiple sclerosis. Science 1990;247:718–21.
[4] Zhang J, Markovic-plese S, Lacet B, et al. Increased frequency of interleukin 2- responsive T cells specific for myelin basic protein and proteolipid protein in peripheral blood and cerebrospinal fluid of patients with multiple sclerosis. J Exp Med 1994;179:973–84.
[5] Stadelmann C, Kerschensteiner M, Misgeld T, et al. BDNF and gp145trkB in multiple sclerosis brain lesions: neuroprotective interactions between immune and neuronal cells? Brain 2002;125(Pt 1):75–85.
[6] Hohlfeld R, Kerschensteiner M, Stadelmann C, et al. The neuroprotective effect of inflammation: implications for the therapy of multiple sclerosis. J Neuroimmunol 2000; 107(2):161–6.

[7] Antel JP, Bar-Or A. Do myelin-directed antibodies predict multiple sclerosis. New Engl J Med 2003;249:107–9.

[8] Committee on MS. Institute of Medicine: Clinical and biological features. In: Joy JE, Johnston RB Jr, editors. Multiple sclerosis: current status and strategies for the future. Washington, DC: National Academy Press; 2001. p. 29–114.

[9] Taylor R. Immunologic aspects of multiple sclerosis. Phys Med Rehabil Clin N Am 1998; 9:525–36.

[10] Prat A, Biernacki K, Lavoie JF, et al. Migration of multiple sclerosis lymphocytes through brain endothelium. Arch Neurol 2002;59(3):391–7.

[11] Hartung HP, Gonsette R, Konig N, et al. Mitxoantrone in progressive MS: a placebo-controlled, double-blind, randomized, multicentre trial. Lancet 2002;360:2018–25.

[12] Kraft G, Bowen J, Cui J, et al. Clinical application of autologous stem cell transplantation in severe MS treated with high-dose immunosuppressive therapy. Neurology 2002;58(Suppl 3): A166.

[13] Yong VW. Differential mechanisms of action of interferon beta and glatiramer acetate in MS. Neurology 2002;59:802–8.

[14] Neuhaus O, Farina C, Wekerle H, et al. Mechanism of action of glatiramer acetate in multiple sclerosis. Neurology 2001;56:702–8.

[15] Chen M, Malenzuela RM, Dhib-Jalbut S. Glatiramer acetate-reactive T cells produce brain-derived neurotrophic factor. J Neurol Sci 2003;215:37–44.

[16] Sorensen PS, Ross C, Clemmesen KM, et al. Clinical importance of neutralizing antibodies against interferon beta in patients with RR MS. Lancet 2003;362:1184–91.

[17] Miller A, Bourdette D, Cohen JA, et al. The significance of neutralizing antibodies in patients treated with interferon. Continuum lifelong learning in neurology: Multiple sclerosis 1999;5(5):107–19.

[18] Rice GPA, Paszner B, Oger J, et al. The evolution of neutralizing antibodies in MS patients treated with interferon beta-1b. Neurology 1999;52:1277–9.

[19] The IFNB Multiple Sclerosis Study Group and the University of British Colombia MS/MRI Analysis Group. Neutralizing antibodies during treatment of MS with interferon beta-1b: experience during the first 3 years. Neurology 1996;47:889–94.

[20] Teitelbaum D, Brenner T, Abramsky O, et al. Antibodies to glatiramer acetate do not interfere with its biological function and therapeutic efficacy. Mult Scler 2003;9:592–9.

PHYSICAL MEDICINE
AND REHABILITATION
CLINICS OF
NORTH AMERICA

ELSEVIER
SAUNDERS

Phys Med Rehabil Clin N Am
16 (2005) 359–381

# Diagnosing Multiple Sclerosis and Its Imitators

## James Bowen, MD

*Department of Neurology, Box 356465, 1959 NE Pacific, University of Washington, Seattle, WA 98195-6465, USA*

The diagnosis of multiple sclerosis (MS) is one of the most difficult in neurology. The disease affects central nervous system white matter at seemingly random locations through a series of attacks that occur at unpredictable times. As a result, there is no typical symptom pattern to help the physician recognize patients. Likewise, there is not a standard set of clinical signs that is indicative of the disease. In the absence of typical findings on history or examination, physicians often turn to laboratory tests. There are no tests for MS that provide sufficient sensitivity and specificity to be used as gold standards for the diagnosis. To provide guidance in this difficult situation, diagnostic criteria have been created to assist with the diagnosis.

## Historical criteria for diagnosis

The combination of clinical attacks that affect different parts of the central nervous system at different times was recognized by Charcot, who generally is credited with unifying previous clinical descriptions with his own observations of the disease under the name "sclerose en plaque." The first widely applied criteria for diagnosis were those of Allison and Millar [1]. This was followed by those of McAlpine et al [2], McDonald and Halliday [3], and Rose et al [4]. The Schumacker et al [5] criteria (1965) required dissemination in time and space, objective abnormalities, and no better explanation. They also defined attacks as lasting for at least 24 hours and occurring at least 1 month apart. The Schumacker criteria were modified by the Poser Committee in 1983 [6]. The Poser criteria allowed dissemination in space to be provided by clinical means or by paraclinical tests, such as imaging, evoked potentials, or

Supported by the National Institute on Disability and Rehabilitation Research (grant no. H133B031129).

*E-mail address:* jbowen@uwashington.edu

doi:10.1016/j.pmr.2005.01.011
*pmr.theclinics.com*

urological testing. Furthermore, separate categories of laboratory-supported MS were established to include cerebrospinal fluid (CSF) testing. The Poser criteria were the primary means of diagnosing MS for nearly 2 decades.

## McDonald criteria

The Poser criteria had several shortcomings, including a complicated scheme of four major categories (definite, probable, possible, and not MS), subdivisions of these categories into clinical and laboratory-supported subcategories, and outdated definitions of attacks and laboratory testing. MRI was not included in the Poser criteria because they predated the advent of this technology. To reassess the diagnostic criteria for MS, an International Panel on the Diagnosis of Multiple Sclerosis was convened in London in 2000 under the auspices of the U.S. National Multiple Sclerosis Society and the International Federation of MS Societies. Chaired by Dr. W.I. McDonald, this committee produced new criteria to diagnose MS that are known as the London or McDonald criteria [7].

The McDonald criteria retain the basic outline of dissemination in space and time that was required by previous diagnostic criteria (Box 1). This includes evidence of two or more attacks (in time), evidence of two or more lesions (in space), and no better explanation than MS. Each of these requirements is discussed in more detail in the sections that follow.

Most patients who do not meet these criteria should be classified as not having MS; however, there are patients who have incomplete evaluations, or whose evaluations suggest MS, but who do not meet the criteria. These patients should be classified as having possible MS and they should be followed closely until the diagnosis is clear.

Although the McDonald criteria generally have been accepted by the medical community, a consensus panel was convened in Fort Worth in 2001 to address additional issues that are related to the diagnosis of MS [8]. One of these issues involves the use of MRI in the diagnosis. It is possible to meet the McDonald criteria based on the clinical presentation alone. This allows the diagnosis of MS to be made in areas without access to imaging

---

**Box 1. McDonald criteria**

All three criteria must be met.
(1) Evidence of two or more attacks
   Two or more clinical attacks OR one clinical attack plus
      dissemination in time by MRI (Box 2)
(2) Evidence of two or more lesions
   Two or more clinical lesions OR one clinical lesion plus
      dissemination in space by MRI (Box 3)
(3) No better explanation than MS

**Box 2. MRI criteria for dissemination in time**

One of the following:

Gadolinium-enhancing lesion at least 3 months following original clinical attack at site different than the original attack OR if the first MRI scan is within 3 months of the original attack, then enhancement on a second scan must be done at least 3 months after the clinical event qualifies

New T2-hyperintense lesion compared to a baseline scan obtained at least 3 months from the original attack OR if the first MRI scan is within 3 months of the original attack, a second scan must be done at least 3 months after the clinical event. This scan serves as the baseline. A new T2 lesion on a scan that was obtained at least 3 months after this baseline scan qualifies.

---

**Box 3. MRI criteria for dissemination in space**

Scans must have three of the following four items:
(1) One gadolinium-enhancing lesion OR nine T2-hyperintense lesions
(2) At least one infratentorial lesion
(3) At least one juxtacortical lesion
(4) At least three periventricular lesions (Fig. 1)

Spinal cord lesions may substitute for one of the nine brain lesions.

In patients who have two to eight MRI lesions, the presence of oligoclonal bands or an elevated IgG index on cerebrospinal fluid analysis constitutes dissemination in space.

---

technology; however, it is strongly recommended that the diagnosis be made only after obtaining MRI imaging if the technology is available. The Fort Worth panel also emphasized that the McDonald criteria were to be used only for diagnosis and not for treatment decisions or determining prognosis. This modification allowed patients who had clinically isolated syndromes and were at high risk of having MS to proceed with treatment. The need for standardization of the MRI and CSF analysis was recognized.

Several studies have been completed to assess the performance of the McDonald criteria. One study of 119 patients who had single attacks of demyelination (clinically isolated syndromes) found that a diagnosis of MS could be made in 20% at 3 months, 48% at 1 year, and 56% at 3 years [9]. This is in contrast to the Poser criteria where criteria were met by 7% at 3

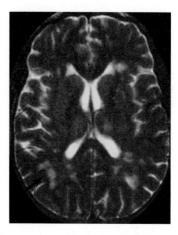

Fig. 1. Periventricular lesions (*arrow*) located in the white matter at the corticomedullary junction are called juxtacortical lesions. They typically outline the cortical ribbon while sparing the cortex.

months, 20% at 1 year, and 38% at 3 years [9]. A second study compared the McDonald and Poser criteria in 139 patients who had clinically isolated events [10]. At 1 year, 37% of the patients had met McDonald criteria, whereas only 11% had met Poser criteria. These patients were followed for 3 years. By the third year, 85% of those who met McDonald criteria at 1 year had gone on to have another clinical attack, whereas only 20% of those who had not met the McDonald criteria at 1 year had another attack [10]. Thus, the McDonald criteria at 1 year predicted the future clinical course. In another study of 76 patients who had possible MS, McDonald and Poser criteria were applied [11]. This study was unusual in that it used MRI changes as paraclinical evidence of dissemination in space for the Poser criteria. Also, lumbar punctures were performed in 75 of the patients to provide data for the laboratory-supported clinically definite MS category of the Poser criteria. Only 38% of patients met Poser criteria for clinically definite MS compared with 52% who met the McDonald criteria for MS. After inclusion of spinal fluid analysis, however, an additional 46% met the criteria for laboratory-supported clinically definite MS. Less than 10% of those who met the criteria for laboratory-supported clinically definite MS also met the McDonald criteria. This group also followed the McDonald definition of dissemination in space that allowed only two MRI lesions if spinal fluid was abnormal. This study underscores the importance of using MRI to identify additional lesions, and of using spinal fluid analysis in cases that do not meet the dissemination in space criteria [12]. Other investigators found that the use of spinal fluid analysis in patients who had fewer than nine MRI lesions increased sensitivity at the expense of specificity and accuracy [10]. Clearly, additional refinements of the McDonald criteria can be expected to improve our ability to diagnose MS [12].

## Definitions used by the McDonald criteria

Attacks (exacerbations, relapses) are defined carefully in the McDonald criteria. They: (1) must include neurologic disturbances "of the kind seen in MS," (2) must last for at least 24 hours, and (3) must not be related to a pseudoattack. Typical neurologic disturbances are not defined in the criteria. Typical symptoms are included in Box 4. Patients who have symptoms that are atypical for MS should receive the diagnosis with caution. By definition, attacks must last 24 hours; however, most attacks last several days or weeks, especially if they have not been treated with corticosteroids. Brief or fleeting symptoms are difficult to attribute to an episode of demyelination because it takes a certain amount of time for the immune attack to cause symptomatic damage to the myelin, and it takes even longer to repair the damage sufficiently to allow signal transmission. People who have MS commonly get fleeting symptoms, especially sensory symptoms. These include Lhermitte's phenomenon, trigeminal neuralgia, brief paresthesias, and restless leg syndrome. Fleeting motor symptoms, such as tonic spasms, may be seen. Autonomic dysreflexia may accompany myelopathy. These fleeting symptoms are evidence of nervous system abnormality, but they should not be mistaken for attacks. An exception is the patient who has the new onset of multiple episodes of transient symptoms that occur over 24 hours or longer. This scenario would represent an attack because a new area of central nervous system damage has occurred that led to symptoms (albeit transient symptoms) that lasted for more than 24 hours. Care should be taken to avoid misdiagnosing pseudoattacks. This refers to a transient worsening of symptoms that is associated with another illness or increased core body temperature. Patients who have infections commonly have a worsening of their underlying

---

**Box 4. Typical symptoms and signs of multiple sclerosis**

Motor: weakness, spasticity, hyperreflexia, Babinski sign
Cerebellar: ataxia, limb or gait; tremor, rubral
Visual: visual loss (optic neuritis), diplopia, nystagmus, internuclear ophthalmoplegia
Sensory: numbness, paresthesias (pins/needles, burning), pain, trigeminal neuralgia, Lhermitte's phenomenon, torso band of tightness, restless leg syndrome
Autonomic: bladder (urgency, hesitancy, frequency); bowel (constipation, urgency); sexual dysfunction
Fatigue
Heat Sensitivity
Cognitive dysfunction

symptoms, even if fevers are absent. Elevations of core body temperature (from fever, inability to dissipate body heat, or increased ambient temperatures) often lead to heightened symptoms. In these cases, the underlying illness or elevated temperature should be addressed.

When attacks follow one another over short time intervals, it can be difficult to determine whether a new attack has occurred or whether the previous attack is responsible for the worsening. The McDonald criteria define new or worsening symptoms that occur within 30 days of the onset of an attack as a single event. A new or worsened symptom that begins more than 30 days from the onset of an attack would constitute a separate event. It should be emphasized that the timing for clinical attacks differs from that for attacks that are defined by MRI. New gadolinium-enhancing lesions or new T2-weighted lesions must be separated from previous attacks by at least 3 months to be considered separate events (see later discussion).

Evidence for dissemination in time and space must be objective. Attacks may consist of objective or subjective events. For example, patients commonly have attacks that consist entirely of subjective symptoms, such as paresthesias or fatigue; however, reliance on subjective symptoms carries risks of misdiagnosis because of problems with inaccurate recall, misinterpretation of symptoms (by patients or physicians), or misleading histories from patients who are seeking answers. Therefore, purely subjective attacks cannot be used to meet the requirements for the diagnostic criteria. The objectivity of symptoms may be demonstrated by current findings on examination; abnormalities demonstrated on previous physical examinations; or findings on tests, such as MRI or evoked potentials.

MRI scanning parameters for imaging patients who have MS vary widely between institutions. Standardization of MRI procedures for evaluating MS was addressed recently by a working group (unpublished at the time of this writing). The guidelines that are recommended by this group emphasize the importance of obtaining standardized images to improve reproducibility and to facilitate comparisons between images that were obtained at different institutions. Recommendations include using field strengths of 1.0 T or greater, obtaining 3-mm slice thicknesses without gaps, obtaining an in-plane resolution of 1 mm × 1 mm, and using the subcallosal line to position patients in a standard manner. Standard brain MRI sequences for MS studies should include a sagittal FLAIR, Axial PD/T2 (proton density and T2-weighted), axial FLAIR, and gadolinium-enhanced T1-weighted images. The detection of gadolinium-enhancing lesions is improved by waiting 5 minutes between the infusion and scanning.

MRI criteria for dissemination in space have been proposed by several groups [13–16]. Those proposed by Barkhof and Tintore had the greatest specificity and accuracy while retaining acceptable sensitivity (see Box 3). Generally, lesions should be 3 mm or larger in size to minimize false positive readings that are due to other conditions, such as enlarged Virchow-Robin spaces. Although not included in the criteria, several additional MRI findings increase the likelihood of MS [13]. These include location (periventricular), shape (ovoid), size (larger than 6 mm), and orientation (perpendicular to the ventricles). Also, lesions that are located in the midline of the corpus callosum are highly suggestive of MS because the redundant blood supply and lack of perforating arteries in this region make vascular explanations less likely. The presence of a mixture of enhancing and non-enhancing lesions suggests lesions of differing ages, although this finding is not sufficient to meet the requirement for dissemination in time [13]. There is little evidence regarding the application of spinal cord lesions demonstrated by MRI to the diagnosis of MS. It was decided arbitrarily that spinal cord lesions could substitute for a single brain lesion in the criteria. Future data may lead to an increased role for spine MRI imaging in the diagnosis [17].

MRI criteria for dissemination in time are shown (see Box 2). The requirements for dissemination in time have not been studied as intensively as those for dissemination in space. An important objective of this requirement is to avoid inclusion of cases with acute disseminated encephalomyelitis (ADEM). Three months has been suggested as an appropriate time requirement to allow differentiation of ADEM and MS [18]. It is likely that future studies will lead to refinement of these criteria [19].

CSF abnormalities may include oligoclonal bands or an elevated IgG index. These tests require matching serum and CSF samples. A consensus panel recently addressed the methods that are used to determine the presence of oligoclonal bands. A recommendation was made to use isoelectric focusing because of high false negative results with other techniques (unpublished data). Up to half of MS cases may have negative results using agarose gel electrophoresis [20]. The preference for using isoelectric focusing also was expressed by other groups [21].

## Primary progressive multiple sclerosis

The diagnosis of primary progressive MS (PPMS) presents unique problems. By definition, PPMS does not include attacks, but has a slow decline in function over months or years. Those patients who have PPMS, therefore, cannot meet the criteria that require dissemination of attacks in time. Patients who become progressively disabled through a series of attacks, yet do not deteriorate outside of acute attacks, have relapsing remitting disease. Those who have attacks currently or in the past, but whose baseline deteriorates in the time between attacks have secondary progressive MS. The clinical subtypes of MS are illustrated in Fig. 2.

Because of the unique feature of PPMS, diagnosis of this form of MS was not included in earlier diagnostic schemes. The McDonald criteria now

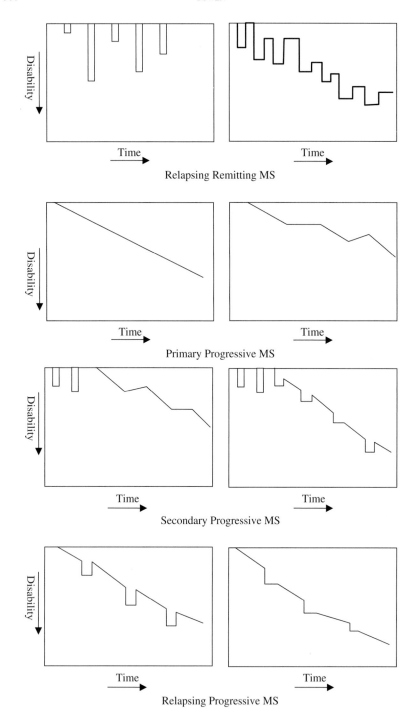

Relapsing Remitting MS

Primary Progressive MS

Secondary Progressive MS

Relapsing Progressive MS

---

**Box 5. Criteria for diagnosing primary progressive multiple sclerosis**

(1) Abnormal CSF
(2) Dissemination in time documented by worsening disability over 1 year or MRI evidence of dissemination in time (see Box 2)
(3) Dissemination in space documented by nine or more brain lesions on MRI; or four to eight MRI brain lesions plus one spinal cord MRI lesion; or four to eight MRI brain lesions plus abnormal visual evoked potential (VEP); or less than 4 MRI brain lesions plus 1 spinal cord MRI lesion plus abnormal VEP; or two or more spinal cord MRI lesions
(4) No better explanation than MS

---

include PPMS. These criteria follow those suggested by Thompson et al [22]. Abnormal CSF is required; however, this will lead to underdiagnosis because many patients who have PPMS have normal CSF. In a recent trial of 943 patients who had PPMS, 20% had normal CSF findings [23]. Aside from the CSF requirement, the diagnosis of PPMS follows the same general pattern of requiring dissemination in time and space (Box 5).

### Pitfalls in the diagnosis of multiple sclerosis

*Errors in the definition of attacks*

The requirement that symptoms from an attack last for at least 24 hours is intended to eliminate several nondemyelinating causes of neurologic symptoms. Most of these causes reflect changes in the electrical physiology of the nervous system rather than structural changes. In general, structural damage to the nervous system takes longer than 24 hours to repair. These conditions may be differentiated from MS by their clinical context and the absence of objective findings on examination. The use of MRI to rule out MS in these patients may be problematic because of frequent false positive findings in the normal population. For example, there is an increased incidence of T2-weighted lesions on brain MRI in people who have migraine [24]. Some diseases that present with attacks of short duration are shown in Table 1.

---

Fig. 2. Clinical subtypes of MS based on clinical course. (*Adapted from* Lublin FD, Reingold SC. Defining the clinical course of multiple sclerosis: results of an international survey. National Multiple Sclerosis Society (USA) Advisory Committee on Clinical Trials of New Agents in Multiple Sclerosis. Neurology 1996;46:907–11.)

Table 1
Diseases presenting with attacks lasting less than 24 hours

| Disease | Comment |
|---------|---------|
| Seizures | Usually stereotyped, simple or complex partial seizures |
| Migraine | Usually, but not always, associated with headache (eg, ocular migraine) |
| Panic disorder/hyperventilation | Often reproducible on voluntary hyperventilation |
| Transient ischemic attack | Vascular risk factors, MRI with grey matter lesions as well as white matter lesions |
| Medications/recreational drugs | Usually sedatives |
| Metabolic derangements | Hyperglycemia, hypoglycemic conditions, sodium derangements, calcium derangements |
| Toxins | Best diagnosed through history of exposure |
| Somatization | Myriad symptoms, excessive concern |

Illustrative case: a 35-year-old woman presents with a tentative diagnosis of MS. She has had recurrent attacks of nonvertiginous dizziness and disequilibrium over the past 3 years. These attacks have a rapid onset, last 10 to 30 minutes, and occur from once a month to several times a week. In addition, she has suffered numerous attacks of paresthesias in her hands, feet, or face. Her MRI shows several punctuate white matter lesions. Her neurologic examination is normal. Her symptoms of dizziness were reproduced after 30 seconds of hyperventilation. On further questioning, she has a past history of panic attacks and a positive family history of panic disorder. A diagnosis of panic disorder associated with hyperventilation was made. Although this patient's symptoms of recurrent dizziness and paresthesias suggest MS, the short duration of the episodes do not meet the definition of MS attacks.

The diagnostic criteria consider events that occur within 30 days to be part of the same attack. Patients may be mistakenly diagnosed with MS if events within a 30-day period are separated into different attacks. Examples of this include stuttering strokes, infectious diseases, and a variety of nervous system tumors. ADEM may be particularly difficult to differentiate from the first attack of MS (vide infra).

*Errors in symptom identification*

Symptoms should be typical of those that are seen with MS (see Box 4). Symptoms that are not typical should be evaluated carefully before attributing them to the disease. These atypical features often offer important clues to the correct diagnosis (Table 2).

Illustrative case (adapted from [25]): a 35-year-old woman developed scintillating scotomata, headache, and personality change. Three months later there was sudden visual loss in the right eye. By the fourth month she required hospitalization for headache, nausea, and acute psychosis. On MRI, she had multiple areas of increased T2 signals without enhancement. Serum

Table 2
Diseases presenting with neurologic symptoms atypical for multiple sclerosis

| Atypical symptom | Disease |
| --- | --- |
| Hearing loss | Susac's disease [25] |
| | Cogan's syndrome [26] |
| Retinitis pigmentosa | NARP (Neuropathy, ataxia, retinitis pigmentosa) [27] |
| | Usher's syndrome [28] |
| Cranial nerve palsies (involvement of the peripheral nervous system portions of these nerves) | Lyme disease [29] |
| | Sarcoid |
| | Whipple's disease [30] |
| | Carcinomatous meningitis |
| Aphasia | Stroke |
| | Tumors |
| Altered mental status | Acute disseminated encephalomyelitis |
| Peripheral neuropathy alone | Guillain-Barre |
| | Chronic inflammatory demyelinating polyneuropathy |
| Peripheral neuropathy with central nervous system changes | B12 deficiency |
| | Adreno leukodystrophy [31] |
| | Metachromatic leukodystrophy [31] |
| | Krabbe's leukodystrophy [31] |
| | Friedreich's ataxia [31] |
| Lower motor neuron disease | Amyotrophic lateral sclerosis [32] |
| | Hereditary motor sensory neuropathy [33] |
| Seizures | Focal brain lesions |
| | Primary seizure disorder |
| Headaches | CADASIL |
| | Migraine |

*Abbreviation:* CADASIL, cerebral autosomal dominant asteriopathy with subcortical infarcts and leukoencephalopathy.

tests for vasculitic diseases were normal. By the fifth month her confusion had improved, but she developed severe bilateral hearing loss and vertigo. Ophthalmologic examinations with fluorescein angiography demonstrated multiple retinal branch artery occlusions. She was diagnosed with Susac's syndrome and improved with appropriate treatment [25]. Susac's syndrome is confused easily with MS; both diseases present with recurrent acute attacks of neurologic dysfunction. It is a vasculopathy that consists of a triad of cochlea, retina, and brain involvement. It typically presents with headache and encephalopathy. The pathology consists of small infarctions that are due to arteriolar occlusion which leads to a variety of central nervous system symptoms. Symptoms often are abrupt in onset. Involvement of the cochlea leads to hearing loss and tinnitus, and vestibular involvement may cause vertigo. Visual symptoms may be present, but many patients have asymptomatic retinal findings. Although most retinal lesions are visible on fundoscopy, fluorescein angiography may be necessary in some cases. The MRI findings in Susac's syndrome resemble those that are seen in MS. The corpus callosum is involved commonly; however, the lesions in Susac's syndrome typically affect the central portions of the corpus callosum, whereas they typically affect the undersurface in MS [34]. This gives them the appearance of multiple small holes in the middle of the corpus callosum on sagittal imaging. The diagnosis is made by identification of clinical symptoms followed by demonstration of the vascular changes on retinal examination. This case illustrates the importance of considering alternative diagnoses in patients who have symptoms that are atypical for MS. The encephalopathy and hearing loss were important clues to the correct diagnosis.

## Errors in requiring objective findings

Basing a diagnosis of MS entirely on subjective symptoms can lead to several errors. For example, patients who have somatization, hyperventilation/panic disorder, seizures, or malingering often have normal examinations. Even more problematic is the patient who has no symptoms, but lesions that are seen on an MRI. These patients should not be diagnosed with MS unless they develop symptoms that are typical of the disease. A considerable proportion of the normal population has lesions on MRI. A recent meta-analysis found white matter lesions in 7% of a control group and 23% of those who had migraine [24]. Four of the seven studies in the analysis selected control subjects to exclude comorbidities that might result in white matter lesions. Fazekas et al [35] found that white matter lesions were common in asymptomatic people and that they increased with age. By age 50, about half of the population has white matter hyperintensities.

Illustrative case: a 29-year-old woman presented with frequent headaches. An MRI was obtained which showed multiple white matter lesions. The radiology report described these as consistent with demyelinating disease. After 6 years of follow-up, she remains stable, clinically and by MRI. This case should not be diagnosed as MS because she did not have objective findings. In addition, she did not have dissemination in time. The cause of the changes on MRI is unknown, but could include several alternative explanations, such as trauma or remote infectious causes.

## Errors in dissemination in time

The requirement for multiple events at different times eliminates diseases that are nonrecurrent. This has important implications, diagnostically and therapeutically. Diseases comprising single events generally do not require long-term treatment. Table 3 includes diseases that may be confused with MS, but which do not have dissemination in time.

Illustrative case: a 42-year-old man had the sudden onset of numbness and weakness in the feet. Over several hours, this progressed to profound weakness in both legs, and numbness to the level of T4. MRI of the spine showed a T2-weighted lesion at T4 that enhanced with gadolinium. Brain

Table 3
Diseases presenting without dissemination in time

| Categories | Disease |
|---|---|
| Demyelinating diseases | Transverse myelitis |
|  | Optic neuritis |
|  | Acute disseminated encephalomyelitis (ADEM) |
| Trauma |  |
| Central nervous system neoplasms | Glioma, lymphomas, metastases |
| Posterior leukoencephalopathy | Associated with chemotherapy |
| Infections | Congenital infections (TORCH [toxoplasmosis, other infections, rubella, cytomegalovirus, and herpes simplex virus infections]) |
|  | Childhood viral infections |

MRI was normal. He improved with steroids, but was left with mild weakness and numbness with paresthesias in the legs. He was diagnosed with transverse myelitis. There is only a single lesion in space and a single lesion in time. His risk of developing MS is much lower given the normal brain MRI [36]. Recurrent bouts of transverse myelitis may occur in patients who do not develop MS [37]. Diagnostic criteria and suggested diagnostic evaluations for transverse myelitis have been published [38].

ADEM is used often to describe a variety of conditions, including perivenous encephalomyelitis, postinfectious encephalomyelitis, postvaccinial encephalomyelitis, and acute hemorrhagic leukoencephalomyelitis. ADEM presents with acute monophasic neurologic dysfunction that varies from mild to severe; however, it may have stuttering symptoms over several weeks and MRI changes over a few months [18]. Rare cases may be recurrent. It often has a younger age of onset than MS and is most common in the pediatric population. It often is preceded by a viral illness, and may have hemorrhagic changes on MRI. If optic neuritis is present, it often is bilateral. Early-onset ataxia suggests ADEM [39]. The clinical symptom that best differentiates ADEM from MS is altered mental status, which is found in 75% of cases of ADEM [40]. The CSF often has elevated numbers of cells and protein, usually lacks oligoclonal bands, and occasionally may be hemorrhagic [40]. The MRI appearance of ADEM may be indistinguishable from that of MS [35]. Because ADEM is a monophasic disease, the lesions often have a similar age. For example, there may be contrast enhancement of all or most lesions [35]; however, additional lesions may appear over time [41]. One study noted that new enhancing lesions in ADEM may appear during the recovery period, and that these may occur up to 4 months after symptom onset [42]. The differentiation of ADEM from MS may be particularly difficult in adults and may require long-term follow-up before a monophasic course can be certain [43].

Demyelinating diseases that have a single episode in time are termed clinically isolated syndromes (CIS). These may represent single events that are unlikely to recur, or they may be the first events of what eventually will be recognized as MS. It is inaccurate to diagnose CIS as MS until a second event is documented, either clinically or by MRI changes. Although CIS technically is not MS, it is appropriate to treat cases with a high risk of having MS. Currently, the best discriminator of those who are at high risk is a brain MRI (even in patients whose symptoms localize to nonbrain areas, such as the eye or spinal cord). In one large series of patients who had CIS, 6% of those with normal brain MRIs and 72% of those with abnormal brain MRIs developed MS within 5 years [44]. Fourteen years after the initial presentation, 19% of those with normal brain MRIs and 89% of those with abnormal brain MRIs developed clinically definite MS. Another 6% had probable MS. The risk for patients who present with optic neuritis may be slightly less than those with other presentations. In patients who have optic neuritis and an abnormal MRI, 56% will develop MS by 10 years, in contrast to 22% of those with normal MRI scans [45]. The number of abnormal lesions on the initial MRI did not indicate a greater likelihood of developing MS; however, larger numbers of lesions may suggest a greater risk of disability over time [36].

*Errors in dissemination in space*

Recurrent episodes of neurologic dysfunction that occur at a single location in the nervous system usually can be explained by some local pathology. In most cases, the pathology is obvious on imaging. Several conditions have lesions on MRI that may mimic MS. These differ in having MRI pathology only at the location of the focal symptom. Table 4 notes some of these diseases.

*Errors in addressing explanations other than multiple sclerosis*

The most difficult aspect of diagnosing MS is addressing other possible explanations. The differential diagnosis includes virtually all diseases that can cause lesions on brain MRI scans. Furthermore, many of these conditions do not have noninvasive screening tests available; many of those that do have simple tests available have unacceptably high false positive rates. The key to diagnosing these cases correctly lies in recognizing nonneurologic clues; however, there are so many possible diseases that it is difficult to address each one systematically in an individual who presents for diagnosis. Therefore, in addition to an extensive past medical history and review of systems, it is necessary to remain constantly vigilant for clues to an alternative diagnosis. A partial outline of these diseases is found in Table 4.

Illustrative case: a 34-year-old woman presents for evaluation of possible MS. At age 33 she presented with weakness of the left leg. Her symptoms progressively worsened over 3 months and led to paraplegia that required a wheelchair. She was diagnosed with transverse myelitis and treated with steroids. She had three additional attacks of transverse myelitis over the

Table 4
Diseases that mimic multiple sclerosis through dissemination in space and time

| Disease | Comments |
| --- | --- |
| Neuromyelitis optica (Devic's) | Spinal cord, optic nerve |
| Multiple small vessel strokes | Vascular risk factors |
| CADASIL | Family history |
| Rheumatologic disorders: | Usually evidence of systemic illness |
|   Lupus vasculitis | |
|   Rheumatoid arthritis vasculitis | |
|   Behcet's disease | |
|   Sarcoidosis | |
|   Sjogren's disease | |
| Central nervous system vasculitis | No serologic markers |
| Infections: | |
|   Progressive multi-focal leukoencephalopathy | Confluent lesion |
|   Human T-cell lymphotrophic virus (HTLV-1) | Endemic areas |
|   Lyme disease [29] | Endemic areas |
|   Syphilis | |
| Mitochondrial diseases: [31] | |
|   Myoclonus epilepsy associated with ragged-red fibers (MERRF) | |
|   Mitochondrial myopathy, encephalopathy, lactic acidosis, stroke-like episodes (MELAS) | |
|   Leber's hereditary optic neuropathy | |
|   Overlapping mitochondrial syndromes | |
| Gastrointestinal diseases: | |
|   Crohn's vasculitis [46] | |
|   Mitochondrial neurogastrointestinal encephalopathy [47] | |

following year. These were treated with steroids, but led to residual weakness in the legs, sensory symptoms in her arms, and a neurogenic bladder. She also was noted to have decreased vision in the right eye. Her brain MRI showed multiple T2- and FLAIR-weighted white matter lesions (Fig. 3). Her spinal cord MRI showed several areas of increased T2 signal and an atrophic spinal cord (Fig. 4). Further history revealed that she had systemic lupus erythematosus (SLE) since age 19 with an antinuclear antibody of 1:2500, positive antiphospholipid antibodies, aseptic necrosis of the hips, and 10 hospitalizations for complications of lupus. Her neurologic condition was attributed to SLE rather than MS. Lupus usually is not mistaken for MS. Generally, patients who have SLE have clinical features that lead to the diagnosis of lupus, with neurologic complications occurring later in the disease course. In one series, only one of nine patients who had transverse myelitis in the setting of lupus had the myelitis at onset; however, that patient had an extensive lesion that stretched from the cervicomedullary junction to T10, which suggested that this was a case of neuromyelitis optica [48]. Screening of patients who are suspected of having MS with serologic

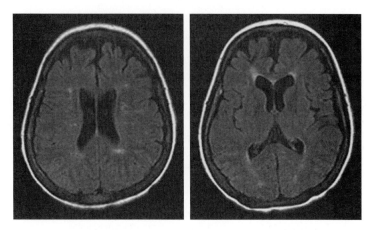

Fig. 3. T2-weighted lesions in the periventricular white matter typical of those seen in demyelinating disease; however, this patient had systemic lupus erythematosus.

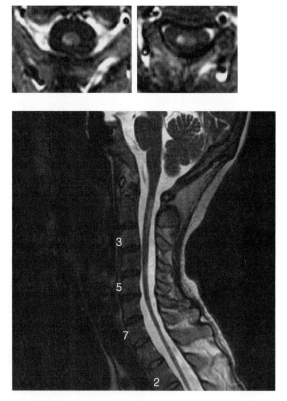

Fig. 4. Extensive T2-weighted lesions in the spinal cord of a woman who has SLE. Note the atrophy in the lower portions of the cord.

tests for lupus has a high false positive rate, does not identify a subset having lupus, and does not identify patients who have MS with different clinical courses [49]. The antiphospholipid antibody syndrome also may present with several central nervous system symptoms; however, most investigators recommend that screening not be performed unless there are other systemic symptoms of the disease [50]. The benefit of indiscriminant screening is doubtful and the false positive rate is high [51].

Illustrative case: a 56-year-old woman presented with a history of MS. At age 53, she developed the abrupt onset of numbness on the left face, arm, and leg. She had a relapsing remitting course of neurologic symptoms that led to disability over 7 months. She had weakness and spasticity of all four limbs, more prominently in the legs. She had numbness and paresthesias in her legs and a neurogenic bladder. She had tremors, memory loss, depression, fatigue, and occasional vertigo. Her brain MRI showed multiple white matter lesions. Because of a history of colitis since age 51, a gastroenterology consult was undertaken. Her colitis was deemed under good control with sulfasalazine and prednisone. During the subsequent 3 years, she continued to have relapses of neurologic dysfunction, despite treatment for MS. She also developed weight loss and prominent wasting of her legs and arms. Two electromyographic examinations were inconclusive. Her arm wasting became more marked. An MRI of the cervical cord and the brachial plexus were unremarkable. A magnetic resonance neurogram was performed which showed a high signal abnormality in the brachial plexus. Her final diagnosis was Crohn's vasculitis, rather than MS. Although her initial course was consistent with MS, the recognition of unusual symptoms that suggested peripheral nerve involvement, and consideration of alternative diagnoses eventually led to the correct diagnosis. MRI lesions have been reported in a high percentage of patients who have Crohn's disease [46].

Several additional diseases provide sufficient diagnostic difficulty to warrant further discussion. Strokes, in particular small vessel strokes, can be difficult to differentiate from MS. Typically, with stroke, the clinical presentation is of more rapid onset, occurring over seconds or minutes rather than hours. The MRI appearance may be similar. Strokes usually spare the subcortical "U" fibers, whereas juxtacortical lesions are seen in 30% of cases of MS [13,27]; however, one recent study found juxtacortical lesions in 80% of patients who had MS and 41% of patients who had symptomatic cerebrovascular disease [52]. Infratentorial lesions were found in 84% of patients who had MS and 35% of patients with who had cerebrovascular disease [43]. Barkhof criteria for MS were met by 12% of cases of cerebrovascular disease [52]. The degree of damage within a lacunar stroke often is more severe than in MS; the center of lacunar lesions tend to appear isodense with CSF [27]. Finding evidence of neurologic disease in the spinal cord or optic nerves increases the likelihood of MS relative to vascular disease because these are locations that are unlikely to suffer silent infarctions. Spinal cord MRI was abnormal in 92% of patients who had MS compared with only 6% of patients who had symptomatic vascular disease [52].

Cerebral autosomal dominant arteriopathy with subcortical infarcts and leukoencephalopathy (CADASIL) frequently presents with dementia, migraine, and strokelike events. It is dominantly inherited, so there often is a positive family history. Migraine may be absent in approximately 35.4% of cases and stroke histories may be absent in 31.2% [53]. More than 90% of patients who have CADASIL have multiple white matter lesions that resemble those of MS [54]. One third do not have the T1-weighted changes that are expected with strokes. Lesions are often in the periventricular and deep white matter. Confluent lesions are seen commonly in the anterior temporal pole and the external capsule (Fig. 5). In one series, moderate or severe involvement of the anterior temporal pole was seen in

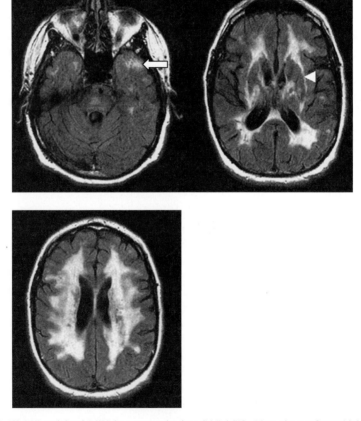

Fig. 5. FLAIR-weighted MRI in a man who has CADASIL. Note the confluent high-signal area in the anterior temporal region (*arrowhead*) and the involvement of the external capsule (*arrow*).

89% of cases, whereas moderate or severe involvement of the external capsule was seen in 93% of cases. Using patients who were less than 60 years of age who had recurrent lacunar strokes and leukoaraiosis as a comparison group, anterior temporal pole lesions had a sensitivity of 89% and a specificity of 86%. Changes in the external capsule had a sensitivity of 93% and a specificity of 45% [53].

Traditionally, neuromyelitis optica (Devic's syndrome) has been viewed as a monophasic acute illness with devastating neurologic symptoms; however, that view has now been called into question [55]. The disease involves the optic nerves and spinal cord. Approximately 32% of patients present with a monophasic course, with 68% having a relapsing course that resembles that seen in MS. Although many of these cases had benign courses, the disease can be aggressive with respiratory failure developing in 25%. Antinuclear antibodies may be found in almost half. The CSF shows a mild pleocytosis in 79% with 35% having more than 50 cells/mm$^3$. The initial brain MRI is normal or near normal, but approximately half of patients develop a few lesions over time. These generally do not meet the MRI criteria for MS. MRI of the spinal cord typically shows confluent lesions that extend across three or more bony levels (Fig. 6). This is in contrast to MS in which each spinal cord lesion typically is confined to fewer than three levels. Diagnostic criteria have been proposed [55].

*Errors in diagnosing primary progressive multiple sclerosis*

Diagnosing primary progressive MS carries all the pitfalls of errors in identifying dissemination in space and time that have already been discussed.

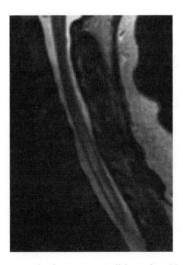

Fig. 6. Spine MRI in a woman who has neuromyelitis optica. Note the extent of the lesion extending beyond three bony levels.

Table 5
Diseases that mimic primary progressive multiple sclerosis

| Disease | Comments |
| --- | --- |
| Spinal dural arteriovenous malformations (AVM) [56] | Enlarged vessels on MRI |
| Vitamin deficiencies (B12, vitamin E) | Check serum levels |
| Paraneoplastic syndromes (cerebellar ataxia, limbic encephalitis, carcinoma-associated retinopathy) | Often with constitutional symptoms |
| Syphilis | |
| Copper deficiency [57] | Excessive zinc intake |
| Hereditary cerebellar ataxias (dominant and recessive) [58] | |
| Hereditary spastic paraparesis [59] | |
| Olivopontocerebellar degeneration | |
| Leukodystrophies [60] | |
| Infectious causes (HTLV-1, progressive multifocal leukoencephalopathy [PML], AIDS) | |
| Compressive myelopathies | MRI findings |
| Central nervous system neoplasms (gliomas, lymphomas) | Constitutional symptoms |
| Vasculitis | Constitutional symptoms |
| Syringomyelia | Found on MRI |

In addition, there is a broad differential of other potential causes that must be addressed. A partial outline of the diseases that must be considered in found in Table 5.

Illustrative case: this 51-year-old woman had a 2-year history of slowly progressive weakness in the legs followed by tingling in her hands and numbness in her lower trunk. An MRI of the brain showed a thin rim of hyperintensity around the lateral ventricles on T2-weighted images. In addition, there were two punctuate lesions in the periphery of the cerebral white matter. Visual and somatosensory evoked potentials were normal and there were no oligoclonal bands in her CSF. She was referred for suspected MS. A cervical MRI showed a compressive myelopathy (Fig. 7). This case illustrates the need to evaluate other causes of slowly progressive neurologic loss, especially in those who have symptoms of myelopathy.

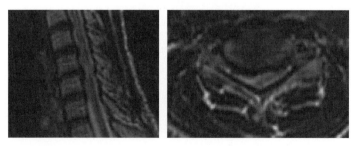

Fig. 7. Compressive myelopathy with a high signal lesion on T2-weighted images. Note the compression on the axial slice.

## Summary

The diagnosis of MS requires central nervous system symptoms that are disseminated in time and space, and that have no better explanation. Dissemination in time and space may be demonstrated clinically or by MRI imaging. The differential diagnosis is broad, and requires the exclusion of several diseases that are described in the text. Following the new guidelines for the diagnosis of MS allows an early and accurate diagnosis of the disease.

## References

[1] Allison R, Millar J. Prevalence of disseminated sclerosis in Northern Ireland. Ulster Med J 1954;23(Suppl 2):1–27.

[2] McAlpine D, Lumsden C, Acheson E. Multiple sclerosis: a reappraisal. Edinburgh (Scotland): Churchill Livingstone; 1973.

[3] McDonald W, Halliday A. Diagnosis and classification of multiple sclerosis. Br Med Bull 1977;33(1):4–9.

[4] Rose A, Ellison GW, Myers L, Tourtellotte W. Criteria for the clinical diagnosis of multiple sclerosis. Neurology 1976;26(6 Pt 2):20–2.

[5] Schumacker G, Beebe G, Kibler R, et al. Problems of experimental trials of therapy in multiple sclerosis. report by the panel on the evaluation of experimental trials of therapy in multiple sclerosis. Ann N Y Acad Sci 1965;122:552–68.

[6] Poser C, Paty D, Scheinberg L, et al. New diagnostic criteria for multiple sclerosis: guidelines for research protocols. Ann Neurol 1983;13(3):227–31.

[7] McDonald W, Compston A, Edan G, et al. Recommended diagnostic criteria for multiple sclerosis: guidelines from the International Panel on the Diagnosis of Multiple Sclerosis. Ann Neurol 2001;50(1):121–7.

[8] Herndon R, Coyle P, Murray T, et al. Report of the Consensus Panel on the New International panel Guidelines for Diagnosis of MS. J Mult Scler Care 2002;4(4):2.

[9] Dalton C, Brex P, Miszkiel K, et al. Application of the new McDonald criteria to patients with clinically isolated syndromes suggestive of multiple sclerosis. Ann Neurol 2002;52(1): 47–53.

[10] Tintoré M, Rovira A, Ryó J, et al. New diagnostic criteria for multiple sclerosis: application in first demyelinating episode. Neurology 2003;60(1):27–30.

[11] Fangerau T, Schimrigk S, Haupts M, et al. Diagnosis of multiple sclerosis: comparison of the Poser criteria and the new McDonald criteria. Acta Neurol Scand 2004;109(6):385–9.

[12] Miller D, Filippi M, Fazekas F, et al. Role of magnetic resonance imaging within diagnostic criteria for multiple sclerosis. Ann Neurol 2004;56(2):273–8.

[13] Barkhof F, Filippi M, Miller D, et al. Comparison of MRI criteria at first presentation to predict conversion to clinically definite multiple sclerosis. Brain 1997;120(Pt 11):2059–69.

[14] Fazekas F, Offenbacher H, Fuchs S, et al. Criteria for an increased specificity of MRI interpretation in elderly subjects with suspected multiple sclerosis. Neurology 1988;38(12): 1822–5.

[15] Paty D, Oger J, Kastrukoff L, et al. MRI in the diagnosis of MS: a prospective study with comparison of clinical evaluation, evoked potentials, oligoclonal banding and CT. Neurology 1988;38(2):180–5.

[16] Tintore M, Rovira A, Martinez M, et al. Isolated demyelinating syndromes: comparison of different MR imaging criteria to predict conversion to clinically definite multiple sclerosis. Am J Neuroradiol 2000;21(4):702–6.

[17] Bot J, Barkhof F, Polman C, et al. Spinal cord abnormalities in recently diagnosed MS patients: added value of spinal MRI examination. Neurology 2004;62(2):226–33.

[18] Dale R, DeSousa C, Chong W, et al. Acute disseminated encephalomyelitis and multiple sclerosis in children. A follow-up study to compare clinical and investigative findings on disease presentation. Brain 2000;123(Pt 12):2407–22.

[19] Dalton C, Brex P, Miszkiel K, et al. New T2 lesions enable an earlier diagnosis of multiple sclerosis in clinically isolated syndromes. Ann Neurol 2003;53(5):673–6.

[20] Lunding J, Midgard R, Vedeler C. Oligoclonal bands in cerebrospinal fluid: a comparative study of isoelectric focusing, agarose gel electrophoresis and IgG index. Acta Neurol Scand 2000;102(5):322–5.

[21] Andersson M, Alvarez-Cermeno J, Bernardi G, et al. Cerebrospinal fluid in the diagnosis of multiple sclerosis: a consensus report. J Neurol Neurosurg Psychiatry 1994;57(8): 897–902.

[22] Thompson A, Montalban X, Barkhof F, et al. Diagnostic criteria for primary progressive multiple sclerosis: a position paper. Ann Neurol 2000;47(6):831–5.

[23] Wolinsky JS, PROMiSe Trial Study Group. The PROMiSe trial: baseline data review and progress report. Multiple Sclerosis 2004;10:S65–72.

[24] Swartz R, Kern R. Migraine is associated with magnetic resonance imaging white matter abnormalities. Arch Neurol 2004;61(9):1366–8.

[25] Papo T, Biousse V, Lehoang P, et al. Susac syndrome. Medicine 1998;77(1):3–11.

[26] Haynes B, Kaiser-Kupfer M, Mason P, et al. Cogan syndrome: studies in thirteen patients, long-term follow-up, and a review of the literature. Medicine 1980;59(6):426–41.

[27] Santorelli F, Tanji K, Shanske S, et al. Heterogeneous clinical presentation of the mtDNA NARP/T8993G mutation. Neurology 1997;49(1):270–3.

[28] Petit C. Usher syndrome: from genetics to pathogenesis. Annu Rev Genomics Hum Genet 2001;2:271–97.

[29] Halperin J, Logigian E, Finkel M, et al. Practice parameters for the diagnosis of patients with nervous system Lyme borreliosis (Lyme disease). Neurology 1996;46(3):619–27.

[30] Marth T, Raoult D. Whipple's disease. Lancet 2003;361(9353):239–46.

[31] Natowicz M, Bejjani B. Genetic disorders that masquerade as multiple sclerosis. Am J Med Genet 1994;49(2):149–69.

[32] Comi G, Rovaris M, Leocani L. Review neuroimaging in amyotrophic lateral sclerosis. Eur J Neurol 1999;6(6):629–37.

[33] Pareyson D. Diagnosis of hereditary neuropathies in adult patients. J Neurol 2003;250(2): 148–60.

[34] Susac J, Murtagh F, Egan R, et al. MRI findings in Susac's syndrome. Neurology 2003; 61(12):1783–7.

[35] Fazekas F, Barkhof F, Filippi M, et al. The contribution of magnetic resonance imaging to the diagnosis of multiple sclerosis. Neurology 1999;53(3):448–56.

[36] Brex P, Ciccarelli O, O'Riordan J, et al. A longitudinal study of abnormalities on MRI and disability from multiple sclerosis. N Engl J Med 2002;346(3):158–64.

[37] Kim K. Idiopathic recurrent transverse myelitis. Arch Neurol 2003;60(9):1290–4.

[38] Transverse Myelitis Consortium Working Group. Proposed diagnostic criteria and nosology of acute transverse myelitis. Neurology 2002;59(4):499–505.

[39] Hynson J, Kornberg A, Coleman L, et al. Clinical and neuroradiologic features of acute disseminated encephalomyelitis in children. Neurology 2001;56(10):1308–12.

[40] Mikaeloff Y, Suissa S, Vallee L, et al. First episode of acute CNS inflammatory demyelination in childhood: prognostic factors for multiple sclerosis and disability. J Pediatr 2004;144(2):246–52.

[41] Kesselring J, Miller D, Robb S, et al. Acute disseminated encephalomyelitis: MRI findings and the distinction from multiple sclerosis. Brain 1990;113(Pt 2):291–302.

[42] Honkaniemi J, Dastidar P, Kahara V, et al. Delayed MR imaging changes in acute disseminated encephalomyelitis. AJNR Am J Neuroradiol 2001;22(6):1117–24.

[43] Schwarz S, Mohr A, Knauth M, et al. Acute disseminated encephalomyelitis: a follow-up study of 40 adult patients. Neurology 2001;56(10):1313–8.

[44] Morrissey S, Miller D, Kendall B, et al. The significance of brain magnetic resonance imaging abnormalities at presentation with clinically isolated syndromes suggestive of multiple sclerosis: a 5-year follow-up study. Brain 1993;116(Pt 1):135–46.

[45] Beck R, Trobe J, Koke P, et al. High- and low-risk profiles for the development of multiple sclerosis within 10 years after optic neuritis: experience of the optic neuritis treatment trial. Arch Ophthalmol 2003;121(7):944–9.

[46] Hart P, Gould S, MacSweeney J, et al. Brain white-matter lesions in inflammatory bowel disease. Lancet 1998;351(9115):1558.

[47] Hirano M, Nishigaki Y, Marti R. Mitochondrial neurogastrointestinal encephalomyopathy (MNGIE): a disease of two genomes. Neurologist 2004;10(1):8–17.

[48] Chan K, Boey M. Transverse myelopathy in SLE: clinical features and functional outcomes. Lupus 1996;5(4):294–9.

[49] Tourbah A, Clapin A, Gout O, et al. Systemic autoimmune features and multiple sclerosis. Arch Neurol 1998;55(4):517–21.

[50] Sastre-Garriga J, Montalban X. APS and the brain. Lupus 2003;12(12):877–82.

[51] Sastre-Garriga J, Reverter J, Font J, et al. Anticardiolipin antibodies are not a useful screening tool in a nonselected large group of patients with multiple sclerosis. Ann Neurol 2001;49(3):408–11.

[52] Bot J, Barkhof F, Nijeholt G, et al. Differentiation of multiple sclerosis from other inflammatory diseases and cerebrovascular disease: value of spinal MR imaging. Radiology 2002;223(1):46–56.

[53] Markus H, Martin R, Simpson M, et al. Diagnostic strategies in CADASIL. Neurology 2002;59(8):1134–8.

[54] Chabriat H, Levy C, Taillia H, et al. Patterns of MRI lesions in CADASIL. Neurology 1998; 51(2):452–7.

[55] Wingerchuk D, Hogancamp W, O'Brien P, et al. The clinical course of neuromyelitis optica (Devic's syndrome). Neurology 1999;53(5):1107–14.

[56] Muraszko K, Oldfield E. Vascular malformations of the spinal cord and dura. Neurosurg Clin North Am 1990;1(3):631–52.

[57] Kumar N, Gross J, Ahlskog J. Myelopathy due to copper deficiency. Neurology 2003;61(2): 273–4.

[58] Schols L, Bauer P, Schmidt T, et al. Autosomal dominant cerebellar ataxias: clinical features, genetics, and pathogenesis. Lancet 2004;3(5):291–304.

[59] McDermott C, White K, Bushby K, et al. Hereditary spastic paraparesis: a review of new developments. J Neurol Neurosurg Psychiatry 2000;69(2):150–60.

[60] Schiffmann R, van der Knaap M. The latest on leukodystrophies. Curr Opin Neurol 2004; 17(2):187–92.

ELSEVIER
SAUNDERS

Phys Med Rehabil Clin N Am
16 (2005) 383–409

PHYSICAL MEDICINE
AND REHABILITATION
CLINICS OF
NORTH AMERICA

# MRI in Multiple Sclerosis

## Jack H. Simon, MD, PhD

*Department of Radiology, University of Colorado Health Sciences Center,*
*4200 East Ninth Avenue, Box A-034, Denver, CO 80262, USA*

MRI provides multiple uses and applications in multiple sclerosis (MS), ranging from diagnosis in individuals to its use as an outcome measure in MS clinical trials. In this article, the basic features of the MRI-detected lesions, including the underlying pathology, are discussed to provide reference for evaluating the extensive literature in the field. MRI allows assessment of the normal-appearing white and gray matter, and neuronal tract and functional system disturbances. An overview of the clinical significance of these MRI measures is included, as a basis for understanding their role as outcome measures in clinical trials. MRI recently assumed greater importance in its role in establishing an earlier diagnosis of MS after a first clinical event, and in monitoring subclinical disease before or subsequent to the formal diagnosis. The background to these applications and practical issues are discussed.

## Basic MRI lesion overview

It is convenient and instructive to classify MS pathology that is detected by direct neuropathologic examination or MRI as focal or diffuse. Focal, classic MS lesions represent a range of pathology from minimal change (eg, edema) to demyelination and axonal injury or loss [1]. The diffuse pathology may be evident by MRI only indirectly (volume loss-atrophy), or based on analyses of the normal-appearing white or gray matter tissue using the advanced quantitative MRI methodologies [2,3]. The normal-appearing white or gray matter may be found to be abnormal [2]. There is mounting evidence that the clinical and cognitive consequences of MS pathology require understanding the focal pathology, yet the diffuse pathology may be equally, if not more, important in contributing to injury.

---

*E-mail address:* jack.simon@uchsc.edu

1047-9651/05/$ - see front matter © 2005 Elsevier Inc. All rights reserved.
doi:10.1016/j.pmr.2005.01.012                          *pmr.theclinics.com*

*Enhancing lesions, the blood–brain barrier, and inflammation*

The first sign of an acute MS lesion using conventional MRI is the focal gadolinium-chelate enhancing lesion, which typically also is associated with hyperintensity on T2-weighted imaging. The focal enhancing lesion reflects abnormal leakage of contrast material across the blood–brain barrier into the interstitial spaces; the blood–brain barrier normally is resistant to passive transport of contrast as a result of the tight junctions of the vascular endothelium. A complex interplay of factors are active at the endothelial level, related to the adhesion molecules, promoting attachment of activated cells, and matrix metalloproteinases which may promote translocation of cells through the endothelial boundaries. These and other factors come into play around the time that antigen-specific T cells enter the central nervous system, recognize antigen, and trigger a cytokine/chemokine cascade that further mediates disruption of the blood–brain barrier [4,5]. There is strong evidence that the macroscopic-enhancing lesion is preceded, by months or years, by tissue changes that are detected in the normal-appearing white matter (NAWM) by multiple quantitative methodologies [6–9], including, most recently, measures of perfusion [10]. When enhancement is detected by conventional MRI in MS, although its basis is the disrupted blood–brain barrier, it functionally serves as a marker of macroscopic inflammation [11–13], and potentially out-of-control inflammation [14].

More specific probes of the cellular migration that occurs at the level of the blood–brain barrier during the inflammatory process are feasible using superparamagnetic iron oxides. After intravenous (IV) injection, these particles concentrate within macrophages, and can be followed in vivo in humans as they enter the compartments of the central nervous system (CNS). The intracellular particles exert a strong influence on the local magnetic field, which is detected as signal loss (eg, using T2*-weighted [pronounced T2-star] pulse sequences) [15,16]. Cell-type specific tagging has been shown to be feasible in animal studies. In this approach, super-paramagnetic tags are introduced out of the body through transfection, then the tagged cells are reintroduced by IV injection [17]. These approaches may contribute to understanding the details of microscopic, so-called smoldering and possibly "good" inflammation in MS [14,18].

Once gadolinium enhancement is observed in an acute MS lesion, enhancement remains visible for a period of approximately 2 to 8 weeks in most cases, but can last from less than 1 week to as long as 16 weeks (Fig. 1) [19,20]. The enhancement pattern (size, rings, shape) may be strikingly variable within, and especially, between patients; this is highly suggestive of heterogeneous pathology that may be related to "host" response, etiology [21,22], or severity [23]. The relationship between the enhancement pattern and pathology and enhancement pattern and clinical outcome is not strong. Enhancement that is seen only after high (triple dose) magnetic resonance contrast infusion tends to be smaller and also may be a less destructive

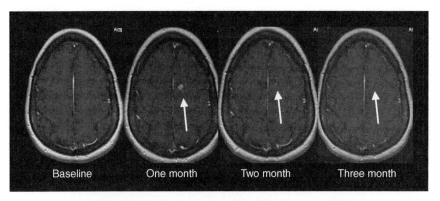

Fig. 1. Time course for enhancing lesion. Serial monthly MRI shows new enhancing lesion after one month, and expected decrease in size over subsequent 2 months which corresponds to reduction in inflammation and return of the integrity of the blood–brain barrier breakdown.

pathology than that detected by single (standard) dose magnetic resonance contrast [24,25].

In addition to harboring an inflammatory pathology, evidence from biopsy and autopsy series suggest that acute MS lesions can be characterized by an impressive degree of axonal injury and axonal transection within the lesion, and less so, along its borders [26]. That axonal injury occurs early in MS is supported by the in vivo magnetic resonance spectroscopy literature which provides evidence that N-acetylaspartate (NAA), a neuronal marker [27], already is reduced in acute lesions and early disease, as it is in later stages of disease [28–30].

The number and volume of enhancing lesions within individual patients who have MS varies over time, as documented most dramatically in high-frequency (monthly and weekly) MRI series [19,20,31]; however general activity patterns often can be recognized, even in individuals. Some individuals, on most monthly enhanced MRI studies, show little or no enhancing lesion activity. Others are more likely than not to have one or more lesions. In population studies, the magnitude of the peak number and the frequency of the enhancement peaks show some stability over time [31,32]; this permits enhancing lesion measures to be informative in natural history studies and MS clinical trials [31].

## The T2-hyperintense (T2) lesion

Most acute, enhancing MS lesions are hyperintense on T2-weighted imaging; the T2-hyperintense area includes and often extends beyond the borders of the enhancement (Fig. 2). The more peripheral areas of T2-hyperintensity most likely represent reversible, perilesional edema. T2-hyperintensity reflects a locally disturbed water environment and is non-specific regarding pathology [1]. Examination of chronic T2-hyperintense

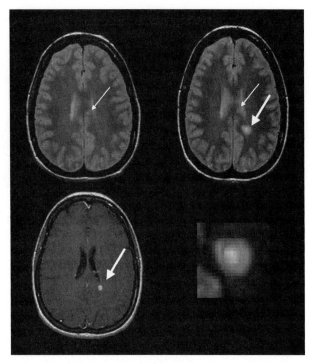

Fig. 2. Development of an acute T2-hyperintense lesion observed by serial MRI. (*Upper left*) Case of relapsing MS with low T2-hyperintense lesion burden, including chronic lesions in the corpus callosum (*dotted arrow*). (*Upper right*) One month later, a new T2-hyperintense lesion develops in the left parietal-occipital white matter (*solid arrow*), whereas the corpus callosum lesions remain completely stable (*dotted arrow*). (*Lower left*) Corresponding enhancement in acute lesion, from blood–brain barrier breakdown and concurrent inflammation. (*Lower right*) Exploded view of the new lesion shows the complex structure, centrally hyperintense (likely mixed pathology); intermediate black ring, possibly related to zone of macrophage infiltration; and outer ring of edema.

lesions under the microscope reveals a great deal of heterogeneity between lesions. In some T2 lesions, demyelination predominates, whereas others suffer more severe injury with axonal loss and severe matrix disruption. This lack of pathologic specificity of the T2 lesion is believed to contribute strongly to the poor association between T2-lesion load in the brain or spinal cord and disability [33].

After reaching a maximal T2-hyperintense lesion size over a period of approximately 4 to 8 weeks, the T2-hyperintensity typically shrinks over weeks to months [34,35]. The smaller residual area of focal T2-hyperintensity is the nonspecific "footprint" of the earlier acute event. Although many T2 lesions will not change over years, activity with expansion may occur along the periphery or centrally. Reactivation, or subsequent events in a focal lesion is an important potential mechanism that is related to more

severe focal injury, through cumulative demyelination or axonal injury, and at least in theory, through loss of capacity for remyelination [36,37].

Over time, in individual patients and in populations, multiple focal T2-lesions in the brain or spinal cord accumulate in number; individual lesions may increase in volume; and overall, the T2-burden of disease (T2-BOD) tends to increase in the absence of treatment. With disease progression, the multiple focal lesions often become confluent; as their borders collide, there is loss of normal intervening tissue, and additional T2-hyperintensity develops through secondary (fiber) degeneration [38,39].

## Chronic T1-hypointense lesions (T1–black holes)

By T1-weighted imaging, chronic MS lesions can be separated into two distinct groups (Fig 3). Most chronic T2-hyperintense lesions are isointense (same signal intensity) relative to normal white matter. A smaller fraction of the chronic T2-hyperintense lesions (~10%–20%) are hypointense (lower signal) relative to normal white matter [40,41]. The chronic T1-hypointense lesion fraction (the classic T1–black hole) is important because it represents white matter enriched for severe injury, with reduction in axonal density and matrix disruption. Consistent with more severe focal injury, the T1-hypintense lesions also show reduced magnetization transfer ratios, elevated diffusion coefficient, and reduced NAA [40].

In evaluating an image, it is important to distinguish acute T1-hypointense areas—which are T1-hypointense on the basis of edema and may show considerable recovery—from chronic T1-hypointense lesions, which are the classic T1–black holes described in the literature. Because

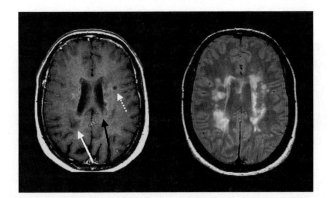

Fig. 3. T1-hypointense lesion terminology. (*Left panel*) In the left frontal white matter, a sharply-defined ring-enhancing lesion (*dotted white arrow*) is T1-hypointense on the basis of acute edema. The posterior right parietal white matter (*solid white arrow*) shows a classic, chronic, nonenhancing region of T1-hypointensity (ie, a T1-black hole), which is an area of more severe injury, as compared with other nonspecific T2-hyperintense regions without corresponding T1-hypointensity (*black arrow*, posterior left parietal-occipital white matter). (*Right panel*) T2-weighted image.

serial studies are not always available to assess the chronicity of a T1-hypointense lesion, chronicity often is assumed based on T1-hypointensity after contrast enhancement. Acute T1-hypointense (edematous) lesions evolve over 3 to 9 months to isointensity to normal white matter or remain hypointense to normal white matter; the latter occurs approximately one third of the time. Transition of an acute MS lesion to normal signal intensity reflects recovery from the edematous stage, and potentially partial re-myelination [36]. There is no specific remyelination MRI measure [37].

T1-hypointense lesion volume (T1-BOD) based on enhanced MRI is being used increasingly in MS clinical trials to measure the fraction of tissue that is more severely and mostly irreversibly injured (compared with the less specific T2-BOD). Another measure is based on following the development of T1–black holes from each individual earlier enhancing lesion to determine if treatment has the effect of decreasing the rate of evolution to severe damage [42,43].

## Distribution of focal lesions in the brain and spinal cord

### Characteristics and distribution of lesions in the brain

T2-hyperintense lesions occur throughout the CNS, with a typical distribution in the periventricular (touching ventricle surface) white matter more so than the peripheral white matter, but they occur commonly in both regions [35]. Within the white matter, T2-lesions may be discrete (separate from ventricle surface), and when peripheral, many touch the gray matter (juxtacortical). Lesions may straddle gray and white matter (juxtacortical-cortical), or rarely, by MRI, may lie entirely within the cortical gray matter (cortical) (Fig. 4). Many periventricular or discrete lesions extend at a right

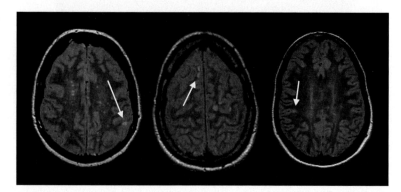

Fig. 4. Cortical MS lesion. Pure cortical gray matter lesions are difficult to identify by conventional MRI (*left panel*), but are not uncommon by histopathology. (*Middle panel*) A lesion that appears to be partly cortical and partly within white matter (juxtacortical-cortical). (*Right panel*) shows a juxtacortical (touching cortex) white matter lesion, a common finding in MS.

angle from the lateral ventricle surfaces and have a characteristic ovoid shape. Corpus callosum lesions are more likely within the inner or deep surfaces. Optic nerve lesions can be seen with high-resolution fat-suppression techniques, acutely, at the time of an optic neuritis, and show strong correlations with visual function and electrophysiologic impairment [44]. Good clinical-MRI correlations also are seen for brainstem lesions that cause an internuclear ophthalmoplegia [45] and for fifth nerve findings, with abnormalities at the root entry zone or more peripherally [46]. Deep gray matter involvement may occur, but disproportionate deep gray matter lesion volume would suggest alternative diagnoses. Deep cerebellar hemisphere, cerebellar peduncle, and brainstem surface lesions are common; the latter is more typical of demyelination than infarction or ischemia.

Another common feature in MS is brain atrophy. Brain atrophy is not a rare or a late event, may progress at a surprisingly rapid pace in some individuals, and can be measured over 1-year intervals in populations [47,48]. CNS atrophy that is detected by MRI in MS can be focal, and affect the central white matter and result in ventricular expansion; may affect the cerebellum or result in sulcal widening; and can cause brain volume loss [49]. Although atrophy is believed to reflect irreversible injury, it is a nonspecific measure that is based on variable loss of axons. The axon accounts for much of the volume of the normal white matter; however, myelin loss and other structural changes (those from astrogliosis) also contribute to atrophy in MS [48].

## Characteristics and distribution of lesions in the spinal cord

Most patients who have early MS have lesions that are detectable within the spinal cord [50,51]. In one study of 115 patients around the time of optic neuritis, only 12% had an abnormal spinal cord MRI when the brain MRI was normal. This increased to 45% when there were nine or more brain lesions; this group has a greater likelihood of MS [52].

Because spinal cord T2-hyperintense lesions are rare incidental findings that typically are not observed with normal aging—in contrast to nonspecific brain T2-hyperintensities—their observation can be helpful in increasing the confidence in a diagnosis of MS [51]. On sagittal imaging, most T2-hyperintense MS lesions in the spinal cord are oriented vertically and are less than 10 mm to 15 mm in height [51]. On axial T2-weighted images, lesion distribution across the spinal cord typically is asymmetric and corresponds to the frequent asymmetric clinical presentation of partial transverse myelitis [53]. Acute spinal cord lesions are expected to enhance; however, for technical reasons (image quality, pulsation artifacts) and possibly related to spinal cord structure, enhancement presence or absence is not reliable. Chronic T1–black holes are rare in the spinal cord in MS. A diffusely swollen, T1-hypointense spinal cord is more characteristic of Devic's neuromyelitis optica [54] or viral or idiopathic myelitis than MS. A focally swollen spinal cord (eg, one segment), although rare, occurs with sufficient frequency in MS at clinical onset that this finding should not discourage consideration of MS as a differential diagnostic consideration. Secondary changes in the spinal cord from MS include focal and diffuse volume loss [51,55,56], with atrophy in focal lesions from demyelination and axonal loss, and more diffuse volume loss from Wallerian degeneration [57–59].

### The normal-appearing white matter

Much of the injury in MS is known—from the pathology literature and increasingly from the MRI literature—to reside within the so-called NAWM and the normal-appearing gray matter (NAGM) [2,60]. Within the NAWM, microglial inflammatory pathology may dominate, rather than the lymphocytic inflammation that is characteristic of focal lesions [2]. In addition to glial pathology, axonal loss and loss or disruption of myelin also are seen in the NAWM [57,58,61–63].

By MRI, abnormalities are detected in the NAWM by all of the advanced quantitative methodologies. These abnormalities are detected readily in secondary progressive MS more so than in relapsing MS, and in primary progressive MS [2,64,65]. For the earliest stages of MS—as defined after a clinically isolated syndrome in individuals who have a positive MRI—abnormal NAWM may or may not be detected, but is more likely in cases that eventually go on to definite MS [2].

The physical basis for the quantitative MRI techniques are summarized in the Appendix. For magnetization transfer imaging, no single pathology is likely to account for the observed changes (ie, decreased magnetization transfer ratio with pathology); however, this method is sensitive to pathology in the NAWM that otherwise would go undetected by conventional imaging [64–67]. Experimental (animal) studies show variable, but modest, correlations for magnetization transfer ratio (MTR) with demyelination and Wallerian degeneration [68,69]. Remyelination has an effect on magnetization transfer [70]. Small changes in MTR can be detected readily in population studies, but MTR measures in individuals are not reliable or informative.

Several water diffusion–based measures detect abnormal NAWM in MS [71,72]. Nonspecific increases in the diffusion coefficient are detected in the NAWM in MS. This contrasts with the more specific decrease in diffusion coefficient (restricted diffusion) that is characteristic of acute infarction. Fractional anisotropy measures are more specific for loss or disruption of physical barriers in organized tissue, and provide an approximation of demyelination, because myelin disruption allows increased diffusion at right angles (transverse diffusion) to the principle fiber direction and a corresponding decrease in anisotropy (directionality). Potentially complicating this working hypothesis for interpreting anisotropy measures in MS is the experimental observation that neurofilament integrity contributes to measured anisotropy in nerve fibers [73,74], and reduction in fractional anisotropy also occurs with disintegration of axonal structure in early CNS Wallerian degeneration, as shown after infarction [75].

The fundamental T1- (longitudinal) and T2- (transverse) relaxation rate measures also are sensitive to the underlying pathology in the NAWM. With specialized pulse sequences, multi-exponential T2–relaxation rates can be observed and analyzed; the short T2-fraction reflects myelin water (myelin water fraction) as opposed to interstitial and free water fractions [76].

By magnetic resonance spectroscopy, abnormally low NAA levels can be detected in the NAWM in relapsing and progressive MS, generally more so in the latter [77,78]; this decrease in NAA indicates that axonal loss or injury may account for more pathology overall than that detected in focal lesions. A progressive decrease in the NAA in the NAWM and in whole brain [79] from axonal loss is accompanied by tissue volume loss; the latter may artifactually stabilize the measured, but not true total NAA content with advancing disease and secondary progressive stages. A recent study suggests that in the early stages of disease, the characteristic signature of the NAWM by MR spectroscopy (MRS) may be increased myoinositol rather than NAA [80]. As in relapsing MS, myoinositol and creatine may be related to changes in glia in the NAWM [2,80,81].

An area of new interest in MS imaging is the importance of microvascular injury as a component of the pathophysiology of focal and diffuse injury, or as a secondary change. The NAWM in relapsing MS already shows diffusely decreased perfusion [82]. How this relates to increased perfusion in the focal pathology that precedes the development of enhancing lesions is not known [10].

In addition to the diffuse abnormality of the NAWM, pathology in the NAWM also can be detected in serial magnetic resonance studies as focal pathology below the sensitivity of conventional T1- or T2-weighted imaging; this precedes the development of classic focal MS lesions by months or years [6–10]. This microscopic pathology has been hypothesized as potentially being the result of low-grade inflammation and related to activated microglia or from microscopic blood–brain barrier leakage [2].

## The gray matter

Focal cortical gray matter MS pathology has been known for some time from the classic neuropathology literature; however, conventional MRI is consistently insensitive to this pathology [83]. By MRI, most cortical gray matter lesions are centered in the adjacent white matter with extension into the gray matter (juxtacortical-cortical). Some of these may appear to be cortical on casual inspection but may be better classified as U fiber lesions that are in a position to affect short association tracts and may have functional consequences [84]. Pure cortical lesions are rare by MRI, not rare by neuropathology, and are recognized increasingly with improved technique by both approaches (Fig. 4).

By neuropathologic examination, most cortical lesions also involve the subcortical white matter. Approximately 15% to 25% are exclusively cortical [85,86], including lesions that extend from the pial surface into the cortex [86,87]. Poor tissue contrast (eg, the signal intensity of lesion relative to adjacent tissue) accounts for the insensitivity of conventional MRI to the focal cortical pathology. The basis for this may be the less inflammatory nature of the active gray matter lesions compared with white matter lesions; the gray matter lesions are characterized by fewer lymphocytes, microglia, and perivascular cuffs [87,88]. However, gray matter lesions do contain transected neurites (axons and dendrites) and loss of neurons from apoptosis [86].

Cortical gray matter is a difficult tissue to evaluate in its entirety by quantitative MRI techniques as a result of its thinness and convoluted shape. Nevertheless, abnormal, normal-appearing cortical gray matter has been described in all MS phenotypes and stages of disease to varying degrees [2]. Deep gray matter is more approachable target, technically, and shows several indications of progressive pathology in MS, including accumulation of iron [89] that is detected as "black T2 signal" with T2*-sensitized sequences, and reduced neuronal fibers by combined structure volume–MRS measures [90]. Although interesting correlations have been noted for deep and cortical gray measures with disability, these are not consistently strong for cognition, fatigue, or disability [2].

**Neuronal tract degeneration**

Although it is convenient to discuss the focal lesional and diffuse (ie, NAWM and NAGM) pathology of MS separately, they are likely related, in part, through several mechanisms, including the processes of retrograde and antegrade degeneration that originate in the focal lesions, with extension into fibers that originate from that lesion or pass through that lesion. Measures of MS tissue based on amyloid precursor protein (increased levels as a result of reduced axonal transport) and confocal microscopy of immunostained material (loss of normal neurofilament and transection indicated by terminal ovoids) directed attention to the important contribution of axonal injury in MS [61,91] and indicated that injuries occur early, in the inflammatory stages, and potentially are an important factor in the progressive stages of disease [92]. Axonal transection can be found within inflammatory tissue samples; one study found approximately 10,000 transections per cubic millimeter [61]. In vivo, acute enhancing (inflammatory) MS lesions can be the source of signal and anatomic changes that are suggestive of secondary Wallerian (fiber) degeneration (Fig. 5) [38,39]. One informative case report links an inflammatory MS lesion in the

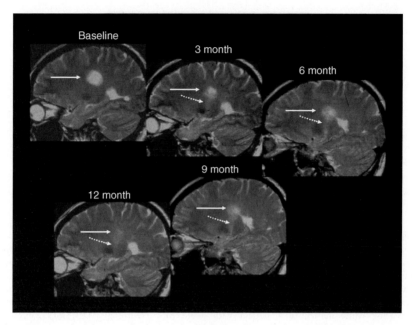

Fig. 5. Temporal and anatomic course of a Wallerian degeneration pattern in vivo by sagittal imaging. Note the contiguous T2-hyperintense lesion (*dashed arrows*) that emanates from the acute lesion (*arrows*) at 3 months that extends along the corticospinal tract. Patient's initial MRI was at the time of a clinically isolated syndrome.

brain stem to distant spinal cord axonal degeneration (Fig. 6) [59]. Further support for neuronal tract degeneration in MS comes from in vivo studies that showed reduced NAA [93] and increased diffusivity that potentially were related to connected lesions [94]; and studies showing reduced fractional anisotropy remote from focal lesions [71] and reduced NAA in visual pathways [95].

Axonal loss can be profound in later stages of disease, from local and distant disease. In one study, there was a 53% reduction in axonal number in the NAWM of corpus callosum, which was proportionate to the reduction in cross-sectional area [96]. Reductions in nerve fiber density also are seen in spinal cord, including in otherwise normal-appearing tissue [58], and likely are related to permanent disability [98].

## Functional MRI, plasticity, and adaptive mechanisms

Functional MRI (fMRI) has become an important methodology to evaluate normal functional systems and is being evaluated as a measure of disease. Interpretation of these studies may be confounded by multiple levels of abnormality and physical limitations in MS. Nevertheless, there is

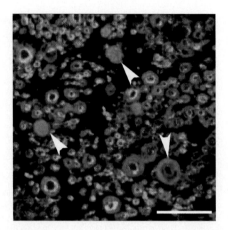

Fig. 6. Case report describing axonal degeneration in the spinal cord secondary to a distant brainstem lesion. Confocal images of the ventral cervical column stained for myelin (*green*) and neurofilaments (*red*). In cross-section, numerous myelin profiles that lack axons (*arrowheads*) are detected among intact myelinated axons. Some appeared as "empty" myelin circumferences, whereas others were composed of collapsed myelin membranes. Signs of primary demyelination were not detected. (*From* Bjartmar C, Kinkel RP, Kidd G, et al. Axonal loss in normal-appearing white matter in a patient with acute MS. Neurology 2001;57(7):1250; with permission.)

consistency in the observation of motor impairment in MS that is associated with fMRI activation over larger cortical regions. Increased activation may include recruitment of greater contralateral networks—the primary and secondary somatomotor cortex and ipsilateral supplementary motor cortex [99]. Several studies suggest that sensorimotor fMRI is sensitive, even in the early stages of disease [100,101]. In secondary progressive MS [102], a strong correlation between cortical activation and injury in the NAWM and NAGM was noted in one study. Cognitive function and information processing also can be evaluated by fMRI [103–105].

Functional disturbances that are detected through fMRI have been the basis for hypotheses that suggest that there may be active compensatory mechanisms in early MS, which initially may compensate for and mask dysfunction. Functional disturbance may become apparent after exhaustion of the adaptive mechanisms [106,107].

## Disease course by MRI

At the time of the first onset of a neurologic event that resembles demyelination, many patients have multiple, previously unsuspected, and widely distributed lesions in the brain or spinal cord, primarily in clinically silent areas of the white matter. Multiple studies suggested that these individuals are at high risk for a subsequent clinical attack or will show MRI evidence for ongoing demyelination; this recently was recognized as indicative of a diagnosis of MS (see later discussion). Alternatively, at the time of a clinically isolated syndrome (CIS), a negative brain (and spinal cord) MRI suggests a low, but not zero, probability of a second clinical attack or MRI disease activity. Most of these individuals will remain categorized as having CIS after long-term clinical follow-up [108].

Although there can be striking interindividual variability, most individuals who have a CIS and a positive MRI have a small number (2 or 3 to 20) and volume (a few cm$^3$) of focal MS lesions [109] compared with the later relapsing (typically 5–15 cm$^3$) and secondary progressive stages (typically 5–25 cm$^3$) [35]. In the earliest stages of disease, focal lesions are counted readily, confluent lesions are rare, T1–black hole volume is low, and most cases show no signs of atrophy by visual criteria. Enhancing lesions in the brain are observed in approximately 30% to 60% of these patients [31]. The literature is not consistent regarding the degree of abnormality of the NAWM in early MS defined at the time of a CIS. Some studies suggest abnormality, whereas others do not; this may reflect patient selection, but also suggests that much of the NAWM may be normal or only minimally abnormal by current criteria, relative to the later stages of disease.

With clinical disease progression or disease duration, as patients progress through relapsing and secondary progressive stages of disease, the focal T1- and T2-lesion volume increases, lesions show an increasing tendency to become confluent, and atrophy may become apparent as thinning of the corpus callosum and enlarged third and lateral ventricles [110]. Some, but not all, studies suggest an increase in the relative T1–black hole lesion volume with an increase in the apparent T1/T2 burden of disease ratio. The likelihood of observing enhancing lesions in relapsing MS is similar to earlier stages and ranges from approximately 53% to 65% in the larger studies [31]. Enhancing lesion number and volume decrease in secondary progressive MS is parallel to the well-known decrease in clinical relapses; however, enhancing lesions are not infrequent with 36% to 48% of patients having one or more enhancing lesions [31].

## Primary progressive multiple sclerosis

Primary progressive MS has several distinct clinical, neuropathologic, and immunologic features compared with relapsing and secondary progressive MS [111–114]. Similarly, although the MRI findings in primary progressive MS overlap with those of other disease phenotypes and are most often indistinguishable [115], several distinctive features can be detected in population studies. Most striking is the decreased number and volume of enhancing lesions which are believed to be related to the less intense inflammation that is observed by histopathology [112,115,116]. Spinal cord pathology was hypothesized to be an important factor in disease progression in primary progressive MS. Although patients may have severe and progressive disability that is localized to the spinal cord, the number or volume of T2-hyperintense spinal cord lesions is not known to account for this difference. Although not a distinguishing feature, observations of an increase in total T2-lesion volume based on expansion of pre-existing lesions—more so than by additional lesions—and more diffuse, rather than focal abnormality of the spinal cord in some patients [51], may be clues to the differing pathophysiologic mechanisms in primary progressive MS. Although total T2-BOD may be lower on average in primary progressive MS, T2 lesion measures, in conjunction with atrophy measures, remain the mainstay of studies and trials [56,117,118].

## The clinical significance of the MRI pathology

Acute relapse in MS essentially is an inflammatory event [119]. Inflammatory, enhancing MS lesions—when they occur in functionally exquisite regions of the CNS—result in imaging findings, symptoms, and electrophysiologic disturbances with a similar time course [120]. MS relapse—many associated with MRI findings—initially may seem to be inconsequential early in the disease, with full clinical recovery; however, relapses frequently leave a residual deficit [121]. More often than not, the correlation between new enhancing lesions and new clinical activity is poor, with approximately 5 to 10 MRI events occurring for every clinical event [122]; 50 to 100 or more MRI events may occur in the absence of any clinical event [123]. Frequent MRI series reinforce the message that substantial, ongoing enhancing, and by inference, inflammatory activity, can, and frequently does, occur during periods when the patient and their physician perceive the disease to be clinically stable.

When results are averaged for a large numbers of subjects, a significant relationship between enhancing lesion number and relapse can be seen; however, this relationship is not strong, with only modest correlations, at best [31]. A meta-analysis that was based on monthly MRI in relapsing and secondary progressive MS found a weak, although significant, relationship between relapse over 1 year and enhancing lesions over 6 months [124].

Over short intervals (years), most studies find no or minimal relationships between enhancing lesions and disability. The relationship between enhancing lesions and significant injury, evidenced by atrophy, was noted in some series but not others, but this too remains only weak at best [31,47]. Factors that may account for this poor clinical (and pathology) relationship, despite pathophysiologic connections, include: (1) the location of lesions (eg, those that occur in white matter that is silent to some degree may have only late effects when critical levels of injury, such as fiber loss, occur, which may take years; (2) the fact that much of the enhancing lesion burden may be missed with conventional imaging that is sensitive only to the macroscopic lesions; and (3) that injury that is associated with enhancement is likely heterogeneous and our measures do not account for this. Nevertheless, enhancing lesions do provide a measure of disease, with pathologic consequences, that would be missed based on clinical evaluation alone.

The correlation between T2-BOD and physical disability in population studies is significant, but poor (on the order of r = 0.2 in the larger series); typically, in individuals, the relationship between lesion burden and disability can be strikingly poor. The magnetic resonance–disability discrepancy most likely is multi-factorial and related to the lack of pathologic specificity of the T2-lesion, imperfections of the disability scoring systems, and limited long-term observations. In the 15-year follow-up of patients who presented with a CIS, modest correlation was seen between increasing T2-lesion load and disability [108]. The relationship between T2-BOD and neuropsychologic impairment also is modest at best, and is poor in most studies [125].

The early literature that evaluated the advanced quantitative MRI measures brought enthusiasm to the field in suggesting stronger correlations with physical disability and cognitive dysfunction. These measures, however, applied in populations provide only modest correlations, at best [2]. The strongest correlations between MRI measures and disability may be those that are provided by atrophy measures [125–127]. Although the limited MRI-functional correlations are discouraging, the poor correlations only may realistically reflect the complex relationships between the pathology, its location, and heterogeneity (severity); the long-term consequences that are not evaluated; and the limited measures of dysfunction (typically physical, rather than cognitive or functional) that usually are used.

## MRI in the diagnosis of multiple sclerosis

Until recently, after a CIS, the diagnosis of MS was dependent on the occurrence of an independent, second clinical event. With the new International Panel Criteria for Diagnosis of MS in 2001 [128], a new MRI event in the setting of dissemination in space (DIS) can be used to establish the diagnosis of MS. This has the effect, in many instances, of expediting the formal diagnosis by months or potentially years [129], to allow for earlier treatment in many instances, better counseling, and support.

The basis for the new criteria were many reports that showed that at the time of the CIS, a negative MRI study was associated with a low (up to ~20%), but not zero, probability of a future second attack, and a diagnosis of MS, whereas a positive MRI was associated with a high probability (~50%–90%) for a second attack and a diagnosis of MS [128]. Operational refinements in the criteria evolved with observations which suggested that the number and volume of lesions at the time of a CIS, and the characteristics of the lesions might be used to increase the predictiveness of the various criteria [128–130]; this would increase accuracy and limit false positive diagnoses at the expense of sensitivity. Because a positive cerebrospinal fluid (CSF) is also known to predict MS after a CIS, in the absence of the DIS criteria with only two MRI lesions, the McDonald criteria permit a positive CSF for diagnosis, provided a second attack or new MRI lesion subsequently develop. Lesions in the spinal cord may be substituted for lesions in the brain. These criteria for diagnosis of MS after a CIS are summarized in Box 1.

An alternative approach that is used by many MS neurologists to initiate therapy is based on a positive MRI after a CIS, with the MRI positive for at least two MRI lesions (periventricular or ovoid), or three or more lesions [131]. The likelihood of ongoing demyelination in carefully selected individuals who had a classic CIS and only a few MRI lesions is supported by results from the placebo arm of the CHAMPS (Controlled High Risk Avonex MS Prevention Study) Trial [132], which found that more than 50% of the patients who did not meet the formal DIS (Barkhof) criteria developed CDMS or had evidence for ongoing demyelination based on new MRI lesions over a short (18 month) follow-up. Consequently, careful magnetic resonance and clinical follow-up may be informative for any patient after a first attack with a positive magnetic resonance study, to reduce the likelihood of delaying diagnosis or treatment in individuals who have early subclinical disease, particularly those who have aggressive disease.

Although relaxed criteria (fewer lesions, less formal anatomic character-istics) increase sensitivity and function well in formal trial settings, their use must be balanced against the possibility, in clinical practice, of increasing false positive diagnoses in patients who have nonspecific findings, including those that are associated with aging and small vessel disease [129,133].

## Monitoring patients in clinical trials and in the clinic

The use of MRI is well-established in clinical MS trials of relapsing or secondary progressive disease. MRI-based measures are the primary outcome measures in phase II trials (most frequently enhancing lesions); MRI contributes secondary outcome measures to phase III trials (eg, T2-BOD); and more recently, MRI has been used as a safety metric (enhancing lesions) in the phase I setting [134]. Atrophy measures are being used increasingly in MS clinical trials as a measure of irreversible injury [47,48,135]; this measure shows good long-term correlation with disability [127,135]. The advanced quantitative methodologies for evaluating the NAWM and NAGM also are being tested in formal trial settings, although their use remains secondary until they are validated in clinical trials setting; these require stringent control of hardware and software, and the necessity for highly specialized quality control [66].

Current therapy that is based on immunomodulatory agents results in measurable change in several MRI measures in population studies; however,

---

**Box 1. MRI criteria**

*For brain abnormality* (Dissemination in space)
Three of four of the following:
   One gadolinium-enhancing lesion or nine T2-hyperintense
      lesions if there is no gadolinium-enhancing lesion.
   At least one infratentorial lesion.
   At least one juxtacortical lesion.
   At least three periventricular lesions.

---

   Note: one spinal cord lesion can be substituted for one brain lesion.

*For dissemination of lesions in time*
If a first scan occurs 3 months or more after the onset of the
   clinical event, the presence of a gadolinium-enhancing lesion is
   sufficient to demonstrate dissemination in time, provided that
   it is not at the site implicated in the original clinical event. If
   there is no enhancing lesion at this time, a follow-up scan is
   required. The timing of this follow-up scan is not crucial, but
   3 months is recommended. A new T2- or
   gadolinium-enhancing lesion at this time then fulfills
   the criterion for dissemination in time.
If the first scan is performed less than 3 months after the onset
   of the clinical event, a second scan done 3 months or more
   after the clinical event showing a new gadolinium-enhancing
   lesion provides sufficient evidence for dissemination in time.
   However, if no enhancing lesion is seen at this second scan,
   a further scan not less than 3 months after the first scan that
   shows a new T2 lesion or an enhancing lesion will suffice.

---

   *Adapted from* McDonald WI, Compston A, Edan G, et al. Recommended
diagnostic criteria for multiple sclerosis: guidelines from the International Panel on
the Diagnosis of Multiple Sclerosis. Ann Neurol 2001;50(1):123; with permission.

---

the effect of these therapies and the use of MRI in monitoring individual
patients is not straightforward. In populations, the β-interferons decrease
enhancing lesions and the percentage of patients who have positive scans;
the response is detectable within weeks after initiation of therapy. There are
only limited data regarding the wash-out of effect after cessation of therapy,
but one study observed wash-out 6 to 10 months after treatment was halted
in two patients who were treated with interferon β-1b [136]. Copaxone
(glatirimer acetate) also suppresses enhancing lesions; the effect increases to
maximum benefit after an interval of approximately 4 to 6 months [137].

More targeted therapies are being tested, including those that are based on disrupting lymphocyte adhesion to endothelium; in phase II trials, this resulted in significant decreases in enhancing lesions and relapse [138].

In the clinic, where monthly MRI is not feasible, MRI activity can be monitored by counting new T2-hyperintense lesions as a measure of interval change, and counting enhancing lesions as a measure of inflammation around the time of the MRI evaluation (Fig. 7). Several initiatives are underway to define criteria for successful or acceptable treatment versus treatment failure—based on clinical and MRI activity—and to standardize MRI to assist in these assessments (see MSCARE.org). Because current therapy is only partially effective, the MRI metrics may be limited, but can provide a means to evaluate aggressive continued subclinical disease that may signal the need for initiation or change in therapy. MRI monitoring

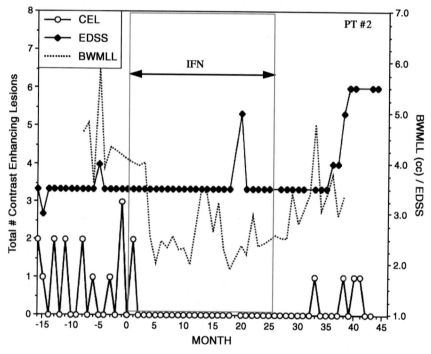

Fig. 7. Following MRI in the clinic? Following the response to therapy may be limited to annual MRI to detect activity trends. In this optimal monthly MRI follow-up, responsiveness to initiation of therapy with interferon-β is apparent, as is return toward baseline activity with cessation of therapy. Because monthly MRI is not practical, counting new T2-lesions over a 1-year interval (not shown) provides a good estimate of intercurrent MRI activity; most new lesions leave a permanent residue—the footprint of previous activity. Enhancing lesions provide estimates of activity trends, and a measure of inflammation around the time of the MRI. (*From* Richert ND, Zierak MC, Bash CN, et al. MRI and clinical activity in MS patients after terminating treatment with interferon beta-1b. Mult Scler 2000;6(2):86–90; with permission.)

may increase confidence in a clinical impression of stable disease or help to discount borderline symptoms or signs and support maintaining the current therapy. Severe MRI activity may support a clinical impression for the need to initiate aggressive and more risky therapy with immunosuppressive agents.

## Appendix 1

*Physical basis for advanced MRI techniques*

*Magnetization transfer imaging*

There are multiple hydrogen proton fractions in CNS tissue, including those from free water and those associated with macromolecules (bound water). Radiofrequency pulses ("off water resonance") are used to irradiate the normally MRI "invisible" bound fractions, which secondarily affects the free water fraction. The latter and its change after "off-resonance" irradiation is measured readily, the change from pre- to postirradiation is reflected in the magnetization transfer ratio (MTR). High MTR ratios are characteristic of intact, normal tissue; decreases on the order of several percent are seen as structure is disrupted (eg, from demyelination); severe damage results in a more fluidlike (low) MTR. CSF has an MTR that is near zero. Methods to evaluate the more fundamental exchange and relaxation properties that are inherent in the MTR more selectively are being developed [139]. Although MTR and relaxation measures are fundamentally independent, in practice, this independence is not achieved using standard magnetization transfer approaches, but can be better approximated based on the newer quantitative magnetization transfer methodologies.

*Water diffusion–based MRI measures*

Water molecule diffusion can be measured in vivo because the motion of water affects the magnitude of magnetic resonance signal that is measured with any given magnetic resonance pulse sequence. For measuring diffusion, the generic pulse sequence is sensitized further to water motion using one or more additional strong transient magnetic field gradients that are sensitive to motion over the intervals of interest. Variation in technique range from diffusion-weighted imaging (useful in detecting restricted diffusion in stroke) to diffusion tensor methods that allow more complete descriptions of the diffusion properties, irrespective of magnet or anatomic reference frames [140]. From the diffusion tensor, multiple analyses can be derived, including a measure of diffusivity (related to the average diffusion coefficient of the water molecules), and measures that describe the strength and principal direction of diffusion. These often are simplified as a fractional anisotropy index, a measure of variance from isotropic (nondirectional) diffusion. From the diffusion tensor, diffusion tractography maps of principal fiber pathways can be derived by several methodologies (Fig. 8) [97].

*Magnetic resonance spectroscopy*

In MRI, a combined hydrogen (proton) signal is displayed for each picture element (pixel) in an image. Water is by far the dominant contributor to signal in the brain. Lipid molecules are much less visible because of their short T2 relaxation time. In proton (1H) magnetic resonance spectroscopy, pulse sequences are modified to suppress the water signal and to allow observation of individual resonances that contribute to signal as a water-suppressed proton spectrum. The dominant peak from a water-suppressed proton magnetic resonance spectrum is from NAA. The NAA peak is a pool of N-acetylated moieties, most likely precursor molecules because they are abundant in brain ($\sim$10 mmol/L). NAA is not strictly a measure of number of axons (neurons) because transient changes in concentration can be seen. Another peak in the 1H spectrum is based on the combined concentration of creatine and phosphocreatine (Cr). The Cr peak is used often as a reference to report ratios, such as NAA/Cr; however, creatine may be a marker for abnormally increased levels of glial cells in the CNS [81]. The choline resonances provide information about membrane

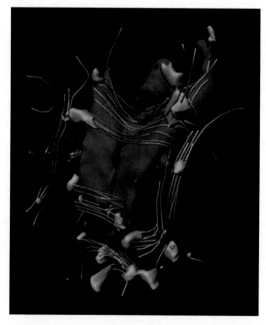

Fig. 8. Diffusion tractography in early, relapsing MS. By using diffusion tractography methods, it is now feasible to determine which fibers travel through focal MS lesions. The potential fibers that are at risk for axonal injury as a result of focal inflammatory MS can be determined. CSF in ventricle (blue); fibers that intersect focal lesions, (pink); focal T2-hyperintense lesions (yellow-green). Collaboration between University of Colorado and Brown University. (Courtesy of David Laidlaw, PhD, and Song Zhang, PhD.)

integrity. The myoinositol resonances also are believed to reflect glial change. Other minor resonances that are more difficult to quantitate with conventional magnetic resonance spectroscopy include glutamine and glutamate, and various pools of amino acids.

## Functional MRI

fMRI is based on blood oxygen level dependent (BOLD) signal changes. Simplistically, this is based on local neuronal activity, secondary increases in the local blood flow, followed by a decrease in deoxyhemoglobin relative to oxyhemoglobin. Deoxyhemoglobin causes decreased signal intensity in the $T2^*$-weighted sequences that are used in fMRI. Consequently, activity, after a short (milliseconds) delay, results in localized increased signal on the order of 1% to 5% that can be detected by conventional high field magnetic resonance systems (typically $\geq 1.5T$). Because these signal changes are small relative to noise, fMRI typically requires multiple measurements that are averaged, processed, and overlaid onto anatomic images such that statistically significant activation is represented with reference to the anatomy of interest.

## References

[1] Simon JH. Pathology of multiple sclerosis as revealed by in vivo magnetic-resonance-based approaches. In: Herndon RM, editor. Multiple sclerosis. Immunology, pathology, and pathophysiology. New York: Demos Medical Publishers; 2003. p. 199–213.

[2] Miller DH, Thompson AJ, Filippi M. Magnetic resonance studies of abnormalities in the normal appearing white matter and grey matter in multiple sclerosis. J Neurol 2003;250(12): 1407–19.

[3] Filippi M, Dousset V, McFarland HF, et al. Role of magnetic resonance imaging in the diagnosis and monitoring of multiple sclerosis: consensus report of the White Matter Study Group. J Magn Reson Imaging 2002;15(5):499–504.

[4] Markovic-Plese S, McFarland HF. Immunopathogenesis of the multiple sclerosis lesion. Curr Neurol Neurosci Rep 2001;1(3):257–62.

[5] Oksenberg JR, Baranzini SE, Hauser SL. Emerging concepts of pathogenesis: relationship to therapies for multiple sclerosis. In: Cohen JA, Rudick RA, editors. Multiple sclerosis therapeutics. 2nd edition. London: Martin Dunitz; 2003. p. 289–322.

[6] Goodkin DE, Rooney WD, Sloan R, et al. A serial study of new MS lesions and the white matter from which they arise. Neurology 1998;51(6):1689–97.

[7] Filippi M, Rocca MA, Martino G, et al. Magnetization transfer changes in the normal appearing white matter precede the appearance of enhancing lesions in patients with multiple sclerosis. Ann Neurol 1998;43(6):809–14.

[8] Pike GB, De Stefano N, Narayanan S, et al. Multiple sclerosis: magnetization transfer MR imaging of white matter before lesion appearance on T2-weighted images. Radiology 2000; 215(3):824–30.

[9] Narayana PA, Doyle TJ, Lai D, et al. Serial proton magnetic resonance spectroscopic imaging, contrast-enhanced magnetic resonance imaging, and quantitative lesion volumetry in multiple sclerosis. Ann Neurol 1998;43(1):56–71.

[10] Wuerfel J, Bellmann-Strobl J, Brunecker P, et al. Changes in cerebral perfusion precede plaque formation in multiple sclerosis: a longitudinal perfusion MRI study. Brain 2004; 127(Pt 1):111–9.

[11] Bruck W, Bitsch A, Kolenda H, et al. Inflammatory central nervous system demyelination: correlation of magnetic resonance imaging findings with lesion pathology. Ann Neurol 1997;42:783–93.

[12] Katz D, Taubenberger JK, Cannella B, et al. Correlation between magnetic resonance imaging findings and lesion development in chronic, active multiple sclerosis. Ann Neurol 1993;34:661–9.

[13] Nesbit GM, Forbes GS, Scheithauer BW, et al. Multiple sclerosis: histopathologic and and/or CT correlation in 37 cases at biopsy and three cases at autopsy. Radiology 1991;180(2): 467–74.

[14] Yong VW. Prospects for neuroprotection in multiple sclerosis. Front Biosci 2004;9:864–72.

[15] Dousset V, Ballarino L, Delalande C, et al. Comparison of ultrasmall particles of iron oxide (USPIO)-enhanced T2-weighted, conventional T2-weighted, and gadolinium-enhanced T1-weighted MR images in rats with experimental autoimmune encephalomyelitis. AJNR Am J Neuroradiol 1999;20(2):223–7.

[16] Rausch M, Hiestand P, Baumann D, et al. MRI-based monitoring of inflammation and tissue damage in acute and chronic relapsing EAE. Magn Reson Med 2003;50(2): 309–14.

[17] Anderson SA, Shukaliak-Quandt J, Jordan EK, et al. Magnetic resonance imaging of labeled T-cells in a mouse model of multiple sclerosis. Ann Neurol 2004;55(5):654–9.

[18] Martino G, Adorini L, Rieckmann P, et al. Inflammation in multiple sclerosis: the good, the bad, and the complex. Lancet Neurol 2002;1(8):499–509.

[19] Lai M, Hodgson T, Gawne-Cain M, et al. A preliminary study into the sensitivity of disease activity detection by serial weekly magnetic resonance imaging in multiple sclerosis. J Neurol Neurosurg Psychiatry 1996;60:339–41.

[20] Cotton F, Weiner HL, Jolesz FA, et al. MRI contrast uptake in new lesions in relapsing-remitting MS followed at weekly intervals. Neurology 2003;60(4):640–6.

[21] Lucchinetti C, Bruck W, Parisi J, et al. Heterogeneity of multiple sclerosis lesions: implications for the pathogenesis of demyelination. Ann Neurol 2000;47(6):707–17.

[22] Wingerchuk DM, Lucchinetti CF, Noseworthy JH. Multiple sclerosis: current pathophysiological concepts. Lab Invest 2001;81(3):263–81.

[23] Morgen K, Jeffries NO, Stone R, et al. Ring-enhancement in multiple sclerosis: marker of disease severity. Mult Scler 2001;7:167–71.

[24] Filippi M, Rocca MA, Rizzo G, et al. Magnetization transfer ratios in multiple sclerosis lesions enhancing after different doses of gadolinium. Neurology 1998;50: 1289–93.

[25] Tortorella C, Codella M, Rocca MA, et al. Disease activity in multiple sclerosis studied by weekly triple-dose magnetic resonance imaging. J Neurol 1999;246:689–92.

[26] Bjartmar C, Trapp BD. Axonal and neuronal degeneration in multiple sclerosis: mechanisms and functional consequences. Curr Opin Neurol 2001;14(3):271–8.

[27] Bjartmar C, Battistuta J, Terada N, et al. N-acetylaspartate is an axon-specific marker of mature white matter in vivo: a biochemical and immunohistochemical study on the rat optic nerve. Ann Neurol 2002;51(1):51–8.

[28] Arnold DL, De Stefano N, Narayanan S, et al. Proton MR spectroscopy in multiple sclerosis. Neuroimaging Clin N Am 2000;10(4):789–98.

[29] Brex PA, Gomez-Anson B, Parker GJ, et al. Proton MR spectroscopy in clinically isolated syndromes suggestive of multiple sclerosis. J Neurol Sci 1999;166:16–22.

[30] Wolinsky JS, Narayana PA. Magnetic resonance spectroscopy in multiple sclerosis: window into the diseased brain. Curr Opin Neurol 2002;15(3):247–51.

[31] Simon JH. Measures of gadolinium enhancement in multiple sclerosis. In: Cohen JA, Rudick RA, editors. Multiple sclerosis therapeutics. 2nd edition. London: Martin Dunitz; 2003. p. 97–124.

[32] McFarland HF, Frank JA, Albert PS, et al. Using gadolinium-enhanced magnetic resonance imaging lesions to monitor disease activity in multiple sclerosis. Ann Neurol 1992;32:758–66.

[33] Filippi M, Rocca MA, Comi G. The use of quantitative magnetic-resonance-based techniques to monitor the evolution of multiple sclerosis. Lancet Neurol 2003;2(6):337–46.

[34] Guttmann CR, Ahn SS, Hsu L, et al. The evolution of multiple sclerosis lesions on serial MR. AJNR Am J Neuroradiol 1995;16:1481–91.

[35] Simon JH. Magnetic resonance imaging in the diagnosis of multiple sclerosis, elucidation of disease, course, and determining prognosis. In: Burks JS, Johnson KP, editors. Multiple sclerosis. Diagnosis, medical management, and rehabilitation. New York: Demos; 2000. p. 99–126.

[36] Barkhof F, Bruck W, De Groot CJ, et al. Remyelinated lesions in multiple sclerosis: magnetic resonance image appearance. Arch Neurol 2003;60(8):1073–81.

[37] Bruck W, Kuhlmann T, Stadelmann C. Remyelination in multiple sclerosis. J Neurol Sci 2003;206(2):181–5.

[38] Simon JH, Kinkel RP, Jacobs L, et al. A Wallerian degeneration pattern in patients at risk for MS. Neurology 2000;54:1155–60.

[39] Simon JH, Jacobs L, Kinkel RP. Transcallosal bands: a sign of neuronal tract degeneration in early MS? Neurology 2001;57:1888–90.

[40] van Walderveen MA, Barkhof F, Pouwels PJ, et al. Neuronal damage in T1-hypointense multiple sclerosis lesions demonstrated in vivo using proton magnetic resonance spectroscopy. Ann Neurol 1999;46(1):79–87.

[41] Van Walderveen MA, Kamphorst W, Scheltens P, et al. Histopathologic correlate of hypointense lesions on T1-weighted spin-echo MRI in multiple sclerosis. Neurology 1998; 50(5):1282–8.

[42] Filippi M, Rovaris M, Rocca MA, et al. Glatiramer acetate reduces the proportion of new MS lesions evolving into "black holes." Neurology 2001;57(4):731–3.

[43] Dalton CM, Miszkiel KA, Barker GJ, et al. Effect of natalizumab on conversion of gadolinium enhancing lesions to T1 hypointense lesions in relapsing multiple sclerosis. J Neurol 2004;251(4):407–13.

[44] Hickman SJ, Toosy AT, Jones SJ, et al. Serial magnetization transfer imaging in acute optic neuritis. Brain 2004;127(Pt 3):692–700.

[45] Frohman EM, Zhang H, Kramer PD, et al. MRI characteristics of the MLF in MS patients with chronic internuclear ophthalmoparesis. Neurology 2001;57(5):762–8.

[46] van der Meijs AH, Tan IL, Barkhof F. Incidence of enhancement of the trigeminal nerve on MRI in patients with multiple sclerosis. Mult Scler 2002;8(1):64–7.

[47] Simon JH. Brain and spinal cord atrophy in multiple sclerosis: role as a surrogate measure of disease progression. CNS Drugs 2001;15(6):427–36.

[48] Miller DH, Barkhof F, Frank J, et al. Measurement of atrophy in multiple sclerosis: pathological basis, methodological aspects and clinical relevance. Brain 2002;125:1676–95.

[49] Pelletier D, Garrison K, Henry R. Measurement of whole-brain atrophy in multiple sclerosis. J Neuroimaging 2004;14(3)(Suppl 3):11S–9S.

[50] Bot JC, Barkhof F, Polman CH, et al. Spinal cord abnormalities in recently diagnosed MS patients: added value of spinal MRI examination. Neurology 2004;62(2):226–33.

[51] Lycklama G, Thompson A, Filippi M, et al. Spinal-cord MRI in multiple sclerosis. Lancet Neurol 2003;2(9):555–62.

[52] Dalton CM, Brex PA, Miszkiel KA, et al. Spinal cord MRI in clinically isolated optic neuritis. J Neurol Neurosurg Psychiatry 2003;74(11):1577–80.

[53] Cordonnier C, de Seze J, Breteau G, et al. Prospective study of patients presenting with acute partial transverse myelopathy. J Neurol 2003;250(12):1447–52.

[54] Filippi M, Rocca MA, Moiola L, et al. MRI and magnetization transfer imaging changes in the brain and cervical cord of patients with Devic's neuromyelitis optica. Neurology 1999;53(8):1705–10.

[55] Lin X, Tench CR, Evangelou N, et al. Measurement of spinal cord atrophy in multiple sclerosis. J Neuroimaging 2004;14(3)(Suppl 3):20S–6S.

[56] Stevenson VL, Ingle GT, Miller DH, et al. Magnetic resonance imaging predictors of disability in primary progressive multiple sclerosis: a 5-year study. Mult Scler 2004;10(4): 398–401.

[57] Bergers E, Bot JC, De Groot CJ, et al. Axonal damage in the spinal cord of MS patients occurs largely independent of T2 MRI lesions. Neurology 2002;59(11):1766–71.

[58] Ganter P, Prince C, Esiri MM. Spinal cord axonal loss in multiple sclerosis: a post-mortem study. Neuropathol Appl Neurobiol 1999;25(6):459–67.

[59] Bjartmar C, Kinkel RP, Kidd G, et al. Axonal loss in normal-appearing white matter in a patient with acute MS. Neurology 2001;57(7):1248–52.

[60] Allen IV, McQuaid S, Mirakhur M, et al. Pathological abnormalities in the normal-appearing white matter in multiple sclerosis. Neurol Sci 2001;22(2):141–4.

[61] Trapp BD, Peterson J, Ransohoff RM, et al. Axonal transection in the lesions of multiple sclerosis. N Engl J Med 1998;338(5):278–85.

[62] Evangelou N, Konz D, Esiri MM, et al. Regional axonal loss in the corpus callosum correlates with cerebral white matter lesion volume and distribution in multiple sclerosis. Brain 2000;123(Pt 9):1845–9.

[63] Coombs BD, Best A, Brown MS, et al. Multiple sclerosis pathology in the normal and abnormal appearing white matter of the corpus callosum by diffusion tensor imaging. Mult Scler 2004;10(4):392–7.

[64] Tortorella C, Viti B, Bozzali M, et al. A magnetization transfer histogram study of normal-appearing brain tissue in MS. Neurology 2000;54(1):186–93.

[65] Filippi M, Inglese M, Rovaris M, et al. Magnetization transfer imaging to monitor the evolution of MS: a 1-year follow-up study. Neurology 2000;55(7):940–6.

[66] Horsfield MA, Barker GJ, Barkhof F, et al. Guidelines for using quantitative magnetization transfer magnetic resonance imaging for monitoring treatment of multiple sclerosis. J Magn Reson Imaging 2003;17(4):389–97.

[67] Filippi M, Grossman RI. MRI techniques to monitor MS evolution: the present and the future. Neurology 2002;58(8):1147–53.

[68] Brochet B, Dousset V. Pathological correlates of magnetization transfer imaging abnormalities in animal models and humans with multiple sclerosis. Neurology 1999; 53(5)(Suppl 3):S12–7.

[69] Lexa FJ, Grossman RI, Rosenquist AC. Dyke Award paper. MR of Wallerian degeneration in the feline visual system: characterization by magnetization transfer rate with histopathologic correlation. AJNR Am J Neuroradiol 1994;15(2):201–12.

[70] Deloire-Grassin MS, Brochet B, Quesson B, et al. In vivo evaluation of remyelination in rat brain by magnetization transfer imaging. J Neurol Sci 2000;178(1):10–6.

[71] Bammer R, Augustin M, Strasser-Fuchs S, et al. Magnetic resonance diffusion tensor imaging for characterizing diffuse and focal white matter abnormalities in multiple sclerosis. Magn Reson Med 2000;44(4):583–91.

[72] Werring DJ, Clark CA, Barker GJ, et al. Diffusion tensor imaging of lesions and normal-appearing white matter in multiple sclerosis. Neurology 1999;52(8):1626–32.

[73] Gulani V, Webb AG, Duncan ID, et al. Apparent diffusion tensor measurements in myelin-deficient rat spinal cords. Magn Reson Med 2001;45(2):191–5.

[74] Beaulieu C. The basis of anisotropic water diffusion in the nervous system—a technical review. NMR Biomed 2002;15(7–8):435–55.

[75] Thomalla G, Glauche V, Koch MA, et al. Diffusion tensor imaging detects early Wallerian degeneration of the pyramidal tract after ischemic stroke. Neuroimage 2004; 22(4):1767–74.

[76] Whittall KP, MacKay AL, Li DK, et al. Normal-appearing white matter in multiple sclerosis has heterogeneous, diffusely prolonged T(2). Magn Reson Med 2002; 47(2):403–8.

[77] Fu L, Matthews PM, De Stefano N, et al. Imaging axonal damage of normal appearing white matter in multiple sclerosis. Brain 1998;121:103–13.

[78] Arnold D, Matthews PM. Measures to quantify axonal damage in vivo based on magnetic resonance spectroscopy in multiple sclerosis. In: Cohen JA, Rudick RA, editors. Multiple sclerosis therapeutics. 2nd edition. London: Martin Dunitz; 2003. p. 193–205.

[79] Gonen O, Moriarty DM, Li BS, et al. Relapsing-remitting multiple sclerosis and whole-brain N-acetylaspartate measurement: evidence for different clinical cohorts initial observations. Radiology 2002;225(1):261–8.

[80] Fernando KT, McLean MA, Chard DT, et al. Elevated white matter myo-inositol in clinically isolated syndromes suggestive of multiple sclerosis. Brain 2004;127(Pt 6):1361–9.

[81] Rooney WD, Goodkin DE, Schuff N, et al. 1H MRSI of normal appearing white matter in multiple sclerosis. Mult Scler 1997;3(4):231–7.

[82] Law M, Saindane AM, Ge Y, et al. Microvascular abnormality in relapsing-remitting multiple sclerosis: perfusion MR imaging findings in normal-appearing white matter. Radiology 2004;231(3):645–52.

[83] Catalaa I, Fulton JC, Zhang X, et al. MR imaging quantitation of gray matter involvement in multiple sclerosis and its correlation with disability measures and neurocognitive testing. AJNR Am J Neuroradiol 1999;20(9):1613–8.

[84] Miki Y, Grossman RI, Udupa JK, et al. Isolated U-fiber involvement in MS: preliminary observations. Neurology 1998;50(5):1301–6.

[85] Kidd D, Barkhof F, McConnell R, et al. Cortical lesions in multiple sclerosis. Brain 1999; 122(Pt 1):17–26.

[86] Peterson JW, Bo L, Mork S, et al. Transected neurites, apoptotic neurons, and reduced inflammation in cortical multiple sclerosis lesions. Ann Neurol 2001;50(3):389–400.

[87] Bo L, Vedeler CA, Nyland HI, et al. Subpial demyelination in the cerebral cortex of multiple sclerosis patients. J Neuropathol Exp Neurol 2003;62(7):723–32.

[88] Bo L, Vedeler CA, Nyland H, et al. Intracortical multiple sclerosis lesions are not associated with increased lymphocyte infiltration. Mult Scler 2003;9(4):323–31.

[89] Bakshi R, Benedict RH, Bermel RA, et al. T2 hypointensity in the deep gray matter of patients with multiple sclerosis: a quantitative magnetic resonance imaging study. Arch Neurol 2002;59(1):62–8.

[90] Wylezinska M, Cifelli A, Jezzard P, et al. Thalamic neurodegeneration in relapsing-remitting multiple sclerosis. Neurology 2003;60(12):1949–54.

[91] Ferguson B, Matyszak MK, Esiri MM, et al. Axonal damage in acute multiple sclerosis lesions. Brain 1997;120:393–9.

[92] Bjartmar C, Wujek JR, Trapp BD. Axonal loss in the pathology of MS: consequences for understanding the progressive phase of the disease. J Neurol Sci 2003;206(2):165–71.

[93] De Stefano N, Narayanan S, Matthews PM, et al. In vivo evidence for axonal dysfunction remote from focal cerebral demyelination of the type seen in multiple sclerosis. Brain 1999; 122(Pt 10):1933–9.

[94] Werring DJ, Clark CA, Droogan AG, et al. Water diffusion is elevated in widespread regions of normal-appearing white matter in multiple sclerosis and correlates with diffusion in focal lesions. Mult Scler 2001;7(2):83–9.

[95] Heide AC, Kraft GH, Slimp JC, et al. Cerebral N-acetylaspartate is low in patients with multiple sclerosis and abnormal visual evoked potentials. AJNR Am J Neuroradiol 1998; 19(6):1047–54.

[96] Evangelou N, Esiri MM, Smith S, et al. Quantitative pathological evidence for axonal loss in normal appearing white matter in multiple sclerosis. Ann Neurol 2000;47:391–5.

[97] Mori S, van Zijl PC. Fiber tracking: principles and strategies—a technical review. NMR Biomed 2002;15(7–8):468–80.

[98] Wujek JR, Bjartmar C, Richer E, et al. Axon loss in the spinal cord determines permanent neurological disability in an animal model of multiple sclerosis. J Neuropathol Exp Neurol 2002;61(1):23–32.

[99] Filippi M, Rocca MA, Mezzapesa DM, et al. A functional MRI study of cortical activations associated with object manipulation in patients with MS. Neuroimage 2004; 21(3):1147–54.

[100] Filippi M, Rocca MA, Mezzapesa DM, et al. Simple and complex movement-associated functional MRI changes in patients at presentation with clinically isolated syndromes suggestive of multiple sclerosis. Hum Brain Mapp 2004;21(2):108–17.

[101] Rocca MA, Mezzapesa DM, Falini A, et al. Evidence for axonal pathology and adaptive cortical reorganization in patients at presentation with clinically isolated syndromes suggestive of multiple sclerosis. Neuroimage 2003;18(4):847–55.

[102] Rocca MA, Gavazzi C, Mezzapesa DM, et al. A functional magnetic resonance imaging study of patients with secondary progressive multiple sclerosis. Neuroimage 2003;19(4): 1770–7.

[103] Mainero C, Caramia F, Pozzilli C, et al. fMRI evidence of brain reorganization during attention and memory tasks in multiple sclerosis. Neuroimage 2004;21(3):858–67.

[104] Audoin B, Ibarrola D, Ranjeva JP, et al. Compensatory cortical activation observed by fMRI during a cognitive task at the earliest stage of MS. Hum Brain Mapp 2003;20(2):51–8.

[105] Staffen W, Mair A, Zauner H, et al. Cognitive function and fMRI in patients with multiple sclerosis: evidence for compensatory cortical activation during an attention task. Brain 2002;125(Pt 6):1275–82.

[106] Cifelli A, Matthews PM. Cerebral plasticity in multiple sclerosis: insights from fMRI. Mult Scler 2002;8(3):193–9.

[107] Filippi M. MRI-clinical correlations in the primary progressive course of MS: new insights into the disease pathophysiology from the application of magnetization transfer, diffusion tensor, and functional MRI. J Neurol Sci 2003;206(2):157–64.

[108] Brex PA, Ciccarelli O, O'Riordan JI, et al. A longitudinal study of abnormalities on MRI and disability from multiple sclerosis. N Engl J Med 2002;346(3):158–64.

[109] CHAMPS Study Group. Baseline MRI characteristics of patients at high risk for multiple sclerosis: results from the CHAMPS trial. Mult Scler 2002;8:332–8.

[110] Simon JH. Brain and spinal cord atrophy in multiple sclerosis. Neuroimaging Clin N Am 2000;10(4):753–70.

[111] Pender MP. The pathogenesis of primary progressive multiple sclerosis: antibody-mediated attack and no repair? J Clin Neurosci 2004;11(7):689–92.

[112] Thompson AJ, Polman CH, Miller DH, et al. Primary progressive multiple sclerosis. Brain 1997;120:1085–96.

[113] Wolinsky JS. The diagnosis of primary progressive multiple sclerosis. J Neurol Sci 2003; 206(2):145–52.

[114] Bruck W, Lucchinetti C, Lassmann H. The pathology of primary progressive multiple sclerosis. Mult Scler 2002;8(2):93–7.

[115] Kremenchutzky M, Lee D, Rice GP, et al. Diagnostic brain MRI findings in primary progressive multiple sclerosis. Mult Scler 2000;6(2):81–5.

[116] Filippi M, Rovaris M, Rocca MA. Imaging primary progressive multiple sclerosis: the contribution of structural, metabolic, and functional MRI techniques. Mult Scler 2004; 10(Suppl 1):S36–44 [discussion S44–5].

[117] Leary SM, Miller DH, Stevenson VL, et al. Interferon beta-1a in primary progressive MS: an exploratory, randomized, controlled trial. Neurology 2003;60(1):44–51.

[118] Stevenson VL, Miller DH, Leary SM, et al. One year follow up study of primary and transitional progressive multiple sclerosis. J Neurol Neurosurg Psychiatry 2000;68(6): 713–8.

[119] McDonald WI. Relapse, remission, and progression in multiple sclerosis. N Engl J Med 2000;343(20):1486–7.

[120] Youl BD, Turano G, Miller DH, et al. The pathophysiology of acute optic neuritis. An association of gadolinium leakage with clinical and electrophysiological deficits. Brain 1991;114(Pt 6):2437–50.

[121] Lublin FD, Baier M, Cutter G. Effect of relapses on development of residual deficit in multiple sclerosis. Neurology 2003;61(11):1528–32.

[122] Barkhof F, Scheltens P, Frequin ST, et al. Relapsing-remitting multiple sclerosis: sequential enhanced MR imaging vs clinical findings in determining disease activity. AJR Am J Roentgenol 1992;159:1041–7.

[123] Jacobs LD, Beck RW, Simon JH, et al. Intramuscular interferon beta-1a therapy initiated during a first demyelinating event in multiple sclerosis. CHAMPS Study Group. N Engl J Med 2000;343:898–904.

[124] Kappos L, Moeri D, Radue EW, et al. Predictive value of gadolinium-enhanced magnetic resonance imaging for relapse rate and changes in disability or impairment in multiple sclerosis: a meta-analysis. Gadolinium MRI Meta-analysis Group. Lancet 1999;353(9157): 964–9.

[125] Benedict RH, Weinstock-Guttman B, Fishman I, et al. Prediction of neuropsychological impairment in multiple sclerosis: comparison of conventional magnetic resonance imaging measures of atrophy and lesion burden. Arch Neurol 2004;61(2):226–30.

[126] Amato MP, Bartolozzi ML, Zipoli V, et al. Neocortical volume decrease in relapsing-remitting MS patients with mild cognitive impairment. Neurology 2004;63(1):89–93.

[127] Fisher E, Rudick RA, Simon JH, et al. Eight-year follow-up study of brain atrophy in patients with MS. Neurology 2002;59(9):1412–20.

[128] McDonald WI, Compston A, Edan G, et al. Recommended diagnostic criteria for multiple sclerosis: guidelines from the International Panel on the Diagnosis of Multiple Sclerosis. Ann Neurol 2001;50(1):121–7.

[129] Miller DH, Filippi M, Fazekas F, et al. Role of magnetic resonance imaging within diagnostic criteria for multiple sclerosis. Ann Neurol 2004;56(2):273–8.

[130] Barkhof F, Filippi M, Miller DH, et al. Comparison of MRI criteria at first presentation to predict conversion to clinically definite multiple sclerosis. Brain 1997;120(Pt 11): 2059–69.

[131] Frohman EM, Goodin DS, Calabresi PA, et al. The utility of MRI in suspected MS: report of the Therapeutics and Technology Assessment Subcommittee of the American Academy of Neurology. Neurology 2003;61(5):602–11.

[132] CHAMPS Study Group. MRI predictors of early conversion to clinically definite MS in the CHAMPS placebo group. Neurology 2002;59(7):998–1005.

[133] Simon JH, Thompson AJ. Is multiple sclerosis still a clinical diagnosis? Neurology 2003;61(5):596–7.

[134] Frank JA, McFarland HF. How to participate in a multiple sclerosis clinical trial. Neuroimaging Clin N Am 2000;10(4):817–30.

[135] Rudick RA. Impact of disease-modifying therapies on brain and spinal cord atrophy in multiple sclerosis. J Neuroimaging 2004;14(3)(Suppl 3):54S–64S.

[136] Richert ND, Zierak MC, Bash CN, et al. MRI and clinical activity in MS patients after terminating treatment with interferon beta-1b. Mult Scler 2000;6(2):86–90.

[137] Comi G, Filippi M, Wolinsky JS. European/Canadian multicenter, double-blind, randomized, placebo-controlled study of the effects of glatiramer acetate on magnetic resonance imaging–measured disease activity and burden in patients with relapsing multiple sclerosis. European/Canadian Glatiramer Acetate Study Group. Ann Neurol 2001;49(3):290–7.

[138] Miller DH, Khan OA, Sheremata WA, et al. International Natalizumab Multiple Sclerosis Trial Group. A controlled trial of natalizumab for relapsing multiple sclerosis. N Engl J Med 2003;348(1):15–23.

[139] Sled JG, Levesque I, Santos AC, et al. Regional variations in normal brain shown by quantitative magnetization transfer imaging. Magn Reson Med 2004;51(2):299–303.

[140] Basser PJ, Jones DK. Diffusion-tensor MRI: theory, experimental design and data analysis - a technical review. NMR Biomed 2002;15(7–8):456–67.

ELSEVIER
SAUNDERS

Phys Med Rehabil Clin N Am
16 (2005) 411–436

PHYSICAL MEDICINE
AND REHABILITATION
CLINICS OF
NORTH AMERICA

# Neuropsychological Evaluation and Treatment of Multiple Sclerosis: The Importance of a Neuro-rehabilitation Focus

Mary Pepping, PhD*, Dawn M. Ehde, PhD

*Department of Rehabilitation Medicine, University of Washington
School of Medicine, 1959 NE Pacific Street, Box 356490, Seattle, WA 98195, USA*

Neuropsychological evaluation is a critical tool in the assessment and management of the neurocognitive and neurobehavioral sequelae that can emerge as features of multiple sclerosis (MS). Careful exploration through testing and observation of the underlying neuropsychological causes of disruption allows for increased understanding of the particular person. This detailed view can identify issues that are likely to be neurologically based, as well as those disruptions in thinking or perception that are more likely to reflect heightened emotional distress or a particular personality style of coping.

Evaluation results also can help the person who has MS and his or her provider and family to identify clearly the patient's long-standing strengths and to use that knowledge to support and maximize overall function. Further, the evaluation creates a data-based template to guide neuro-rehabilitation treatment interventions that can target key obstacles to improved real-life function efficiently.

Neuropsychological evaluation in the hands of a competent clinician can create an important opportunity to establish a therapeutic alliance with an individual who is suffering the effects of MS. Informed and compassionate discussion and support from an experienced provider who can understand and describe the person's range of abilities and their key vulnerabilities can provide clarity, a plan for improvement, and a sense of hope that something practical can be done to improve function.

This work was supported in part by the National Institute on Disability and Rehabilitation Research grant #H133B031129-04.

* Corresponding author.

*E-mail address:* mpepping@u.washington.edu (M. Pepping).

1047-9651/05/$ - see front matter © 2005 Elsevier Inc. All rights reserved.
doi:10.1016/j.pmr.2005.01.009

*pmr.theclinics.com*

This article describes the components of a neuropsychological evaluation and some of the primary indications for its use in MS. We also detail the kinds of neurocognitive and neurobehavioral problems that are cited commonly in the relevant literature and seen in the clinical setting. We provide a brief overview of the brain structures that are affected commonly by MS, and their implications for neuropsychological function. We have included an overview of some of the current medications that are used to target cognitive and emotional symptoms that can be a direct result of the disease. We also present four representative case examples of composite patients, and briefly review the ways in which neuropsychological evaluation and neuro-rehabilitation treatments can help people who have MS.

## What is neuropsychological evaluation?

Neuropsychological evaluation (NPE) is a type of assessment that is conducted by psychologists who have extensive specialty training in the understanding of brain-behavior relationships. This training includes graduate and postgraduate education in the areas of brain anatomy, neurophysiology, and neuropathology and extensive review of the specific brain regions and relationships that are known to be associated with higher-level human capacities.

Neuropsychologists also receive extensive training in the theory and practice of psychometric testing, including test development and test stan-dardization procedures. Psychologists, as a group, also are well-grounded in statistical theory and practice. Their clinical psychology training should include a thorough understanding of normal and problematic personality features. This provides further context in which to understand fully a given patient's cognitive and interpersonal style, strengths, weaknesses, and the impact of all this on the person's ability to cope.

A comprehensive NPE ultimately should provide detailed information about a person's thinking, behavior, and emotions, especially as these are related to intact versus impaired brain function. All of this information needs to be viewed in the context of the person's particular personal history. In a rehabilitation context, the NPE also should provide detailed recommendations regarding treatment for the deficits that are noted on examination.

## The evaluation data reviewed by neuropsychologists

The neuropsychologist collects, reviews, and integrates the following information to arrive at a summary, conclusion, and set of recommendations for each person evaluated:

Pertinent medical records
Relevant school or employment records

Detailed interview of the person being evaluated, including their current symptoms and complete past psychosocial history

Interview of the spouse or other important family members

Test data from a selected battery of standardized tests

Informed observation of relevant neurobehavioral signs (eg, agitation, emotional lability, impulsivity, or social and interpersonal difficulties)

Informed observation and evaluation of reactive emotional concerns (eg, anxiety, depression, sadness or frustration)

## Test content areas

Although more will be said later in this article about specific test batteries, test content areas should assess, at simple and complex levels:

Attention and concentration (eg, ability to maintain focus, to screen out distraction, to juggle multiple bits of information mentally)

Speed of information processing

Memory acquisition, storage, and retrieval

Verbal and nonverbal reasoning

Executive functions; these can include problems with:

Tangentiality (straying from the topic)

Flexibility of thinking

Perseveration (the tendency to persist in following a particular approach on a problem-solving task, when the approach that worked initially is no longer effective)

Trial and error reasoning (ie, trouble modifying one's performance on the basis of feedback)

Planning and organization

Initiation of an action or task

Completion of an action or task

Goal-directed behavior

Strategy development

Ability to generalize ideas learned in one circumstance to a different but relevant situation

Fine motor speed

Psychological issues, including reactive emotional concerns, such as anxiety or depression, as well as more enduring personality features.

Quantitative (eg, test scores) and qualitative (eg, person's method or approach to solving problems) features of performance are considered. The NPE results for any given person are compared with a large test data set of individual scores from these same measures for people of their age and education. Systematic clinical observations of behavioral issues for people who do and do not have MS also provide points of comparison.

All of this information should allow the neuropsychologist to produce a thoughtful and thorough review of the person's cognitive, emotional, behavioral, characterologic, and interpersonal strengths and vulnerabilities, especially as these relate to the person's disease. In addition, the review and integration of the evaluation findings in a follow-up meeting with the patient and family, and in a written report, should allow the patient to understand the nature of his or her abilities and difficulties better. Ideally, the report also provides a clear foundation for the development of neuro-rehabilitation treatment (eg, guides the focus or emphasis of cognitive rehabilitation interventions and provides valuable information to the physician, speech therapist or occupational therapist, the clinical psychologist who is providing psychotherapy, the vocational rehabilitation counselor, and other providers).

## Why is a neuropsychological evaluation important in the evaluation and treatment of people who have multiple sclerosis?

Perhaps less well-known or appreciated than the motor and sensory changes that are associated with MS is the fact that many people who have MS experience at least mild-to-moderate neurologically-based changes in their thinking or behavior at some point in their disease process. Current estimates of the prevalence of neuropsychological problems are approximately 50% [1,2].

Neuropsychological evaluation is especially important in the care of patients who have MS, because for some patients, the combination of subtle cognitive and neurobehavioral symptoms are likely to prove most troublesome to successful adjustment. Left unidentified and untreated, these problems may have a greater adverse impact upon work and personal life than does the range of physical difficulties that is recognized and associated more commonly with MS.

Particular patterns of neurocognitive and neurobehavioral problems are characteristic of MS in the subgroup of patients who experiences changes in their thinking. These changes may occur in the absence of any major physical problems, or they can coexist with sensory and motor disturbances. There also are some patients who have MS whose primary difficulties are subtle physical problems, without much cognitive change.

Every person has his or her own unique set of life-long abilities and limitations in various areas of thinking, emotion, personality, and behavior. It is essential to obtain a good history that details previous education, work, leisure interests, coping history, and life accomplishments. Although the primary questions that are addressed by the evaluation may be, "Are there deficits, and if so, in what areas and to what extent?" we also want to know as much as possible about who the person has always been and what their strengths and weaknesses might have been before the onset of their disease.

For example, some people never have had a sense of direction, or good mechanical or visual-spatial ability. For them, low levels of tested visual-spatial skills need not be a sign of acquired, MS-related disturbance in that area of cognitive function; however, if the patient were a mechanical engineer, draftsmen, carpenter, or radiologist, then mildly impaired visual-spatial abilities would be noteworthy. Another example includes patients with a history of poor academic performance or verbal learning disability. Low average levels of reading or spelling on the neuropsychological evaluation for such a person of average intelligence otherwise would not necessarily be a concern in this instance. Even mild difficulties with proverb interpretation or higher-level verbal tasks may not signal a change in performance for such persons.

Although one can never know completely and exactly how the person functioned before the onset of the disease in every domain of interest, some reasonable estimates of premorbid skills can be determined. This is based, in part, upon research and identification of factors that are known to be associated with level of education and age. For example, certain test scores (eg, vocabulary knowledge, reading of single words correctly) do not tend to change much with time or the possible effects of relapsing/remitting MS, but are correlated highly with the level of premorbid verbal IQ.

In addition, the tests that are used in evaluating patients who have MS have been given to thousands of people who do not have MS, as part of the test standardization process. Using these data for comparison allows neuropsychologists to determine how similar or dissimilar their patient's performance is to the wide range of normal scores.

The person who has MS may develop new difficulties in their thinking (eg, trouble with mental juggling or reduced speed of thinking, or with memory retrieval). They also might experience a neurologically-based worsening or intensification of premorbid cognitive or personality vulnerabilities, although the underlying area of difficulty is not completely new. For example, some people who never have been particularly good at organization note more significant difficulty with organization in the months or years following the onset of their MS. Others who always have noted a tendency to be a bit impulsive or outspoken may find that they now have less control (ie, an even stronger tendency to blurt out comments they might have previously and appropriately kept to themselves when the situation warranted this caution). Although the tendency toward disorganization or bluntness is not new, the degree to which the person's life and function is affected adversely by a higher level of the problem is a significant change for them.

There is an emotional risk associated with neuropsychological assessment for some patients who have MS. Test results that document areas of neurocognitive or neurobehavioral difficulty can add another source of worry for patients who already are struggling with a myriad of symptoms and concerns. It is important not to overwhelm the person with information that is likely to increase their stress or diminish their coping abilities. For many people, it is psychologically easier to tolerate changes in sensory and motor functions than changes in important aspects of thinking or personality that constitute what many believe are essential elements of the self.

With the above caution in mind (ie, "do no harm"), if testing and review of test results is approached properly, we believe that almost all patients can derive far more benefit than negative impact. People who have MS often have noticed disruptions in their thinking, but are not sure what is wrong, or why, and do not know what to do about it. The changes can make them feel "crazy," guilty, or frightened, and can intensify psychological reactions unwittingly. These heightened psychological reactions, which can occur within or outside of conscious self-awareness for some patients, often disrupt the person's actual thinking abilities further. The person's alterations in thinking and behavior can be a source of considerable stress to family members and are difficult to understand if the patient's verbal skills are otherwise well-preserved (eg, "Why is a person who looks and sounds bright acting so scattered?").

Having cognitive and behavioral issues clarified can relieve the person of guilt, reduce family members' frustration and anger, and in many instances, reduce anxiety and depression for the patient. They can redirect all energy that was spent previously in confusion and free-floating stress into improved coping. It has been our clinical experience that when people understand why they are having the problems that they experience, are educated about their numerous areas of skill, and are taught to use effective compensatory techniques, it allows a sense of hope and mastery that serves well the patient and family.

Neuropsychological evaluations can help to address several specific concerns and questions in MS, for the patient and the provider. A list of common questions is found in Box 1. For example, NPE is useful in monitoring outcomes of treatment and the course of cognitive recovery or decline. Although a comprehensive evaluation can delineate areas of difficulty in a manner that maximizes the chance to treat the problems effectively, the evaluation can illuminate cognitive or emotional strengths that can be used to facilitate adaptation to deficits. Comprehensive evaluations also can lead to specific recommendations for return to work, maintenance of current employment, independent living, and other health and life goals.

### Areas of the brain that are affected commonly by multiple sclerosis and resulting neuropsychological sequelae

The pathophysiology of white matter disease and its impact upon central nervous system sensory and motor functions has been well-described elsewhere in this issue and will not be repeated here. It is important, however, to appreciate the specific impact that cerebral white matter changes that are caused by MS can have upon neuropsychological functions.

---

**Box 1. Common questions that a neuropsychological evaluation may address**

What are the specific cognitive and behavioral losses or
   disruptions that are caused by MS?
What is the nature and extent of these difficulties?
What is the range and nature of the person's residual strengths?
What are the implications for treatment, everyday functioning,
   health, work, or school?
Knowing the strengths and weaknesses, what practical
   suggestions can be made to improve the situation?
How can rehabilitation help the person to function better
   (eg, return to work, school)?
How likely is the person to be able to return to work or school
   in the near future?
The patient is applying for disability benefits. Might the
   cognitive difficulties be a factor in his/her overall disability
   due to MS?
This patient is having difficulties at work—why might this be?
The patient will be starting a new MS immunomodulation
   therapy—what is their cognitive baseline before treatment?
What role are reactive emotional issues playing in the person's
   overall level of function?

---

The regions of the brain that lie within the deep white matter areas include the limbic system, the midbrain, brain stem, and cranial nerves. These structures form the main highways of transmission to, and communication from, the higher-level cortical regions throughout the brain. The limbic system components, in particular (cingulate gyrus, fornix, hypothalamus, thalamus, amygdala, hippocampus), have important reciprocal connections to the frontal, temporal, and parietal lobes, and vice versa.

Thus, although cortical gray matter may be well-preserved in MS, the basic information it receives to interpret and act upon may be inaccurate or faulty, because white matter structures and systems that are critical to the transmission and integration of various sources of information may be flawed. General speed of information processing and memory retrieval systems, in particular, are especially vulnerable to disruption, as are a kind of higher level inference and executive oversight.

White matter structures also have their own unique functions, such as the thalamic role in sensory relay; the hypothalamic role in regulation of temperature, appetite, thirst, and the endocrine system; the amygdala's role in rage reactions; and the hippocampal role in memory storage. Any or all of these particular structures and functions may be affected by MS.

Deep brain structures in the brain stem also allow for autonomic nervous system control, like regulation of cardiac and respiratory functions. The reticular activating system in the brainstem is crucial for sleep and wake cycles, and for maintenance of "cortical tone" or readiness to respond to incoming information.

Damage to the periventricular white matter that underlies the frontal lobes, and to frontal-subcortical systems, can produce problems in executive function (see later discussion). Difficulties with the production or regulation of behavioral and affective responses also can be linked to frontal-limbic system dysfunction.

Specific psychiatric difficulties that are seen in some people who have MS can include development of intense emotional responses, including rapid mood swings, rage reactions, inappropriate laughing or crying, and development of bipolar disorder features. Problems with impulse control and judgment as well as increased irritability may be seen. Sometimes the person becomes more childlike in their personal and social behavior. Some people develop "la belle indifference" syndrome, a neurologically-based pathologic lack of concern that affects the patient's view of self and others.

People who have MS also can have focal deficits in function that are associated with the location of specific lesions, so that sensory and motor changes can occur on a particular body side or to a particular limb. Lesions in the periventricular white matter that underlies a specific lobe of the brain also can lead to specific problems (eg, lesions in the white matter that underlies the parietal or temporal lobe can lead to specific disruptions in certain kinds of memory or visual perceptual skills).

## Cognitive functions that are impacted most commonly by multiple sclerosis

### Attention and concentration

Attention refers to several related processes that have to do with how an individual receives and begins to process stimuli. It includes the ability to focus or direct one's attention to the matter at hand, to concentrate or sustain a focus beyond the initial moments of attention, and to hold information in mind for initial processing. It may involve alternating or shifting focus back and forth between different stimuli or tasks, or tracking several pieces of information at the same. It also may involve screening out distracting information.

In clinical practice, it is common for persons who have MS to report attentional problems. Although there has been some variability in the results depending on the patient sample studied, in general, the scientific literature suggests that the immediate span of attention typically is intact in persons who have MS [3]. As the attentional task becomes more difficult (eg, one must juggle several bits of information, sustain a focus, or remain free from competing distractions), impairments in attention often are seen. When compared with neurologically-intact controls, persons who had MS exhibited more difficulties on tests of alternating and divided attention [2,4–7]. Attentional capacity also can vary under different conditions that are not caused directly by neurological problems. For example, fatigue, depression, pain, and stress can reduce attention in neurologically-intact adults [8] and also likely impact attention negatively in persons who have MS.

*Information processing speed*

A cognitive function that is discussed often in conjunction with attention is information processing speed, which is the rate at which an individual is able to perform a mental activity. Someone who has a slowed processing speed might complain of feeling "slow" or may notice that it takes them more time to complete cognitive activities. Numerous studies have documented that persons who have MS can have deficits in this area [5,6,9–11]. A recent case-control study cited speed of information processing deficits as a central cognitive issue (ie, specific attention and memory performances are affected more adversely by a decline in simple underlying speed of information processing than may have been appreciated previously) [12].

*Memory functioning*

Memory function has been the most extensively studied cognitive deficit in the MS literature; most studies examined declarative or explicit memory (ie, ability to remember stories, word lists, designs that are presented for memorization by the patient). Relative to neurologically-intact controls, persons who had MS commonly had memory impairment [3,13,14]. Earlier in the literature, several studies suggested that the impairment primarily was the result of retrieval failures (ie, individuals who had memory problems secondary to MS had difficulty retrieving the previously learned information from long-term memory storage) [15,16]. These studies reported that the acquisition of new information (encoding and storage) was intact. More recently, this notion was challenged; several studies showed that memory impairment may be more global in nature, including impairment in explicit, recognition, and working memory [14]. Procedural, implicit, and remote memory seem to be spared more in MS [14,16,17].

*Communication and language*

Typically, intact communication involves several language and speech production abilities. Language includes the ability to comprehend and express information through written and spoken formats. Communication also includes several nonverbal and behavioral aspects, including turn taking, use of gestures, and organization of content.

To understand how MS may impact communication, it is important to distinguish communication problems that are due to language deficits from those that are caused by speech deficits. Motor-speech problems, such as dysarthria, cause difficulties in the production of speech and are common in persons who have MS [13]. Although someone who has slurred, dysarthric speech may seem to be impaired cognitively, motor-speech problems may not predict cognitive impairment in MS [13]. Similarly, language skills (eg, reading, writing, comprehension of language) may be intact in someone who has motor-speech impairment. Severe abnormalities of language, such as aphasia, alexia, and agraphia are rare [18].

Subtle difficulties in language may be present, however [3]. In addition, impairments in verbal fluency are common [2,4,10]. Verbal fluency is the ability to generate words rapidly when given a specific category (eg, animals) or letter ("name all the words you can think of that begin with the letter "F"). The ability to generate words rapidly involves several cognitive functions in addition to language, including memory retrieval and information processing speed. Finally, many patients who have MS complain of word-finding or word-retrieval problems [19] throughout their daily activities.

*Visuoperceptual processing*

Visual perception or visuoperceptual processing involves one's ability to recognize and discriminate between visual stimuli and to interpret these stimuli through association with earlier experiences. Although this cognitive domain has received little investigation in the literature, existing studies suggest that persons who have MS often show difficulties on measures of visuoperceptual processing [2,13].

Several complicating factors likely affect performance in the visual-spatial domain. Being able to see objects is one issue, and we know that impaired sight that is due to blurred or double vision is a well-recognized problem with MS.

Even people who have reasonably intact sight may not have the kind of intact cerebral processing abilities that allow them to perceive lines and angles accurately, to interpret other people's facial expressions correctly, or to gauge accurately the speed and relative position of oncoming cars. Disruptions in planning and organizing can lead to inaccuracies in visual-spatial problem solving. Deficits in conceptual reasoning, such as that needed to recognize figure-ground relationships, may lead to errors in visual-perceptual discrimination, even thought eyesight is intact. Subtle inattention or misperception of the contralateral side of space, which usually occurs outside of the person's awareness, can lead to inaccuracies in final conclusions or reproductions (eg, the person did not notice all of the information that should have been taken into account when developing a solution). They also may have chronic difficulty with mislaying needed objects around the home, more so than the average person does; persons who have MS may find themselves in search of their glasses, a coffee cup, or a piece of needed paperwork. Because visual perceptual skills are necessary in several daily and work activities, a better understanding of them through research is warranted.

### Executive functions, complex problem solving, and adaptive reasoning

The highest form of cognitive processing involves complex problem solving, adaptive reasoning, and executive functions. These abilities refer to a variety of loosely related higher-order cognitive processes that include initiation, goal setting, planning, organization, sequencing of steps or events, hypothesis generation, concept formation, decision-making, problem solving, cognitive flexibility, self-regulation, and judgment. The ability to generate solutions to novel problems and adjust to corrective feedback also is included in this broad definition. These functions enable individuals to pursue independent, purposive behaviors and to adapt to their circumstances as needed. They are critical to all aspects of everyday life, including home, work, and relationships.

Although executive functioning often is included within the domain of cognitive functioning, it may be conceptualized better as a multi-dimensional construct that includes aspects of cognition, emotion, and behavior. Of particular note for patients who have MS is the fact that it is possible to have significant impairment in executive functions, but no major changes in the person's general intellectual abilities as measured by IQ.

Research that examined the various components of problem solving and executive functioning suggests that they often are impaired in persons who have MS [20]. For example, compared with controls, persons who have MS are less efficient and make more errors on tasks that examine their ability to plan and to sequence actions [21,22]. They also have difficulties with concept formation [23] and regulating their own behavior [13].

### Patterns of impairment

Just as the physical symptoms of MS vary from patient to patient as well as within individuals, so do the cognitive changes. For some, difficulty may be circumscribed to one area (eg, memory), whereas for others it may be more global. Despite this variability, specific domains of cognition are impacted more commonly than others. Most commonly impaired are memory, verbal fluency, reasoning, complex attentional processes, and speed of information processing [2,14,22,24–27]. Of the domains that typically are affected, well-learned skills, such as language and simple span of attention, are the least common areas for impairment; executive functions and visual perception fall in the middle of the continuum.

### Degree of impairment

Cognitive impairment that is seen in persons who have MS can range from mild or minimal to severe. For example, one individual may have occasional difficulties with word finding with little impact on everyday functioning, except understandable annoyance when such difficulties occur. Another person may exhibit significant impairments across all cognitive domains that result in the inability to care safely for oneself, work, or drive. For most of the nearly half of all persons who have MS and cognitive dysfunction, the degree of impairment typically is mild to moderate [2]. The likelihood of mild to moderate (versus significant) impairment also seems to vary as a function of the type or stage of MS.

For some individuals, cognitive impairment may be so significant that it warrants a diagnosis of dementia. The term "dementia" in this instance is used to describe a broad clinical syndrome that is characterized by deterioration in cognitive ability of sufficient severity to interfere with social or occupational functioning.

According to the clinical diagnostic criteria in the revised fourth edition of the *Diagnostic and Statistical Manual of Mental Disorders* (DSM-IV), the cognitive manifestations of dementia must include memory impairment in conjunction with impairment in aphasia (severe language deficits), apraxia (impaired ability to carry out motor activities despite intact motor function), agnosia (failure to recognize or identify objects despite intact sensory function), or executive function. The DSM-IV criteria also require that a specific organic factor (in this case, MS) is presumed to be the cause of the cognitive disturbance. Finally, in dementia it is assumed that the cognitive impairments represent a decline in functioning from previous levels (ie, before the MS). Exact rates of DSM-IV–diagnosed dementia are not known because this diagnostic schema is reported rarely in the MS literature.

We prefer not to use the term "dementia" in describing the difficulties that are associated with MS, and generally advise against its use for patients who have MS, in all but the most extreme circumstances of decline. One important reason is that aphasia, apraxia, and agnosia are rare in MS; the use of a term, such as dementia, to describe memory and executive problems alone overstates the difficulties that are present. Further, it can create confusion in the minds of the person who has MS, their families, and providers regarding the nature of cognitive, emotional, and behavioral changes that are present, as well as those to be anticipated. The pattern and severity of impairments that are characteristic of most patients who have MS are different than patterns of deficits and disease course that are associated with the cortical dementias, such as Alzheimer's disease, frontal-temporal dementia, or multi-infarct dementia.

## Medications for cognitive impairment in multiple sclerosis

A variety of medications has been used to address cognitive problems and mental fatigue in people who have MS.

## Donepezil hydrochloride (Aricept)

Donepezil hydrochloride is a piperidine-based acetylcholinesterase inhibitor that is efficacious and safe in the treatment of memory deficits that are due to Alzheimer's disease and has been approved for use in this disease. Donepezil hydrochloride showed promise in a few uncontrolled, open-label studies that targeted MS-related memory impairment [28,29]. Although it did not seem to be effective at a lower dosage, a more recent trial that used 10-mg dosages showed some positive benefit [30].

## Amantadine (Symmetrel)

Although typically used to treat MS-related fatigue, amantadine showed mild improvements in attentional abilities in one study [31] but not in another [32].

## Methylphenidate (Ritalin)

For some time, methylphenidate has been used commonly to treat attentional difficulties in children and adults who have attention deficit disorders. More recently, it showed promise in improving attentional functioning in adults who had acquired brain injury [33,34]. Methylphenidate has not been studied in persons who have MS.

## Immunomodulating medications

Early studies of the immunomodulating medications did not include measures of cognitive functioning, although such trials typically now include thorough neuropsychological test batteries. As such, the literature on their effects on cognition is small. The few studies that have been conducted had mixed results. For example, in a study of Betaseron in the treatment of relapsing-remitting MS, memory for visual information, and to a lesser extent, attention, improved in the treatment group [35]. In another sample of patients who had relapsing-remitting MS, subjects who received interferon β-1a (Avonex) showed modest improvements in memory, information processing, visuospatial abilities, and executive functions relative to subjects who received placebo [36]. In another study of a different agent, glatiramer acetate (Copaxone) failed to improve cognitive function [37]. Inclusion of neuropsychological tests in future clinical trials may reveal additional benefits of such treatments.

## Antidepressant medications

Given the prevalence of major depressive disorder in persons who have MS, as well as the potential for depression to disrupt cognition, the pharmacotherapy of depression warrants mention. In medical specialty settings, the efficacy of pharmacologic treatments of persons who had major depressive disorder was well-established by randomized clinical trials [38,39]. Of the variety of antidepressant medications that is available, the selective serotonin reuptake inhibitor (SSRI) antidepressants often are the first-line medication in treating depression for several reasons. SSRIs have supplanted tricyclic antidepressants as the drug of choice in the treatment of depression in the general population and are effective in treating anxiety [40]. They can be dosed once a day and do not require serum level monitoring or dietary restrictions. Antidepressants with significant anticholinergic side effects, such as tricyclic antidepressants, may exacerbate some of the primary symptoms of MS, including cognitive impairment [41]. The SSRIs were reported to be well-tolerated in persons who had MS [42]. SSRIs are used widely in clinical practice in neurology and rehabilitation medicine settings, but no controlled trial that evaluated their efficacy in treating depression in MS has been published.

Finally, it is important to appreciate that some features of the neuropsychologic issues that are common to patients who have MS, including the neurocognitive, the neurobehavioral, and the relevant useful medications for cognitive disruptions, also may be seen among people who have other forms of brain injury or neurologic disease. For example, people who survive severe traumatic brain injuries often suffered a high degree of axonal shearing in the white matter of the brain; this can produce some overlap with the cognitive and behavioral effects that are seen in the demyelinating effects of MS. People who have severe anoxic brain injuries often suffer damage to white matter structures in the brain, and can have profound memory retrieval impairments. Some patients who have traumatic brain injury or other forms of acquired brain dysfunction also benefit from medications to improve memory or mood.

Indirect disruptions in brain function also can occur with tumor, stroke, MS, or traumatic brain injury. Brain regions that are not affected directly by lesions still may suffer from reduced input from those areas that are affected, or by lack of needed neuronal response from an affected area. Thus, communication among brain structures may be disrupted and lead to secondary problems in how the entire brain is able to process information.

Yet the nature of white matter disease in MS, versus other causes of brain dysfunction, has important neuropsychologic and psychologic implications for the affected person. Although we do not want to minimize the profound and life-altering effects of traumatic brain injury, an aneurysm rupture, or a benign brain tumor, individuals who have those injuries or illnesses can expect to improve and stay improved, after the initial onslaught of symptoms, and changes in how they function. It may be a long, slow course of recovery and they have to work hard to achieve gains; however, once achieved, those are gains that they can count on for their future function.

People who have MS must face the additional burden of a progressive neurologic disorder. In its early stages, it is characterized by waxing and waning of symptoms. The patient may not be able to predict, on any given day, how s/he is going to be feel and function. For many patients, MS tends to be accompanied by a profound fatigue or increased sensitivity to heat. Both issues can make regular and beneficial levels of exercise difficult. The fatigue can limit greatly the person's productivity and activities that bring income, pleasure, or both to life.

As the disease progresses, new symptoms and limitations are added to the list of difficulties that the person already was trying to manage. If the patient is using disease-modifying therapies, s/he may have flulike symptoms as side effects to treatment with which to contend on a regular basis, or inflammation at injection sites.

Understanding the nature of MS-related neuropsychological changes also has important implications for areas of function that are likely to be well-preserved, and that can continue to function as sources of strength and adaptation, long into the disease process.

## Specific test batteries

There are several legitimate approaches to the neuropsychological evaluation of patients who have MS. These can include the use of brief screening instruments to identify possible broad areas of concern initially, as well as administration of a specific set of tests that is known to be sensitive to the cognitive domains that are affected by MS.

In an ideal world of unlimited resources and time, every person who was newly diagnosed with MS, as well as those who had experienced subjective losses or improvements in functioning, would obtain a comprehensive neuropsychological evaluation. Because of limitations in resources, time, and other factors, comprehensive examinations of all patients often are impractical. Thus, a compromise is to have a systematic approach to identify patients who may benefit from more comprehensive neuropsychological assessment.

Some health care providers administer what often are called "bedside" cognitive screens, such as the Mini-Mental Status Examination (MMSE) [43] to screen for cognitive impairment. The advantages of such measures are that they are brief (eg, take 5 to 10 minutes to administer), easily scored, and do not require extensive training in their administration. Research has documented repeatedly that bedside screens, including the MMSE, are insensitive to the cognitive deficits that are seen in MS, with the exception of the deficits that are seen in severely impaired patients [2,17,44]. When such assessments are used, cognitive impairments are likely to go undetected. Any measure that purports to assess cognitive impairment in MS in only a few minutes should be viewed with considerable skepticism.

Recently, a consensus panel of 16 experts [45] in neuropsychologic assessment of MS recommended a test battery that was designed, in part, to fill the gap between brief neuropsychologic screening batteries and comprehensive neuropsychological evaluations, which can prove too lengthy or impractical for routine use. The Minimal Assessment of Cognitive Function in MS (MACFIMS) [45] is a neuropsychological test battery that was designed to detect neuropsychologic impairment in persons who have MS and to monitor changes in those functions over time.

Domains of cognitive functioning that are assessed by the MACFIMS include processing speed/working memory, learning/memory, visual-spatial processing, executive functioning, and word retrieval. The measures that are included in the MACFIMS are: (1) Paced Auditory Serial Addition Test-Rao Version [46]; (2) Symbol Digit Modalities Test [2]; (3) California Verbal Learning Test-II; (4) Brief Visuospatial Memory Test-Revised; Delis-Kaplan Executive Function System (D-KEFS) Sorting Test; (5) Judgment of Line Orientation Test [47]; and (6) Controlled Oral Word Association Test [48]. The battery takes approximately 90 minutes to be administered, with additional time needed for record review; clinical interview; and, if warranted, administration of any self-report measures of psychological functioning. A detailed description of the battery, including the consensus methodology and measure criteria can be found in the panel's paper [45].

In our outpatient neuro-rehabilitation treatment settings, we found that more comprehensive evaluations often are necessary to answer fully the questions that are asked as part of the referral. In the rehabilitation setting, the neuropsychological evaluation results are needed only, in part, to document the pattern and severity of neurocognitive and neurobehavioral difficulty. Equally importantly, evaluation results are used to identify as wide a range as possible of residual abilities.

It also is essential that the results allow detailed understanding of subtle disruptions in thinking that may not qualify as "impairments," but are below average performances for the patient. These neurologically-based inefficiencies, in combination with sensory motor problems, fatigue, and other areas of mild to moderate cognitive deficit, are highly likely to affect, directly and adversely, real world function at work and within home, family, and personal relationships.

The neuropsychological evaluation in the outpatient neuro-rehabilitation circumstance also serves as a blueprint for the treating speech therapists, occupational therapists, clinical psychologists or neuropsychologists, and vocational rehabilitation counselors. They will be able to identify the primary obstacles to improved function, and address these effectively, with full knowledge of the patient's neuropsychological resources.

Comprehensive NPE results also serve as a source of advice and guidance to the patient and family in practical matters, such as division of responsibilities within the home. Test results from comprehensive evaluations also provide the kind of detailed information that is needed for appropriate accommodations in the workplace or at school.

At times, a comprehensive NPE is necessary to allow full documentation of deficits when applying for disability income or medical retirement. In some legal circumstances in which questions of the person's competency may have arisen, a comprehensive battery of tests can allow the fairest and most thorough understanding of strengths and weaknesses, and lead to optimal judgments regarding the person's needs and capacities.

## Neuro-rehabilitation interventions

A well-integrated and experienced interdisciplinary team of rehabilitation therapists can provide several helpful supports and strategies to people who have MS. In this kind of model for treatment, although the specific disciplines vary (eg, speech therapy, physical therapy, occupational therapy, neuropsychology, rehabilitation psychology, vocational rehabilitation, social work) depending upon the patient's clinical needs, the major treatment themes to be addressed are known to all of the therapists that are involved.

Cognitive issues typically are addressed by way of some combination of speech therapy, neuropsychology input, or occupational therapy. These interventions can be delivered as part of individual and group therapies. Compensatory techniques also are integrated into job stations and the patient's home, by way of therapist engagement with family members and employers, with the patient's permission.

Physical problems are addressed directly by way of physical therapy, with a general emphasis upon functional strength, stamina, pacing, and cooling. If there are particular mobility problems, or other specific physical limitations, those are delineated carefully and treated. Other therapists make sure that the patient is using the strategies, positions, or assistive devices properly throughout all hours of the treatment day, not just the physical therapy hour.

In occupational therapy, higher level activities of daily living, such as bill paying, money management, efficient errand running and grocery shopping, and fine motor function can be addressed, as well as any needed titrations for improved fine motor function. In our setting, occupational therapy and vocational counselors often work together closely on any needed assistive technologies (eg, upper extremity limitations that affect functional word processing speed on a keyboard can be addressed by software programs that allow the patient to speak what needs to be typed).

Neurobehavioral changes, such as increased impulsivity, changes in judgment, or emotional lability are treated during individual, family, and group psychotherapy that is provided by clinical psychologists with a specialty in rehabilitation. The person's normal emotional reactions, such as sadness, frustration, depression, anxiety, and increased irritability, also are addressed. Because the patient is being seen weekly by the psychologist, it is a good time to monitor the effectiveness of any current or needed psychotropic medications.

The impact of MS upon employment can be enormous, and a good vocational rehabilitation counselor is a critical member of any complete treatment team. He or she can help patients and employers to work out effective negotiations regarding job duties, so that people who have MS can maintain appropriate employment. The counselor can advise patients regarding family medical leave or other long-term disability issues with respect to work. A good counselor also can function as the intermediary between a treating team and an employer to improve the chances for work success, and between the patient and employer, to help maximize the chances for an appropriate work outcome.

Once a patient's major hurdles to improved adjustment are identified (eg, problems with memory retrieval, planning and organizing, fatigue, and emotional lability), compensatory techniques are taught to the patient by the aforementioned therapists. Those issues and techniques for a particular patient also are reviewed weekly by the entire team, including the physician. Feedback is given to the patient in each of his or her treatment sessions, to help improve performance and generalize the use of appropriate strategies. For example, the physical therapist may remind the patient to jot down exercises in a memory book, and the physician may have reason to remind the patient to use strategies for controlling emotional tone.

## Clinical cases

(Please note: cases reflect composites of several people, blended to preserve the key teaching issues while preserving privacy and confidentiality).

For patients who present with, or develop, neurocognitive or neurobehavioral changes, one usually can see four broad categories of difficulty, clinically speaking, that often are linked to disease type and phase.

### Early relapsing remitting multiple sclerosis

People in the early stages of relapsing remitting MS (RRMS) who have cognitive symptoms usually present with a few areas of mild difficulty (eg, reduced efficiency of memory retrieval under complex circumstances, reductions in complex attention and in highly speeded information processing). They may have subtle fine motor and sensory changes. This group of patients usually can maintain current work or personal responsibilities with some modifications in approach and in environmental factors (eg, some quiet time to tackle complex tasks), and more consistent use of effective strategies.

CASE: 33-year-old married, right-handed woman, with a baccalaureate degree in business and a full-time job doing marketing. She had two young children. She had been diagnosed with RRMS 3 years before her NPE, which was ordered secondary to the patient's complaints of memory disturbance, which was affecting job performance and creating added stress for her. Testing revealed a wide range of intact abilities, but mild disruptions in complex attention, speed of information processing and complex verbal memory retrieval.

She participated in outpatient neuro-rehabilitation treatments, including outpatient speech therapy, rehabilitation psychology, and vocational counseling. The speech therapist helped her to develop and use strategies to improve complex attention skills and memory acquisition strategies, and helped with review and restructuring of her daily routine to allow pacing and prep time. The patient also worked closely with a vocational rehabilitation counselor. A few simple, but key, accommodations were made in the work place (eg, critical information was not given to her breezily by others while passing her in the hall, but was e-mailed to her so there was a written record of it, and so she could read and review the material at times that worked best for her). The treating psychologist met with the patient and her husband to review ways in which some home duties might be reorganized and in some cases, reassigned, to allow each partner some needed rest. With strategies in place, better support and understanding at work and at home, and reassurance regarding a wide rage of intact abilities, the patient has done well.

*Later relapsing remitting multiple sclerosis*

For people who are 10 or more years into their RRMS disease process, one often can find the addition of executive functions disruption as well as mild neurobehavioral changes (eg, increased tangentiality, hyperverbality). Although there is a large degree of variability among patients with respect to the pattern or severity of cognitive problems, it is not uncommon to see some mild to moderate worsening in attention, memory, and speed of thinking, as well. There may be some worsening of fine motor speed or precision, along with increased fatigue. Overall subtle reductions in general health as affected by the MS symptoms may be present (eg, numbness and tingling in the legs at night, leading to reduced sleep, and psychological weariness and reactive emotional concerns may be contributing further to problems). These patients often, although not always, are doing fairly well from an overall motor standpoint (ie, they are ambulatory, even if canes are needed, or wheelchairs used for long distance traverses) and they otherwise are independent in daily activities.

CASE: 48-year-old, single, right-handed woman, with an M.A. in Fine Arts, and with a 13-year history of MS. She was working full-time as a secretary at the time of her NPE, and had accepted the job 10 years earlier because the excellent health benefits and flexible work hours were positive features and she had not been able to find work in her field at that time. She never had intended to stay this long as a secretary and wanted to upgrade her career path. She was considering applying for a position as a curator at a local art museum, which would have required a level of organization and planning, and ongoing rapid oversight of multiple complex projects and of many employees that was at odds with the patient's poor performance on measures of executive function. Yet she was bright, well-educated, and bored with her current job.

With the support and guidance of her neuropsychologist and the vocational rehabilitation counselor, the patient was able to develop a long-range plan. Initially, she obtained a volunteer position at the museum to help with special projects and reduced her hours as a secretary to 32 per week. An opportunity arose at the museum after a year of volunteer work—when a grant was funded—for her to apply for a part-time position as a project assistant. She was hired and had a series of structured tasks to carry out every day, all related to one specific art project at a time, and provided art education for the public.

Speech therapy was called in for consultation to assist the patient in setting up organizational and memory systems that were tailored to her new workplace. She reduced her secretarial job to 24 hours a week, the minimum required to keep all of her health benefits and stable employment intact. She augmented that stable and familiar routine with the more challenging, tiring, but more satisfying work in her chosen field. The patient felt secure in the knowledge that her disease-modifying therapies would continue to be covered by her long-time insurance through her long-time employer, but also was able to look forward every week to stimulating art-related tasks in the museum setting.

### Primary progressive multiple sclerosis

For these individuals, physical symptoms often are the most challenging aspects of the disease at onset. Clinically, patients who have primary progressive MS tend to have well-preserved cognitive function accompanied by mild brain MRI burden of disease. Because much of their disease burden is in the spinal cord, their well-preserved cognitive function often is surprising, considering their severe physical disability. There are some exceptions, as follows.

CASE: 45-year-old, single, right-handed man, college educated, former high school English teacher. At the time that this gentleman came for testing, he essentially was wheelchair bound, with significant motor involvement, including widespread weakness and spasticity (lower extremities worse than upper extremities) along with significant problems with balance, and with ambulation related to all of the above. He was increasingly incontinent of urine. He did not have a history of urinary tract infections. For safety reasons, he always had to be accompanied to the toilet, and assisted in transferring safely to use it.

His speech was mildly dysarthric, but of most concern was his increasingly poorly self-regulated behavior in the assisted living facility where he wished to remain. The patient was well-liked by the staff, but they had major concerns about his safety because he recently had begun to exit his wheelchair impulsively, and therefore, was experiencing multiple falls.

He could not remember to request help first. He also was accidentally bumping into other patients in the hallways with his wheelchair when he attempted to navigate the corridors.

This man had been diagnosed with MS 20 years previously, at the age of 25, when he had been working as a high school English teacher for 3 years and was engaged to be married. With the diagnosis, the engagement was broken by his fiancée and he never married. He lived independently for several years, with his parents for several years, and then with a brother for a few years. Eventually, he needed more care than family could provide to him and he had been in an assisted living setting for approximately 5 years.

Test results revealed a man of high average verbal intelligence overall (which was believed to reflect some mild decline for him, based upon school achievement and family description of premorbid accomplishments). He was able to demonstrate new learning ability, but only when a multiple choice format was used (ie, his spontaneous recall was poor), but he was 100% accurate in selecting items that he had seen previously and attempted to memorize. His visual-perceptual problem-solving skills were extremely poor, to a degree that suggested higher-level cognitive problems, rather than vision limitations. His constellation of reduced awareness of deficit, poor motor planning skills, increased impulsivity, and tangentiality were major challenges to his safe function. He did not consider himself to be cognitively impaired or unsafe in any way.

A review of the neuropsychological test findings was undertaken with the patient and his family. Although the patient had done well in many areas of old, well-learned verbal knowledge, when he heard how poor his memory retrieval skills were, he broke down sobbing. His family never had witnessed this reaction (eg, he often seemed to be blithely unconcerned about his deficits). This led to an opportunity to discuss directly with the patient the grief that he felt over many of his losses. It also allowed his family to tell him the many assets that they saw and loved in him, and also why the staff at the assisted living facility was prepared to do everything that they could to help keep him there, but that he had to help them.

Although the patient's spontaneous recall of the discussion was poor later, with frequent reminders and reframing, he cooperated with updated occupational therapy, physical therapy, and speech evaluations. A treatment plan was developed to try and train the patient to refrain from exiting his chair unsafely.

In the process of this intensive training and several hours of interaction and observation each day by his team of therapists and brother, they were able to learn by questioning the patient at the moment that he was starting to exit his chair, that he suddenly needed to urinate, and was afraid that he would wet himself if he did not get to the toilet immediately. He had so little warning time from his neurogenic bladder that there was no way that regular staff could get to him in time, if he called or buzzed for their help. An indwelling catheter was requested by the patient's family and this particular problem largely was resolved (eg, he went from 7 falls in 3 months to zero falls in 3 months).

In this case, the NPE told us that this was a verbally bright man who had significant impairment, but some preserved new learning ability. The test results provided justification for a specific and well-orchestrated rehabilitation attempt, in a circumstance where continuity and quality of his living situation was at stake.

It was not so much the rehabilitation treatment interventions, as careful observation by the therapists and family which occurred during treatment time, that allowed a cause and effect relationship to be established for the patient's unsafe behavior. An appropriate medical solution was able to resolve what primarily seemed to be a behavioral problem. This man was impulsive and unsafe in the way in which he exited his wheelchair; however, a more direct and simpler fix was the solution.

*Secondary progressive multiple sclerosis*

People who have made the transition to secondary progressive MS often seem to have islands of preserved skill. The person who has secondary progressive MS may have well-preserved overall IQ, but increases in executive disruption; sensory-motor impairments; fatigue; and the usual speed, memory, and concentration issues.

CASE: 45-year-old, married, left-handed, college-educated high school social studies teacher, father of three, first diagnosed with MS at age 22. This pleasant and conscientious teacher had done well for many years with his MS, with no reported cognitive difficulties, and mild to moderate sensory motor symptoms that did relapse but then remit. He was highly energetic and well organized, by all reports. He had elected not to use any of the disease-modifying therapies because the side effects of the two he had tried were troublesome and his MS symptoms had been mild.

In the 4 years before his NPE, he began to experience a significant increase in physical symptoms, including severe burning sensations in both legs which resulted in sleep disturbance and greatly increased physical fatigue. He reported increased irritability and occasional tearfulness, corroborated by his wife; both of which reportedly were out of character for him. He also had changes in his gait that did not improve with time or treatment. He was referred for testing because he had begun to notice difficulty with topic maintenance when teaching, especially following any interruptions by his students. He also noticed problems with word retrieval when teaching, and that it was taking him longer to learn all of the names of his new students. Initially, he believed that this was the result of some sleep deprivation and increasing age, but it was worsening to a degree that his other, 40-something teacher colleagues did not experience.

On formal NPE, this man had well-preserved verbal and visual-spatial intellectual skills overall, but problems with complex attention, especially when he had to screen out distracting information. Fatigue was likely a contributing factor, but probably was not the only factor. He also was experiencing a few intrusions on memory retrieval tasks (ie, information that was similar or related to the target information was coming to mind, rather than the exact information to be recalled), along with mild word-finding problems in general. His higher-level reasoning was excellent on well-structured tasks, such as those that required deductive reasoning. When he had to draw inferences or discern implied meanings, or when he had to create a new and relevant conceptual structure to house seemingly unrelated ideas, he had more difficulty than expected.

The test results were reassuring to him on two levels—his areas of widespread skill were apparent and the specific reasons for his cognitive difficulties could be identified, and therefore, addressed in treatment. He worked closely with a speech therapist, the vocational counselor, the neuropsychologist, his wife, his school principal, and two fellow teachers to develop a treatment plan, a return-to-work plan, lesson plans, and back-up plans during the summer before the next fall semester.

All concerned agreed to the following:

The patient began disease modifying therapy, hoping to slow rate of further progression

He took an antidepressant to help with sleep and mood

He brought in typical kinds of classroom materials and tasks to his speech therapy hours, and worked to improve his systems of teaching

He was assigned a part-time paraprofessional aide in his classroom, who could assist if needed with topic maintenance and with grading of tests and papers

He made use of more small group tasks to help the students discuss and explore issues initially, then they brought lists of key ideas back to the main classroom discussion, which helped keep everyone on track

He was allowed to reduce some of his extra committee work, to preserve energy for teaching

He and another social studies teacher are exploring the option of a job share in another year, so that each would teach part-time, while still maintaining full health benefits

One does not always achieve this kind of ideal outcome. In our experience, however, the chances for optimal outcomes are increased when one is armed with the kind of specific and thorough knowledge that can be obtained from a good NPE. Accompanied by informed and compassionate medical care and the focused interventions of experienced interdisciplinary neuro-rehabilitation teams, patient function in the world of home, work and, community outside of the clinic often can be maximized.

# References

[1] Heaton RK. Neuropsychological findings in relapsing-remitting and chronic-progressive multiple sclerosis. J Consult Clin Psychol 1985;53:103–10.

[2] Rao SM, Leo GJ, Bernardin L, et al. Cognitive dysfunction in multiple sclerosis I. Frequency, patterns, and prediction. Neurology 1991;41:685–91.

[3] Fischer JS. Cognitive impairment in multiple sclerosis. In: Cook SD, editor. Handbook of multiple sclerosis. 3rd edition. New York: Marcel Dekker; 2001. p. 233–55.

[4] Ryan L, Clark CM, Klonoff H, et al. Patterns of cognitive impairment in relapsing-remitting multiple sclerosis and their relationship to neuropathology on magnetic resonance images. Neuropsychology 1996;2:176–93.

[5] Camp SJ, Stevenson VL, Thompson AJ, et al. Cognitive function in primary progressive and transitional progressive multiple sclerosis: a controlled study with MRI correlates. Brain 1999;122:1341–8.

[6] DeLuca J, Gaudino EA, Diamond BJ, et al. Acquisition and storage deficits in multiple sclerosis. J Clin Exp Neuropsychol 1998;20:376–90.

[7] D'Esposito M, Ohishi K, Thompson H, et al. Working memory impairments in multiple sclerosis: evidence from a dual task paradigm. Neuropsychology 1996;10:51–6.

[8] Lezak MD. Neuropsychological assessment. 3rd edition. New York: Oxford University Press; 1995.

[9] Beatty WW, Goodkin DE, Monson N, et al. Anterograde and retrograde amnesia in patients with chronic progressive multiple sclerosis. Arch Neurol 1988;45:611–9.

[10] Beatty WW, Goodkin DE, Monson N, et al. Cognitive disturbances in patients with relapsing remitting multiple sclerosis. Arch Neurol 1989;46:1113–9.

[11] DeLuca J, Johnson SK, Natelson BH. Information processing efficiency in chronic fatigue syndrome and multiple sclerosis. Arch Neurol 1993;50:301–4.

[12] DeLuca J, Chelune GJ, Tulsky DS, et al. Is speed of processing or working memory the primary information-processing deficit in multiple sclerosis? J Clin Exp Neuropsychol 2004; 26(4):550–62.

[13] Beatty WW. Multiple sclerosis. In: Adams RL, Parsons OA, Gulbertson JL, et al, editors. Neuropsychology for clinical practice: etiology, assessment, and treatment of common neurological disorders. Washington, DC: American Psychological Association; 1996. p. 225–42.

[14] Thornton AE, Raz N. Memory impairment in multiple sclerosis: a quantitative review. Neuropsychology 1997;11:357–66.

[15] Rao SM, Leo DO, St. Aubin-Faubert P. On the nature of memory disturbance in multiple sclerosis. Journal of Clinical and Experimental Neuropsychology 1989;11:699–712.

[16] Rao SM, Grafman J, DiGiulio D, et al. Memory dysfunction in multiple sclerosis: its relation to working memory, semantic encoding, and implicit learning. Neuropsychology 1993;7(3):364–74.

[17] Beatty WW, Goodkin DE. Screening for cognitive impairment in multiple sclerosis: an evaluation of the Mini-Mental State Examination. Arch Neurol 1990;47:297–301.

[18] Mahler ME, Benson DF. Cognitive dysfunction in multiple sclerosis: a subcortical dementia? In: Rao SM, editor. Neurobehavioral aspects of multiple sclerosis. New York: Oxford University Press; 1990. p. 88–101.

[19] Larocca NG, Kalb RC. Psychosocial issues in multiple sclerosis. In: Halper J, Holland NJ, editors. Comprehensive nursing care in MS. New York: Demos Vermande; 1997. p. 83–107.

[20] Basso MR, Beason-Hazen S, Lynn J, et al. Screening for cognitive dysfunction in MS. Arch Neurol 1996;53:980–4.

[21] Arnett PA, Rao SM, et al. Executive functions in multiple sclerosis: an analysis of temporal ordering, semantic encoding, and planning abilities. Neuropsychology 1997;11:535–44.

[22] Foong J, Rozewicz L, Quaghebeur G, et al. Executive function in multiple sclerosis: the role of frontal lobe pathology. Brain 1997;120:15–26.

[23] Grigsby J, Kravcisin N, Ayarbe SD, et al. Prediction of deficits in behavioral self-regulation among persons with MS. Arch Phys Med Rehabil 1993;74:1350–3.

[24] Rao S, Leo G, Bernardin L, Unverzagt F. Cognitive dysfunction in multiple sclerosis: I. Frequency, patterns and prediction. Neurology 1991;41:685–91.

[25] Rao SM. Neuropsychology of multiple sclerosis. Current Opinion in Neurology 1995;8: 216–20.

[26] Klonoff H, Clark C, Oger J, et al. Neuropsychological performance in patients with mild multiple sclerosis. J Nerv Ment Dis 1991;179:127–31.

[27] Kujala P, Portin R, Ruutiainen J. Memory deficits and early cognitive deterioration in MS. Acta Neurol Scand 1996b;93:329–35.

[28] Krupp LB, Christodoulou C, Melville P, et al. Donepezil improved memory in multiple sclerosis in a randomized clinical trial. Neurology 2004;63(9):1579–85.

[29] Greene YM, Tariot PN, Wishart H, et al. A 12-week, open trial of donepezil hydrochloride in patients with multiple sclerosis and associated cognitive impairments. J Clin Psychopharmacol 2000;20:350–6.

[30] Krupp LB, Christodoulou C, Melville P, et al. Donepezil improved memory in multiple sclerosis in a randomized clinical trial. Neurology 2004;63(9):1579–85.

[31] Cohen RA, Fisher M. Amantadine treatment of fatigue associated with multiple sclerosis. Arch Neurol 1989;46:676–80.

[32] Geisler MW, Sliwinski M, Coyle PK, et al. The effects of amantadine and pemoline on cognitive functioning in multiple sclerosis. Arch Neurol 1996;53:185–8.

[33] Kaelin DL, Cifu DX, Matthies B. Methylphenidate effect on attention deficit in the acutely brain-injured adult. Arch Phys Med Rehabil 1996;77:6–9.

[34] Plenger PM, Dixon CE, Castillo RM, Frankowski RF, Yablon SA, Levin HS. Subacute methylphenidate treatment for moderate to moderately severe traumatic brain injury: a preliminary double-blind placebo-controlled study. Arch Phys Med Rehabil 1996 Jun; 77(6):536–40.

[35] Pliskin NH, Hamer DP, Goldstein DS, et al. Improved delayed visual reproduction test performance in multiple sclerosis patients receiving interferon B-1b. Neurology 1996;47: 1463–8.

[36] Fischer JS, Priore RL, Jacobs LD, et al. Neuropsychological effects of Avonex in relapsing multiple sclerosis. Neurology 1998;50:A33.

[37] Weinstein A, Schwid SR, Schiffer RB, et al. Neuropsychological status in MS after treatment with glatiramer acetate (Copaxone). Arch Neurol 1999;56:319–24.

[38] Agency for Health Care Policy and Research. Depression in primary care: detection, diagnosis, and treatment. Clin Pract Guidel Quick Ref Guide Clin 1993;5:1–20.

[39] Williams JW Jr, Mulrow CD, Chiquette E, et al. A systematic review of newer pharmacotherapies for depression in adults: evidence report summary. Ann Intern Med 2000;132(9):743–56.

[40] Elliott TR, Frank RG. Depression following spinal cord injury. Arch Phys Med Rehabil 1996;77:816–23.

[41] Minden SL, Moes E. A psychiatric perspective. In: Rao SM, editor. Neurobehavioral aspects of multiple sclerosis. New York: Oxford University Press; 1990. p. 230–50.

[42] Scott TF, Price TR, McConnell H, et al. Characterization of major depression symptoms in multiple sclerosis patients. J Neuropsychiatry Clin Neurosci 1996;8:318–23.

[43] Folstein MF, Folstein SE, McHugh PR. "Mini-Mental State": a practical method for grading the cognitive state of patients for the clinician. Journal of Psychiatric Research 1975; 12:189–98.

[44] Swirsky-Sacchetti T, Field HL, Mitchell DR. The sensitivity of the mini-mental state exam in the white matter dementia of multiple sclerosis. J Clin Psychol 1992;48:779–86.

[45] Benedict RHB, Fischer JS, Archibald CJ, et al. Minimal neuropsychological assessment of MS patients: a consensus approach. Clin Neuropsychol 2002;16:381–97.

[46] Rao S, Leo G, Ellington L, et al. Cognitive dysfunction in multiple sclerosis: II. Impact on employment and social functioning. Neurology 1991;41:692–6.

[47] Benton AL, Sivan AB, Hamsher K, et al. Contributions to neuropsychological assessment. (2nd Ed.). New York: Oxford University Press; 1994.

[48] Benton AL, Hamsher K. Multilingual Aphasia Examination. Iowa City: AJA Associates; 1989.

ELSEVIER
SAUNDERS

Phys Med Rehabil Clin N Am
16 (2005) 437–448

PHYSICAL MEDICINE
AND REHABILITATION
CLINICS OF
NORTH AMERICA

# Depression in Persons with Multiple Sclerosis

Dawn M. Ehde, PhD*, Charles H. Bombardier, PhD

*Department of Rehabilitation Medicine, Box 356490,*
*University of Washington School of Medicine,*
*Seattle, WA 98195-6490, USA*

Depressive symptomatology is quite prevalent among persons with multiple sclerosis (MS) [1–3]. Numerous descriptive and correlational studies have examined the prevalence, risk factors, and impact of depression on individuals with MS. However, considerably less empirical attention has been given to its treatment. Nor do we have a good understanding of the biopsychosocial protective factors that may prevent a large number of individuals with MS from developing a depressive disorder. The purpose of this article is to provide a critical review of what is currently known concerning the nature and scope of depression in persons with MS. It begins with a discussion of relevant terminology, which is followed by a summary of the research literature concerning the prevalence, severity, risk factors for, and impact of depression in MS. Assessment issues are also reviewed. Gaps in the literature on the treatment of depression in persons with MS are also discussed. The article concludes with a discussion of future directions that will improve our understanding not only of depression and its treatment, but also factors that enhance emotional resilience in the face of this serious neurologic condition.

## Terminology

Clinicians and researchers often use the term *depression* interchangeably and imprecisely to describe any of a number of psychologic experiences that

Supported by grant #H133B980017 from the Department of Education's National Institute of Disability and Rehabilitation Research.

* Corresponding author.
*E-mail address:* ehde@u.washington.edu (D.M. Ehde).

may develop when facing a neurologic illness such as MS. *Depression* may refer to diagnosable disorders, subclinical mood symptoms, and distressed or tearful mood. Individuals with MS can experience any of a number of diagnosable mood disorders, including but not limited to mood disorders (eg, major depressive disorder, dysthymia), adjustment disorders, and anxiety disorders. Accurate diagnosis is important to differentiate these disorders from one another and from subclinical levels of symptomatology.

To illustrate the importance of precise terminology, we offer the diagnostic criteria for a major depressive episode (MDE) [4] so that these might be contrasted against the more imprecise label of *depression*. An MDE involves much more than depressed mood, anhedonia, or distress. The symptoms of an MDE are:

Depressed mood
Significantly diminished pleasure or interest in activities (sometimes referred to as anhedonia)
Decreased or increased appetite or significant weight loss or weight gain
Insomnia or hypersomnia
Psychomotor agitation or retardation
Decreased concentration or indecisiveness
Decreased energy or fatigue
Feelings of excessive guilt or worthlessness
Recurrent suicidal ideation with or without a plan or recurrent preoccupation with death

To be diagnosed with an MDE, an individual must have a minimum of five of the nine symptoms, one of which must be depressed mood or anhedonia. In addition, the symptoms must be experienced most of the time for a minimum of 2 weeks. These symptoms must also cause impairment in functioning and must not be attributable to a medical condition or medications. If a person experiences at least one MDE, they meet the diagnostic criteria for a major depressive disorder (MDD) [4].

As pointed out by others [5], too often in research self-report measures of depressive symptoms (eg, Beck Depression Inventory [6], Center for Epidemiological Studies–Depression [7]) are thought to provide a measure of a diagnosable MDD. Many of these self-report measures do not include adequate time referents or measures of the functional impairment that are key to diagnosing an MDD, however. Although such self-report measures are quite valuable for describing the severity and characteristics of psychologic distress and depressive symptoms, they do not constitute a diagnosis of MDD. As noted by Elliott and Frank [5], these self-report measures of depressive symptoms may be better viewed as measures of depressive symptoms or psychologic distress. Diagnosis of an MDD is best obtained through a clinical interview that includes an assessment of the specific MDD criteria, including the impairment in functioning that is required by the *Diagnostic and Statistical Manual of Mental Disorders, 4th*

*Edition* (DSM-IV) [4]. In psychiatric research, the norm is to use standardized diagnostic interviews, which are typically administered by a mental health professional or someone else trained in the administration of the tool.

Although it is beyond the scope of this article, a number of authors [5,8,9] have pointed out the importance of distinguishing depressed mood, depressive symptoms, and MDD from one another and the semantic, conceptual, theoretical, and clinical problems that can arise when such distinctions are not made. Thus we will use the term *depressed mood* when referring to a mood state characterized by feeling depressed, blue, sad, or empty. We will use MDD to represent a DSM-IV–based diagnosis of this mood disorder. For all other subthreshold levels of depressive symptoms, we will use the term *depressive symptoms*. We will use the term *depression* only when discussing literature that does not distinguish between depressive symptoms and MDD.

## Prevalence and impact of the problem

MDD and depressive symptoms are increasingly recognized as highly prevalent and disabling comorbid conditions in persons with MS. The lifetime risk of MDD is between 22.8% and 54%, while the point prevalence of MDD is 27%–54% in people with MS [10–13]. A recent study funded in the previous cycle of our MS Rehabilitation Research and Training Center showed that 29.1% of subjects from a large community sample of persons with MS reported moderate to severe depressive symptom severity [1]. In one of the few epidemiologic studies, the most common mood disorder in MS, MDD, had a 12-month period prevalence of 15.7% in persons with MS, nearly double the prevalence in persons without MS (7.4%) [2]. This same study also reported an age effect: in adults ages 18 to 45 who had MS, prevalence was 25.7%. These rates are in sharp contrast to the lifetime frequency of major depression in the general population [14] and other comparable disorders with similar levels of functional impairment, including other neurologic conditions [3,15,16].

Depressive symptomatology has been associated with greater MS-related disability, and it is suspected that depression can magnify a person's suffering by amplifying symptoms, adding to functional impairments and making it more difficult to manage the disease [17]. An example of how depressive symptomatology may impact functioning can be found in the area of cognitive functioning. In samples of individuals without any known neurologic disorders, MDD has been linked to objective cognitive difficulties, in particular attention and memory impairment [18]. Unfortunately, the relationship between depression and cognitive impairment in persons with MS is not well understood at this time. One study [19] found that persons with MS who were depressed performed significantly worse on working memory tasks than nondepressed controls. It has also been highly associated with subjective reports of poor cognitive functioning, including memory complaints [20]. Although MDD cannot account solely for poor cognitive performance in persons with MS, it likely does contribute to poor cognitive performance as well as a decreased subjective sense of cognitive abilities. More research is needed in this area.

## Issues in the assessment and recognition of depression in persons who have multiple sclerosis

Given the prevalence of depressive disorders in MS, it is important for MS health care professionals to include a measure of depressive symptoms in their overall workups of patients with MS. A variety of self-administered measures are available that purport to assess depressive symptomatology, several of which are listed in Table 1 [7,21–23]. Because self-report measures do not yield a diagnosis of MDD, cutoff scores can be used to indicate the need for a diagnostic evaluation.

One additional measure that warrants consideration for use in the MS population is the Patient Health Questionnaire (PHQ) [21]. The PHQ is a short questionnaire that was developed to assess several mental disorders, including MDD, that are commonly seen in medical populations. It is a flexible measure in that the clinician can elect to have the patient complete the entire 3-page questionnaire, a 2-page version, or a 1-page version depending on what mental disorders the clinician wishes to assess. An MS practitioner may wish to administer only the 1-page PHQ, which screens for MDD as well as panic disorder. In addition to its brevity, a strength of this measure is that it covers the DSM-IV diagnostic criteria for MDD, and by doing so can greatly expedite the subsequent diagnostic process. To date this measure has not been studied in the MS population, but it has been shown to have good sensitivity and specificity for MDD among medical patients

Table 1
Brief measures useful for screening for depression

| Depression measure | Primary reference | Comments |
| --- | --- | --- |
| Patient Health Questionnaire | Spitzer et al [21] | Provides both a diagnosis of MDD and an index of depression severity |
| Chicago Multiscale Depression Inventory | Nyenhuis et al [22] | Provides a depression severity score Developed for use in medical populations |
| Beck Depression Inventory-II | Beck et al [23] | Provides a depression severity score Perhaps the most widely known depression scale May overestimate depression due to somatic items |
| Center for Epidemiological Studies Depression Scale | Radloff [7] | Fewer somatic items, and thus useful in medical populations Provides a depression severity score |

and can be easily integrated into routine medical care [21]; It therefore warrants consideration.

A concern often raised when assessing depressive symptoms in persons with a medical condition such as MS is that somatic and cognitive symptoms secondary to the condition spuriously inflate scores. This is particularly problematic for persons with MS, given that several common MS complaints are also symptoms of depression, including fatigue, concentration difficulties, and sleep disturbance [24]. Thus practitioners may want to consider using a measure that was specifically developed for use in medical populations (including MS): the Chicago Multiscale Depression Inventory (CMDI) [22]. The CMDI is a 24-item self-report measure that has three subscales: mood, evaluative, and vegetative. Although this measure, like most others, does not diagnose an MDE, it shows considerable promise as a measure of depressive symptomatology that partials out the effects of potentially confounding vegetative symptoms.

On the other hand, research among other neurologically affected patients suggests that somatic symptoms such as sleep disturbance, anergia, and appetite change are specific for major depression and should not be ignored [25,26]. In the broader literature on depression among medical patients, the inclusive approach to depression diagnosis, which counts depressive symptoms regardless of etiology, is more reliable and sensitive than the etiologic approach, which counts symptoms only if they are not clearly and fully accounted for by a medical condition [27]. Research examining the use of these two approaches in accurately detecting MDD in persons with MS is needed.

It is important to note that screening alone is unlikely to improve depression care or outcomes. For example, studies performed in primary care populations show that without broader systems change, MDD screening programs do not lead to increased rates of antidepressant treatment or referrals for mental health services. On the other hand, institutions that add collaborative treatment protocols that include case management services have been shown to improve outcomes in other medical populations [28–30]. Given the prevalence and impact of MDD in persons with MS, specialty centers should develop systems to improve care for MDD.

## Treatment

In other medical specialty settings, the efficacy of pharmacologic and psychotherapeutic treatments of persons with MDD has been well established by randomized clinical trials [31,32]. In contrast, the literature on the treatment of MDD in MS is extremely limited and largely anecdotal. Using a meta-analysis, Mohr & Goodkin [33] concluded that both psychotherapy and pharmacotherapy are very effective for decreasing depressive symptoms on persons with MS. Although encouraging, only five studies were of sufficient methodological rigor (ie, randomized clinical trial, objective measure of depression used) to be included in their meta-analysis. Of these, only one study [34] was a randomized clinical trial of an antidepressant medication, desipramine.

Since 1999, only one additional study of MDD treatment could be found in the literature [35]. This study of 63 subjects compared the efficacy of three 16-week interventions for depression with MS and MDD: individual cognitive-behavioral therapy (n = 20), supportive/expressive group psycho-therapy (n = 22), and the antidepressant sertraline (n = 21). The individual cognitive-behavioral therapy treatment (CBT) and the group interventions met weekly for 16 weeks. Treatment assignment was not completely random, as blocks of subjects were used to form groups, with others being randomly assigned to either setraline or CBT. Sertraline was initiated at 50 mg per day and increased by 50 mg every 4 weeks until a dosage of 200 mg was reached or until full remission of symptoms occurred. This study found that depressive symptoms decreased significantly during treatment and that these improvements persisted at a 6-month follow-up. Analyses also showed the CBT and sertraline were significantly more efficacious than group therapy. When examining clinically significant change, defined as at least a 50% decrease in symptoms and symptom severity using the Hamilton Rating Scale of Depression [36], Mohr and Goodkin [33] reported that 24% of those in the sertraline condition showed clinically significant improve-ments, as compared with 50% in the CBT condition and 14% in the group therapy condition. Attrition occurred at the rate of 5%, 18%, and 29% for the CBT, group therapy, and setraline conditions, respectively.

Selective serotonin reuptake inhibitor (SSRI) antidepressants are the drugs of choice for studying the pharmacologic treatment of depressive symptomatology in MS for a variety of reasons. SSRIs have supplanted tricyclic antidepressants as the drug of choice in the treatment of depression and are also effective in treating anxiety [5]. They can be dosed once a day and do not require serum level monitoring or dietary restrictions. Medications with significant anticholinergic side effects, such as tricyclic antidepressants, may exacerbate some of the primary symptoms of MS, including cognitive impairment [37]. SSRIs are generally well tolerated in persons with MS [38] and are widely used in clinical practice in primary care as well as rehabilitation settings; however, to our knowledge, controlled trials evaluating their efficacy in MS have not been published.

Medications or traditional individual psychotherapy may not be feasible or acceptable forms of treatment for some people with MS and MDD. Therefore, alternative means of treating depressive symptoms and MDD are still needed to extend effective treatments to as many people as possible. A recent study that used an 8-week telephone-administered CBT for depressive symptomatology in persons with MS is an example of such an alternative approach [39]. In this study, individuals with MS were randomly assigned to either the telephone cognitive-behavioral intervention or to a usual-care control condition. Depressive symptomatology decreased significantly in the telephone CBT compared with the usual care condition. Furthermore, adherence to MS disease-modifying medications was significantly better at follow-up among those who participated in the telephone CBT compared with those in the usual care condition. Interventions such as this one is this study are promising because they are likely to minimize potential barriers to treatment such as transportation and may also be cost-effective relative to traditional psychopharmacologic or psychotherapeutic interventions.

Exercise holds promise as a means of treating MDD and depressive symptoms in people with MS for many reasons. First, exercise has already been shown to be safe and to improve cardiorespiratory fitness and strength in people with MS [40,41]. Second, exercise has been shown to result in widespread positive effects among people with MS, such as improvements in the areas of mood, quality of life, sexual functioning, recreation, pain, fatigue and psychosocial functioning (see Sutherland & Anderson, 2001 for review) [40]. Third, a number of studies have shown that exercise is an effective form of treatment for MDD. Though not yet studied in MS, the effect of exercise on depressed mood, depressive symptoms, and MDD has been studied in healthy human subjects, persons with psychiatric conditions, and older adults [42–44]. Exercise appears to be more beneficial than no treatment and as effective as other treatments including standard antidepressant medication and psychotherapy [45]. Exercise also is associated with lower depression relapse rates compared with pharmacotherapy, possibly due to continued exercise after the trial ended [44,46]. While most depression and exercise studies have focused on aerobic exercise, some studies suggest that nonaerobic exercise such as weightlifting [47] also improves mood [48]. Moderate exercise, defined as walking 20 minutes a day at 60% maximum heart rate, has been shown to be even more effective than vigorous exercise in decreasing the anxiety and stress components of depression and is associated with fewer dropouts [49,50]. Both group and individual exercise programs have been found to be successful [50]. Because there is no clear relationship between the amount or type of exercise and mood improvement, any exercise within Petajan's activity pyramid [39] (from aerobic to passive range of motion) may be beneficial, making exercise a possibility for the whole range of persons with MS.

Finally, persons with MS tend to be extremely interested in exercise. Somerset and colleagues [51] reported that the single most requested type of medical information was advice about exercise, with 41% requesting such information. At our center, a survey of 739 community-residing people with MS showed they were more interested in exercise than any other health-promoting activity [52]. Eighty-six percent of the total sample was very or somewhat interested in learning more about ways to safely exercise. Surprisingly, the group with significant depressive symptoms ($\geq 16$ on the Center for Epidemiological Studies-Depression scale [CES-D]) was significantly more likely to be interested in exercise (90.5%) than those subjects without depressive symptoms (82.4%). Finally, exercise is appealing because it is inexpensive in terms of health care use, is universally available (if successful, the paradigm could be easily adopted in many settings), takes advantage of the benefits of self-management (in which people with MS are provided with the skills to live an active and meaningful life), and can be used adjunctively with other MDD treatments [53].

Several other forms of depression treatment should be considered for people with MS. Interpersonal therapy [54] is an evidence-based treatment for depression that focuses on grief, role disputes, role transitions, or interpersonal deficits as the framework for therapy. This therapy model is relatively brief (16 weeks), addresses interpersonal topics likely to be relevant for people with MS, and has been shown to be effective among people who have other chronic, debilitating illnesses such as HIV infection [55] and coronary artery disease [56]. Behavioral activation approaches treat depression by increasing access to pleasant events and positive reinforcers as well as decreasing the intensity and frequency of aversive events and consequences [57]. Behavioral activation is thought to be as effective as cognitive therapy [58] and may be especially appealing to people with MS who have responded to relapses or disease progression by relinquishing too many of their important responsibilities or most enjoyable hobbies. Another behavioral therapy for treating depression has been designed for people with significant cognitive impairments [59]. In this approach caregivers are trained in ways to encourage pleasant activities, redirect and refocus the person away from depression thoughts, increase social activities, and eliminate sources of conflict and frustration. This model may hold promise for treating depression among people who have more advanced MS or when cognitive impairment is prominent.

**Future directions**

Many future directions are evident from this review. First, longitudinal research is needed to describe the natural history, risk factors, and protective factors of MDD and depressive symptoms in persons with MS. Research on the availability, quality, and effectiveness of mental health care for persons with MS is also needed. Treatment studies examining the efficacy of existing treatments for MDD are necessary, as are studies examining novel approaches. Mohr and colleagues' recent study showing the efficacy of a telephone-administered cognitive behavioral treatment for depressive symptoms is an example of an empirically based approach being adapted to address barriers, such as transportation and access, to persons with MS and MDD [39]. Across areas of inquiry, research should not only focus on individual risk and protective factors (eg, MS disease, demographic, personality, cognitive styles) but also on environmental factors (eg, societal attitudes, physical barriers, financial challenges, the health care system) that may influence depressive symptoms, behavior, treatment, and quality of care. In addition, research on other mental disorders such as panic disorder and bipolar disorder in persons with MS is also needed.

In the MS literature, very little has been studied or written about the large number of persons with MS who do not suffer from MDD or significant psychologic distress. In the broader health psychology literature, research has shown that many individuals not only persevere but thrive in spite of adversity, trauma, tragedy, loss, or serious medical illness. This process of adapting well to or bouncing back from significant life challenges has been termed *resilience*. It involves the ability to maintain healthy levels of psychologic well-being and functioning in the face of adversity. Another construct that has been examined in the psychology literature is *post-traumatic growth*, defined as positive psychologic changes resulting from or in response to a challenging circumstance such as a traumatic event or onset of a chronic or life-altering disease [60]. Posttraumatic growth can be manifested in a variety of ways, including but not limited to having an increased appreciation for life, feeling increased personal strength, experiencing improved interpersonal relationships, changing life priorities, gaining positive spiritual changes, or finding new meaning and purpose in life. Other terms for such positive changes exist in the literature and include stress-related growth [61], positive adjustment, positive adaptation, thriving, and adversarial growth [62]. All of these share the notion that positive changes can come from a challenging or adverse life experience, an idea that is important but underrecognized in the MS literature.

We hypothesize that many individuals with MS show not only a lack of psychologic distress but also evidence of positive responses such as resilience, positive emotions, and posttraumatic growth, both during and after the diagnosis of MS. Given that the rates of psychopathology are higher in MS samples, it is also likely that an important subset of individuals with MS will suffer considerable psychologic distress that interferes with their functioning. Nonetheless, research examining those people who do not become depressed, but who thrive while living with MS, is needed.

## References

[1] Chwastiak L, Ehde DM, Gibbons LE, et al. Depressive symptoms and severity of illness in multiple sclerosis: epidemiologic study of a large community sample. Am J Psychiatry 2002; 159:1862–8.
[2] Patten SB, Beck CA, Williams JV, et al. Major depression in multiple sclerosis: a population-based perspective. Neurology 2003;61:1524–7.
[3] Rao SM, Huber SJ, Bornstein RA. Emotional changes with multiple sclerosis and Parkinson's disease. J Consult Clin Psychol 1992;60:369–78.
[4] American Psychiatric Association. Diagnostic and Statistical Manual of Mental Disorders, 4th edition. Washington, DC: American Psychiatric Association; 1994.
[5] Elliott TR, Frank RG. Depression following spinal cord injury. Arch Phys Med Rehabil 1996;77:816–23.
[6] Beck AT, Steer RA, Ball R, et al. Use of the Beck Anxiety and depression inventories for primary care with medical outpatients. Assessment 1997;4:211–9.

[7] Radloff LS. The CES-D scale: a self-report depression scale for research in the general population. Applied Psychological Measurement 1977;1:385–401.

[8] Patterson DR, Everett JJ, Bombardier CH, et al. Psychological effects of severe burn injuries. Psychol Bull 1993;113:362–78.

[9] Trieschmann RB. Spinal cord injuries: psychological, social and vocational rehabilitation. New York: Demos; 1988.

[10] Joffe RT, Lippert GP, Gray TA, et al. Mood disorder and multiple sclerosis. Arch Neurol 1987;44:376–8.

[11] Minden SL, Orav J, Reich P. Depression in multiple sclerosis. Gen Hosp Psychiatry 1987;9: 426–34.

[12] Sadovnick AD, Ebers GC. Epidemiology of multiple sclerosis: a critical overview. Can J Neurol Sci 1993;20:17–29.

[13] Patten SB, Metz LM, Reimer MA. Biopsychosocial correlates of lifetime major depression in a multiple sclerosis population. Mult Scler 2000;6:115–20.

[14] Wells KB, Golding JA, Burnam MA. Psychiatric disorder in a sample of the general population with and without chronic medical conditions. American Journal of Psychiatry 1988;145:976–81.

[15] Minden SL, Schiffer RB. Affective disorders in multiple sclerosis. Archives of Neurology 1990;47:98–104.

[16] Schubert DS, Foliart RH. Increased depression in multiple sclerosis patients. A meta-analysis. Psychosomatics 1993;34(2):124–30.

[17] Katon W, Ciechanowski P. Impact of major depression on chronic medical illness. J Psychosom Res 2002;53:859–63.

[18] King DA, Caine ED. Cognitive impairment and major depression: Beyond the pseudodementia syndrome. In: Grant I, Adams K, editors. Neuropsychological assessment of Neuropsychiatric Disorders (2nd Edition). New York: Oxford University Press; 1996. p. 200–17.

[19] Arnett PA, Higginson CI, Voss WD, et al. Depression in multiple sclerosis: relationship to working memory capacity. Neuropsychology 1999;13(4):546–56.

[20] Benedict RH, Fischer JS, Archibald CJ, et al. Minimal neuropsychological assessment of MS patients: a consensus approach. Clin Neuropsychol 2002;16:381–97.

[21] Spitzer RL, Krocnke K, Williams JB. Validation and utility of a self-report version of PRIME-MD: the PHQ primary care study. Primary Care Evaluation of Mental Disorders. Patient Health Questionnaire. JAMA 1999;282(18):1737–44.

[22] Nyenhuis DL, Luchetta T, Yamamoto C, et al. The development, standardization, and initial validation of the Chicago Multiscale Depression Inventory. Journal of Personality Assessment 1998;70:386–401.

[23] Beck AT, Steer RA, Brown GK. Manual for the Beck Depression Inventory-II. San Antonio, TX: The Psychological Corporation; 1996.

[24] Nyenhuis DL, Rao SM, Zajecka JM, et al. Mood disturbance versus other symptoms of depression in multiple sclerosis. J Int Neuropsychol Soc 1995;1(3):291–6.

[25] Jorge RE, Robinson RG, Arndt S. Are there symptoms that are specific for depressed mood in patients with traumatic brain injury? J Nerv Ment Dis 1993;181(2):91–9.

[26] Bombardier CH, Richards JS, Krause JS, et al. Symptoms of major depression in people with spinal cord injury: implications for screening. Arch Phys Med Rehabil 2004;85(11): 1749–56.

[27] Williams JW, Noel PH, Cordes JA, et al. Is this patient clinically depressed? JAMA 2002; 287:1160–70.

[28] Unutzer J, Katon W, Callahan CM, et al. Collaborative care management of late-life depression in the primary care setting: a randomized controlled trial. JAMA 2002;288: 2836–45.

[29] Callahan CM. Quality improvement research on late life depression in primary care. Med Care 2001;39:772–84.

[30] Katon WJ, Unutzer J, Simon G. Treatment of depression in primary care: where we are, where we can go. Med Care 2004;42:1153–7.

[31] Agency for Health Care Policy and Research. Depression in primary care: detection, diagnosis, and treatment. Clin Pract Guide Quick Ref Guide Clin 1993;5:1–20.

[32] Williams JW Jr, Mulrow CD, Chiquette E, et al. A systemic review of newer pharmacotherapies for depression in adults: evidence report summary. Ann Intern Med 2000;132(9):743–56.

[33] Mohr DC, Goodkin DE. Treatment of depression in multiple sclerosis: review and meta-analysis. Clinical Psychology: Science and Practice 1999;6(1):1–9.

[34] Schiffer RB, Wineman NM. Antidepressant pharmacotherapy of depression associated with multiple sclerosis. Am J Psychiatry 1990;147(11):1493–7.

[35] Mohr DC, Boudewyn AC, Goodkin DE, et al. Comparative outcomes for individual cognitive-behavior therapy, supportive-expressive group psychotherapy, and sertraline for the treatment of depression in multiple sclerosis. J Consult Clin Psychol 2001;69(6):942–9.

[36] Hamilton M. Development of a rating scale for primary depressive illness. Br J Soc Clin Psychol 1967;6:278–96.

[37] Minden SL, Moes E. A psychiatric perspective. In: Rao SM, editor. Neurobehavioral aspects of multiple sclerosis. New York: Oxford University Press; 1999. p. 230–50.

[38] Scott TF, Nussbaum P, McConnell H, et al. Measurement of treatment response to sertraline in depressed multiple sclerosis patients using the Carroll scale. Neurol Res 1995;17(6):421–2.

[39] Mohr DC, Likosky W, Bertagnolli A, et al. Telephone-administered cognitive-behavioral therapy for the treatment of depressive symptoms in multiple sclerosis. J Consult Clin Psychol 2000;68:356–61.

[40] Sutherland G, Andersen MB. Exercise and multiple sclerosis: physiological, psychological, and quality of life issues. J Sports Med Phys Fitness 2001;41:421–32.

[41] Petajan JH, Gappmaier E, White AT, et al. Impact of aerobic training on fitness and quality of life in multiple sclerosis. Ann Neurol 1996;39:432–41.

[42] Martinsen EW. Benefits of exercise for the treatment of depression. Sports Med 1990;9:380–9.

[43] North TC, McCullagh P, Tran ZV. Effect of exercise on depression. Exerc Sport Sci Rev 1990;18:379–415.

[44] Blumenthal JA, Babyak MA, Moore KA, et al. Effects of exercise training on older patients with major depression. Arch Intern Med 1999;159:2349–56.

[45] Martinsen EW. Physical activity and depression: clinical experience. Acta Psychiatr Scand Suppl 1994;377:23–7.

[46] Babyak M, Blumenthal JA, Herman S, et al. Exercise treatment for major depression: maintenance of therapeutic benefit at 10 months. Psychosom Med 2000;62:633–8.

[47] Doyne EJ, Ossip-Klein DJ, Bowman ED, et al. Running versus weight lifting in the treatment of depression. J Consult Clin Psychol 1987;55:748–54.

[48] Brosse AL, Sheets ES, Lett HS, et al. Exercise and the treatment of clinical depression in adults: recent findings and future directions. Sports Med 2002;32:741–60.

[49] Brown MA, Goldstein-Shirley J, Robinson J, et al. The effects of a multi-modal intervention trial of light, exercise, and vitamins on women's mood. Women Health 2001;34:93–112.

[50] Castro CM, King AC, Brassington GS. Telephone versus mail interventions for maintenance of physical activity in older adults. Health Psychol 2001;20:438–44.

[51] Somerset M, Campbell R, Sharp DJ, et al. What do people with MS want and expect from health-care services? Health Expect 2001;4:29–37.

[52] Blake K, Bombardier C, Cunniffe M, et al. Health promotion in multiple sclerosis: problems and desire for help [abstract]. Int'l Journal MS Care, vol. 4. Chicago: Consortium of MS Centers annual meeting; 2002:89.

[53] Lorig K. Self-management education: more than a nice extra. Med Care 2003;41:699–701.

[54] Klerman GL, Weissmann MM. Interpersonal psychotherapy (IPT) and drugs in the treatment of depression. Pharmacopsychiatry 1987;20(1):3–7.

[55] Markowitz JC, Kocsis JH, Fishman B, et al. Treatment of depressive symptoms in human immunodeficiency virus-positive patients. Arch Gen Psychiatry 1998;55(5):452–7.

[56] Koszycki D, Lafontaine S, Frasure-Smith N, et al. An open-label trial of interpersonal psychotherapy in depressed patients with coronary disease. Psychosomatics 2003;45(4): 319–24.

[57] Hopko DR, Lejuez CW, Ruggiero KJ, et al. Contemporary behavioral activation treatments for depression: procedures, principles, and progress. Clin Psychol Rev 2003;23(5):699–717.

[58] Jacobson NS, Dobson KS, Truax PA, et al. A component analysis of cognitive-behavioral treatment for depression. J Consult Clin Psychol 1996;64(2):295–304.

[59] Teri L, Logsdon RG, McCurry SM. Nonpharmacologic treatment of behavioral disturbance in dementia. Med Clin North Am 2002;86(3):641–56, viii.

[60] Tedeschi RG, Calhoun LG. Posttraumatic growth: conceptual foundations and empirical evidence. Psychological Inquiry 2004;15:1–18.

[61] Park CL, Cohen LH, Murch RL. Assessment and prediction of stress-related growth. J Pers 1996;64:71–105.

[62] Linley PA, Joseph S. Positive change following trauma and adversity: a review. J Trauma Stress 2004;17:11–21.

PHYSICAL MEDICINE
AND REHABILITATION
CLINICS OF
NORTH AMERICA

ELSEVIER
SAUNDERS

Phys Med Rehabil Clin N Am
16 (2005) 449–466

# A Practical Approach
# to Immunomodulatory Therapy
# for Multiple Sclerosis

## Jack S. Burks, MD[a,b,c,d],*

[a]University of Nevada School of Medicine, Reno, NV, USA
[b]Multiple Sclerosis Association of America, Cherry Hill, NJ, USA
[c]Multiple Sclerosis Alliance, Englewood, CO, USA
[d]Burks & Associates, 4925 Pinebluff Trail, Reno, NV 89509, USA

In multiple sclerosis (MS), the pathogenesis of the disease and the mechanism of an action of immunomodulating therapies (IMTs) are not fully understood [1–3]. Genetic predispositions, socioeconomic influences, sex (women:men = 2:1), infectious agents, and other environmental factors have been implicated [4,5]. Identifying treatment has been challenging because the discovery of a successful therapy usually begins with a solid understanding of the pathogenesis of the disease. Despite a lack of complete understanding of the pathogenesis, four immunomodulating drugs and one immunosuppressive drug have received Food and Drug Administration (FDA) approval for the treatment of MS since 1993.

This article provides a current overview of the definition and pathogenesis of the disease, the different types of MS, a new diagnostic criteria, the rationale for early therapy, a review of the approved MS therapies, the strategies to evaluate ongoing treatment efficacy, the management of "suboptimal" treatment responders, and the prospects for future therapies.

The article's emphasis is on relapsing remitting MS (RRMS) because most of the therapeutic data deal with RRMS. No IMTs have been FDA approved for primary progressive MS (PPMS) or secondary progressive MS (SPMS) without relapses.

One immunosuppressive, antineoplastic agent, mitoxantrone (Novantrone), also has FDA approval for "worsening MS." Its role as a "rescue therapy" for suboptimal responders to IMTs is also discussed.

---

* Burks & Associates, 4925 Pinebluff Trail, Reno, NV 89509.
   *E-mail address:* jack@jackburks.com

1047-9651/05/$ - see front matter © 2005 Elsevier Inc. All rights reserved.
doi:10.1016/j.pmr.2005.01.007
*pmr.theclinics.com*

**The definition and pathogenesis of multiple sclerosis: a reappraisal**

The traditional definition of RRMS states, "MS is a relapsing remitting disease of central nervous system myelin secondary to a T-cell mediated inflammatory process." Although the definition is partially accurate, newer research findings indicate that the disease is much more complex. The following is a reanalysis of the definition based on recent data concerning the clinical and pathologic processes in RRMS.

*"A relapsing remitting disease" course*

This concept is only partially correct. Clinically, MS first appears as a relapsing and remitting disease course in 80% to 85% of patients. After an exacerbation, clinical recovery of all or partial function is likely. This recovery is followed by clinical stability until the next exacerbation. Between relapses, however, MRI demonstrates ongoing dynamic changes, even when clinical worsening is not obvious [6]. As many as 10 new MRI lesions are seen for each new clinical relapse. These new MRI events may last from a few weeks to months or may result in permanent MRI lesions such as increasing T2 burden of disease or "black holes." In addition, most patients initially presenting as RRMS transition to SPMS after 10 years [7,8]. In other words, most people with RRMS will end up with SPMS without treatment, even if they are "normal" between early attacks. Therefore, the concept of "relapsing remitting" is misleading because of continued damage evidenced by MRI and the transition to SPMS in most patients.

Other clinical types of MS include PPMS and progressive relapsing MS [9]. PPMS accounts for 10% to 15% of all MS patients and usually occurs after age 40. The clinical course is best characterized as steadily progressive disability beginning in the lower extremities without acute attacks [10]. The spinal cord is the primary target and MRI scans may show little evidence of acute inflammation. Progressive relapsing MS is uncommon (<5% of MS patients) and follows a progressive course with occasional interspersed attacks.

"Benign" MS accounts for 10% to 25% of RRMS patients [11]. The diagnosis of benign MS is difficult prospectively because many young people seem to fit the benign criteria yet transition to progressive disease (SPMS) after several years. Benign MS is characterized by infrequent, mild attacks with primarily sensory symptoms and little or no long-term disability. The benign diagnosis is only confirmed after 15 to 25 years. It is unfortunate that when the benign condition transitions to SPMS, the opportunity to treat effectively is diminished. Early damage, which might have been prevented with treatment, is not likely to be reversible. For example, patients on placebo for 2 to 3 years in clinical trials did not "catch up" to the therapeutic benefits of patients treated from the onset [12]. What is lost early appears to be lost forever.

*"Disease of central nervous system myelin"*

Myelin damage has been the hallmark of MS pathology. Newer data, however, indicate that although myelin is one target of the immune system dysfunction, oligodendroglia cells (myelin-producing cells), axons, and neurons can also be damaged [13–18]. This damage can be dramatic, occur early in the disease, lead to permanent disability, and may account for the cognitive dysfunction seen in over 50% of MS patients. In fact, cognitive dysfunction may not closely correlate with motor dysfunction such as walking and balance problems. A more accurate MS definition would not restrict the disease to damage of myelin but would include damage to several components of the central nervous system.

*Disease is "secondary to a T-cell mediated inflammation process"*

The immunopathogenesis of MS is undergoing intense scrutiny. Do T cells really initiate the damage in all (or any) types of MS? Do antibodies play any role in MS damage? Is MS only one disease?

New research indicates four distinct types of immunopathology [19]. Type I involves activated T cells and macrophage- and cytokine-mediated multifocal damage of myelin. This pathologic description was thought to be the major pathology in MS. Recent data, however, suggest that less than half of MS patients demonstrate this pathology. Type II involves B cells (antibody) and complement-mediated multifocal damage. Type III is a more diffuse low-grade inflammation with loss of myelin-associated glycoprotein and apoptosis of oligodendrocytes (versus myelin). Type IV appears to involve degeneration (noninflammation induced) of oligodendroglia cells. In summary, T-cell–mediated damage predominates in type I only. Further, the four types may be mutually exclusive; that is, if a patient has one type of pathology, then the other three types are not present. If these observations withstand scientific scrutiny, then MS would not be regarded a single disease entity. Instead, a syndrome with four distinct pathogenic mechanisms would be a more accurate definition, which implies that different treatments may be needed for different types of MS. This diverse pathology may help to explain the diversity of therapeutic responses to IMTs.

Leading MS authorities have evidence that the initial destructive event in MS may be oligodendroglia cell death, which is unrelated to inflammation [20]. In this case, inflammation may be a response to damage and not the cause of central nervous system damage. If correct, this model might drastically change our treatment approach. In any event, recent pathologic data may lead the way to more targeted treatments resulting in even better outcomes.

**New diagnostic criteria for early multiple sclerosis: implications for therapy**

Despite the challenges to the definition and pathologic understanding of MS, certain observations are apparent. First, IMTs can modify the disease course in RRMS. Second, early RRMS treatments produce more favorable outcomes compared with delayed therapy. Furthermore, data demonstrate that IMTs initiated after the first neurologic events are associated with a prolongation of time to the next episode and "clinical definite MS" and with a reduction of MRI lesions [21,22]. Therefore, the trend is to treat before the second clinical neurologic episode if the MRI indicates ongoing activity, after other illnesses are excluded. In fact, a new MS diagnostic criterion has been adopted to take advantage of earlier diagnosis and treatments [23].

The McDonald Criteria for the diagnosis of MS incorporates MRI findings and other tests into an earlier MS diagnosis [23]. For example, if an initial event or "clinically isolated syndrome" is associated with an abnormal MRI and a follow-up MRI after 3 months shows new lesions, then a diagnosis of RRMS may be established before the occurrence of a second clinical episode.

## The rationale for early treatment

As stated earlier, favorable outcomes are seen with early treatment, whereas delaying treatment has less favorable outcomes [12,24]. For example, IMTs in patients with SPMS who no longer have acute attacks are unlikely to delay the progression of disability [25]. This lack of IMT benefit on disease progression comes at a time when the treatments may still have a positive effect on the inflammatory process as measured by MRI and the reduction of exacerbations. In other words, a vigorous IMT anti-inflammation response in early RRMS reduces attacks and delays disease progression, whereas IMTs in later SPMS may reduce inflammation but have little effect on disease progression [26]. Why?

One theory may help explain these data. Although inflammation is robust early in RRMS, a degenerative process, which is noninflammatory, predominates later. Because this later degeneration or apoptosis process is not mediated by acute inflammation, IMTs are unlikely to be beneficial. The mechanism producing degeneration is unclear, and no treatment has been demonstrated to be very adequate in this degenerative process.

A link between early inflammation and later degeneration is plausible, however. For example, early in MS when inflammation is prominent, many cells are damaged but may not be destroyed. These cells may recover or other adjacent cells may expand their capacity to remyelinate axons. Consequently, patients recover from their acute attack after weeks or months. These repaired but distressed cells may function well initially but may be programmed to die earlier than if they were not distressed. Therefore, these cells may only live for 5, 10, or 20 years before apoptosis occurs. Because their eventual cell death is not immediately related to acute inflammation, IMTs at that later time would have no effect. If IMTs effectively reduced inflammation and subsequent early damage, however, the cell would not have become distressed and programmed to die early in the disease course.

Therefore, early anti-inflammatory IMTs may help prevent the degeneration/apoptosis seen later if they reduce the number of central nervous system cells damaged in the first place. The American Academy of Neurology (AAN), the Multiple Sclerosis Council for Clinical Practice Guidelines (MS Council), and the National Multiple Sclerosis Society all support early treatment with IMTs [27,28].

## Immunomodulating therapeutic options for multiple sclerosis

Since 1993, four IMTs and one immunosuppressive agent have receive FDA approval for the treatment of MS. Three of the IMTs (Betaseron, Avonex, and Rebif) fall in the class of interferon-βs, whereas the fourth, glatiramer acetate (GA; Copaxone), is a polypeptide comprising four randomly sequenced amino acids. A detailed review of these drugs is beyond the scope of this article, which focuses on the practical considerations with each of the treatments. In addition, the emphasis is on an evidence-based medicine approach regarding class I clinical trial data as reviewed by independent investigators (ie, not sponsored by the pharmaceutic industry) [28–30].

Defining class I scientific trials requires a careful analysis of the methodology [28]. Class I trials must be randomized, prospective, and adequately controlled. Patients need not be blinded to treatment modalities, but the evaluating clinicians should not be aware of the treatment status of the patients. The AAN/MS Council conducted an evidence-based medicine review of the four IMTs based on their pivotal trial data and other class I scientific studies. In addition, two Cochrane Review committees have conducted independent evidence-based medicine reviews using meta-analysis of interferon and GA data [17,30]. This article attempts to summarize these independent evaluations along with class I head-to-head clinical trials to aid in the understanding of each drug's role in MS therapy.

### Mechanisms of action

The mechanisms of action of the IMTs are not fully understood. Interferon-βs, however, have a number of actions that are beneficial in MS. These actions include reduction of proinflammatory cytokines such as interferon-γ, increased secretion of anti-inflammatory cytokine such as interleukin 10, increased suppressive T-cell activity while prohibiting the proliferation of lymphocytes, down-regulation of antigen presentation crucial for the activation of lymphocytes, and inhibition of lymphocyte trafficking through the blood-brain barrier to the central nervous system [26]. GA binds to major histocompatibility complex class II molecules and creates competition with myelin basic protein, which promotes the transformation of $T_H1$ lymphocytes (producer of proinflammatory cytokines) to $T_H2$ lymphocytes (producer of anti-inflammatory cytokines) in the peripheral blood. GA-specific cells also appear to have positive effects within the brain parenchyma, including expression of interleukin 10, transforming growth factor β, and brain-derived neurotrophic factor [31].

*Interferon beta-1b (Betaseron/Betaferon)*

In 1993, interferon beta-1b became the first FDA-approved IMT for MS. The standard dose is 250 μg every other day, administered subcutaneously. The initial pivotal trial in RRMS demonstrated a 33% reduction in the overall relapse rate and a 50% reduction in moderate to severe relapses [32,33]. The MRI data revealed a dramatic (83%) reduction in gadolinium-enhanced lesions. In addition, there was a reduction in total T2 lesion burden by MRI at 2 years [34]. A trend toward reduction in progression of disease was not statistically significant.

The second class I study with interferon beta-1b involved SPMS [35,36]. The drug increased the time to confirmed disability and time to wheelchair while decreasing exacerbation rates, MRI lesions, hospitalization, and steroid use. A second class I study in SPMS demonstrated the drug's effectiveness in reducing relapses and MRI lesions but did not demonstrate an effect on disease progression [25]. These contrasting results are best explained by the fact that the first study was done in early SPMS, whereas the second study was done in later SPMS. These findings re-enforce the concept that earlier treatment is more likely to be effective in delaying disability than later treatment.

Based on these two studies of SPMS, the FDA approved the use of interferon beta-1b in "relapsing forms" of MS, which would include early SPMS when patients are still having relapses.

Interferon beta-1b for RRMS was evaluated in Italy in an independent (no pharmaceutic company sponsor) head-to-head trial versus weekly interferon beta-1a (Avonex, 30 μg/wk) [37,38]. This trial (Independent Comparison of Interferon; INCOMIN) was rated as class I for MRI outcomes but only class III for clinical parameters because the physicians evaluating the clinical outcomes were not blinded. Clinical and MRI outcomes demonstrated a clinically significant benefit of interferon beta-1b over interferon beta-1a in the 2-year study. The MRI parameters were approximately 50% different, whereas the clinical parameters were between 35% and 50% different—all favoring interferon beta-1b. This trial supported the previous AAN/MS Council recommendation of a probable dose-response effect, with higher-dose interferon-β being more effective than lower-dose [28].

The newest data of MS interferon beta-1b efficacy are intriguing. Two recent studies indicate that increasing the dose of interferon beta-1b is well tolerated and has a further positive effect on the MRI [39,40]. Potentially, this finding indicates that interferons may be more effective at even higher doses. A class I clinical trial is currently underway comparing double-dose interferon beta-1b versus the standard dose. A third arm of this trial is a comparison with GA because there has never been a class I study comparing the effects of interferons versus GA.

Initially, one of the biggest practical issues with interferon beta-1b was lack of tolerability. Flulike side effects were common, and skin reaction including occasional skin necrosis prevented many patients from continuing therapy [32]. It is fortunate that with changes in treatment protocols (dose escalation and prophylactic ibuprofen or acetaminophen), the use of autoinjectors, and targeted nurse support systems, the drop-out rate for interferon beta-1b due to side effects is only about 5% in the first year of therapy [41].

*Interferon beta-1a (Avonex)*

Weekly, 30-μg intramuscular interferon beta-1a was approved by the FDA in 1996 for the reduction of relapses and the progression of disability in RRMS versus placebo [42]. In addition, there was a 50% reduction in gadolinium-enhanced MRI activity. There was no statistically significant difference in T2 lesion burden on MRI. A subsequent class I study that doubled the dose of interferon beta-1a weekly did not show increased efficacy. These results support a statement by the AAN/MS Council that suggests that increasing the frequency (and dose) of interferon-β injections may also be important.

In a study of MS patients with clinical isolated syndrome treated with weekly interferon beta-1a versus placebo, a significant delay in the time to a second relapse (clinical definite MS) and a reduction of MRI lesion were found with interferon beta-1a [21].

In a class I trial in SPMS, interferon beta-1a weekly did not prolong the time to progression of disability using the standardized Expanded Disability Status Scale (EDSS) [43]. Using the MS Functional Composite Scale, however, a difference from placebo was noted in one of the three subscales (9-hole peg test) [44]. No significant difference was found compared with placebo on the cognitive test or the ambulation index. Weekly interferon beta-1a has not been FDA approved for the treatment of SPMS.

The side effect profile of weekly interferon beta-1a administered intramuscularly is similar to the other interferons, although skin reactions are less frequent because of the intramuscular injection. Neutralizing antibodies (NAbs) are least likely with weekly interferon beta-1a versus the other interferons [45].

Weekly interferon beta-1a has been evaluated in two head-to-head trials versus higher-dosed, more frequently administered interferon-βs. The INCOMIN study, with interferon beta-1b versus interferon beta-1a, has been reviewed. A second head-to-head trial also compared weekly interferon beta-1a versus thrice-weekly subcutaneous interferon beta-1a (Rebif).

This class I trial EVIDENCE (EVidence for Interferon Dose-response: European-North American Comparitive Efficacy) demonstrated that the higher-dosed, more frequently administered interferon beta-1a (Rebif) was clinically superior on MRI and on the percentage of relapse-free patients over a 24-week period. The trial was extended to 48 weeks, and the clinical superiority was maintained.

*Interferon beta-1a (Rebif)*

Based on the previously described EVIDENCE trial [46] and the pivotal trial PRISMS (Prevention of Relapses and disability by Interferon beta-1a Subcutaneously in MS), where Rebif interferon beta-1a (44 µg three times per week, subcutaneously) vs. placebo resulted in approval by the FDA for RRMS in 2002. The PRISMS study was the first pivotal trial of any IMT that demonstrated a favorable impact over a 2-year period on all four of the study outcomes viewed by neurologists as most important: reduced relapse rate, prolonged time to progression of disability, reduction of T2 burden of disease on MRI, and reduction of gadolinium-enhanced lesions on MRI. Four-year and 8-year results were also positive [47,48]. In addition, a randomized study in clinically isolated syndrome and early RRMS showed a delay to clinically definite MS (time to next relapse) and reduced MRI lesions compared with placebo Early Treatment of MS Study (ETOMS) [22]. A follow-up from the pivotal trial in RRMS has shown continuing benefit of therapy up to 8 years in RRMS patients still on high-dose interferon beta-1a therapy.

A class I clinical trial of high-dose interferon beta-1a in SPMS (Secondary Progressive Efficacy Trial of Recombinant Interferon Beta-1a in MS) [49] did not demonstrate a difference in prolonging time to progression of disability by the EDSS scale; however, a reduction in relapse rate and MRI activity were noted. A post hoc analysis that categorized patients with or without relapses showed a favorable effect on prolonged time to progression of disability in patients with relapses versus patients without relapses in this SPMS study. The FDA, however, has not approved interferon beta-1a for SPMS.

The side effect profile is similar to interferon beta-1b, except that some people report more burning at the subcutaneous injection site with interferon beta-1a [50]. As with interferon beta-1b, newer treatment protocols (dose escalation and prophylactic ibuprofen or acetaminophen) reduce the flulike side effects. The immunogenicity of high-dose interferon beta-1a is greater than low-dose weekly interferon beta-1a but less than interferon beta-1b. Again, the clinical significance of NAbs is uncertain.

*Neutralizing antibodies*

NAbs to interferon beta-1b are produced in 25% to 45% of treated patients. The relevance of this finding is discussed later. The production of NAbs to interferon-βs and their clinical relevance is hotly disputed [45,51–53]. The data on NAbs are conflicting and the AAN/MS Council concluded that the utility of measuring NAbs is uncertain. NAbs have not been shown to affect progression of disability, although there are mixed data on MRI and relapse rates. Most of these data are not class I. In addition, NAbs are often transient. One study surveyed suboptimal responders to interferon beta-1b and found that only 7% of these patients had high levels of NAbs and about 80% of suboptimal responders had no detectable NAbs. In the Italian head-to-head trial (INCOMIN) of interferon beta-1b versus interferon beta-1a, no effects of NAbs on clinical or MRI outcomes were found [37]. In the pivotal trial of weekly interferon beta-1a, no significant difference was found in clinical outcomes of NAb-positive versus NAb-negative patients, although gadolinium-enhanced MRI lesions were more numerous (but not significant) in NAb-positive patients. NAb-positive patients, however, had a slightly lower relapse rate (but not significantly different). No change in EDSS was noted between the two groups [54].

In the author's opinion, when a patient is doing well clinically and by MRI but is NAb-positive, the patient should continue on interferon. On the other hand, when a patient is responding suboptimally, even if no NAbs are found, a change in therapeutic regimen should be considered. Emphasizing the patient's clinical response to therapy and not the results of a controversial test seems prudent at the present time. The author, therefore, does not use NAb testing.

## An overview of interferon β therapy

Interferon βs have similar mechanisms of action and similar side effects depending on the route of administration. All can be associated with hematologic and liver function abnormalities and are all rated as class C for safety in pregnancy. None are recommended for women who are pregnant or are contemplating pregnancy in the near future. It is fortunate that women who have become pregnant while on interferons have not demonstrated an increased risk of fetal abnormalities; however, interferons have been shown to be abortifacient in animal studies. Regular blood work for liver function abnormalities and hematologic abnormalities are recommended. Significant abnormalities may necessitate lowering the dose, a drug holiday, or discontinuation of therapy. Depression may be seen with any of the interferons; however, MS patients have an increased risk of depression even without therapy. Nonetheless, patients who are depressed should be treated before the initiation of interferon therapy, and when depression develops during IMT, an evaluation of the potential role of IMT is indicated and discontinuation of therapy may be justified.

A major differentiating factor in interferon beta-1a therapy is efficacy. The higher-dose, more frequently administered interferons (Betaseron, Rebif) have been demonstrated to be more effective than weekly Avonex in two class I head-to-head trials. The two high-dose interferons are more immunogenic (ie, higher NAbs) than the lower-dose, weekly interferon beta-1a, but the clinical relevance is uncertain. Another difference is that interferon beta-1a drugs are available in a prefilled syringe but must be refrigerated and may cause injection-site burning. Interferon beta-1b must be mixed with the diluent before injection but does not require refrigeration or have the frequency of injection-site pain compared with subcutaneously administered interferon beta-1a.

*Glatiramer acetate*

GA, 20 mg daily, given subcutaneously in a prefilled syringe (refrigeration required) is FDA approved for the treatment of RRMS based on a pivotal trial that showed a reduction of relapse rate compared with placebo [55]. There was no difference in EDSS scores in the two groups, and an MRI component was not done. A subsequent class I MRI study demonstrated a positive effect on MRI [56].

No class I studies of SPMS using GA have been published. A recently completed class I study of GA versus placebo in PPMS was discontinued because of apparent lack of efficacy of therapy. On further analysis, some effect of GA in men with PPMS was noted. In any event, the FDA has not approved GA for the treatment of PPMS or SPMS. A class I placebo-controlled trial of oral GA did not demonstrate efficacy.

GA is generally well tolerated, with most patients having only a mild skin reaction. One study showed a high incidence of dimpling of the skin secondary to loss of fatty tissue (lipoatrophy) in women on GA. In addition, 15% of patients in the pivotal trial had a brief systemic reaction to at least one injection of GA. Patients experienced chest tightness, flushing, palpitation, and anxiety lasting for a few minutes, but no serious long-term sequelae were seen. The etiology of the reactions is unknown, but patients need to be warned. No routine blood work is required for patients on GA. A major issue with GA is its lack of class I data to indicate affect on progression of disability.

NAbs to GA have not been identified. Almost all patients on GA produce antibodies. One study suggests that some of these antibodies have a deleterious effect on efficacy [57]; however, other studies have not shown this to be the case [58] and it has been postulated that the antigen antibody complex formed by the GA may be part of the positive therapeutic effect of the drug (B. Arnason, personal communication, 2004). Conflicts about NAbs abound. Commercial tests for antibodies to GA are not available.

*Long-term effects of immunomodulating therapy*

No scientifically robust studies have been conducted on the long-term effectiveness of IMTs. Most of the class I studies have been limited to 2 years; however, long-term follow-up data of patients on therapy are encouraging. Long-term studies indicate that patients on interferon beta-1b for 12 years have an improvement of T2 burden of disease from baseline. Patients treated with GA for 10 years have relatively stable relapse rates and show little progression of disability. Eight-year follow-up data on high-dose interferon beta-1a are positive, as are 5-year data on low-dose weekly interferon beta-1a. The problem with interpretation of these data is that patients who stay on therapy may be a subpopulation of "responders" or patients who would have a benign disease course without therapy. These long-term data do not provide insight to the superiority of one product over another. Nonetheless, newly diagnosed patients may find it encouraging to know that other patients on therapy for over 10 years are still doing well.

*Immunomodulating therapy effect on cognition*

The initial interferon beta-1b trial demonstrated a positive effect on some cognitive tests in patients on interferon beta-1b versus placebo [59]. The pivotal trial of weekly interferon beta-1a showed positive effects on cognitive outcomes [60]. One study with GA did not show a positive effect on cognition [61]; however, these results are not sufficient to favor one drug over another. It may reassure patients to know, however, that some data indicate that IMTs have a beneficial effect on cognition. Future head-to-head trials are comparing efficacy of therapy on cognition, which may make drug comparisons more meaningful.

**Practical evaluation of effectiveness of immunomodulating therapies**

Although the four IMTs have FDA approval for RRMS, differences exist in efficacy and in individual responses to the various therapies. All treatments are only partially effective. Patients may respond better to one drug versus another drug; however, measuring a suboptimal therapeutic response is imprecise [62]. Setting rigid criteria for defining a suboptimal response may not be appropriate for an individual patient.

For example, assume that a patient had two moderate exacerbations of MS within 1 year. Is this a suboptimal response? If a patient had five exacerbations in the previous year, the physician may consider this a reasonable response to therapy and continue the patient on the treatment. If, however, the patient had no attacks on therapy for 4 years and then had two moderate attacks in 1 year, most physicians would consider this a suboptimal response and consider changing their treatment regimen.

For another example, assume that three new MRI lesions in 1 year is adopted as a criterion for a suboptimal response. If a patient had 10 new MRI lesions the year before treatment and only 3 new MRI lesions in the last year, would this be considered a suboptimal response? By contrast, if the patient had no new MRI lesion for 3 years while on therapy and now has developed 3 new MRI lesions, most physicians would be concerned.

One practical approach to defining a suboptimal response is to establish caution signs for individual patients. Looking for increasing clinical disease activity is the most reliable determination of a suboptimal response. No increase in exacerbations and no progression of disease are ideal. In addition, some physicians order yearly or biyearly MRI scans to help evaluate for suboptimal response. A consensus conference of MS experts, however, did not recommend the routine use of MRI to evaluate therapeutic efficacy; these experts recommended MRI scans only when the physician is contemplating a change in therapy. Despite this recommendation, many treating physicians use MRI in their ongoing evaluation of efficacy of therapy. Some treating physicians use NAb testing as a measure of suboptimal response; however, it is the position of the AAN/MS Council that the utility of measuring NAbs is uncertain [28].

## Managing suboptimal treatment responders

If a patient is found to be a suboptimal responder to an IMT, increasing the dose or switching therapies is appropriate. For example, if the patient is on low-dose weekly interferon beta-1a, switching to a higher-dose interferon is reasonable. Switching to GA is another alternative. Another approach might be to add additional treatments, although no class I scientific evidence exists for this approach. Pulse steroids [63], azathioprine, and methotrexate are potential add-on therapies.

In suboptimal responders to interferons, switching to GA or adding an additional therapy is appropriate. Suboptimal responders on interferon beta-1b may benefit by increasing the dose by 50% to 100% based on recently presented data [40,54].

The use of mitoxantrone (Novantrone) is appropriate in patients who have suboptimal responses [64]. Mitoxantrone is an anthracenedione derivative, antineoplastic agent approved by the FDA for worsening MS (RRMS and SPMS). It kills T cells, B cells, and macrophages while enhancing suppressive T-cell functions, inducing apoptosis of antigen-presenting cells and decreasing proinflammatory and anti-inflammatory cytokines [65]. The standard dose is 12 $mg/m^2$ every 3 months intravenously up to a maximum of 140 $mg/m^2$. Although scientific, long-term studies are lacking, many MS experts add mitoxantrone to the current IMT. Patients tolerate this combination well. The issues with mitoxantrone include a blue tint to the skin and sclera, amenorrhea (which may be permanent), increased risk of infections, cardiotoxicity, and a remote chance of an increased risk of leukemia. Amenorrhea and cardiotoxicity are the most immediate potential problems. Although most patients do not get permanent amenorrhea, this potential risk should be explained to the patient. Cardiotoxicity is evaluated by measuring the left ventricle injection fraction and, if it is reduced, then mitoxantrone should be discontinued. Cardiotoxicity may be irreversible and precipitate heart failure.

## Future therapies

A number of potential MS therapies are currently undergoing clinical trials: natalizumab, intravenous immunoglobulin (IVIG), alemtuzumab (Campath), cladribine, T-cell vaccination, and perphenidone. The most likely to be approved soon is natalizumab [66].

Natalizumab (Tysabri) is an $\alpha_4$ integrin in the class of selective adhesion molecule inhibitors. It binds to integrin on T cells to prevent adhesion to the blood-brain barrier endothelial cells and subsequent migration of these cells into the brain parenchyma. A short-term phase 2 study has shown a reduction of attacks and MRI lesions versus placebo [67]. A recent company press release on a phase III trial with 1-year data indicates a 66% reduction of relapse rate compared with placebo in RRMS.

## Summary

IMT has made marked improvements in the lives of many MS patients over the last 11 years. Although these treatments are only partially effective and their use must be continued to maintain maximum effectiveness, they have improved the disease course, improved care, and stimulated research that will ultimately result in new treatments that are likely to be even more effective. All of the treatments have side effects, of which most can be prevented or managed. Recent scientific reviews and studies have begun to differentiate efficacy between the therapies. Efficacy has taken on new importance because new data have revealed that the disease is much more complex, with early (often subclinical) damage that can lead to short- and long-term negative consequences. The emphasis on early treatment with the most efficacious therapies is a reflection on new research findings. Focusing on IMTs alone, however, is focusing on lymphocytes rather than the patient. IMTs are not substitutes for caring health care providers, symptom management, and aggressive rehabilitation in the integrated care of MS patients.

## Conclusion: a practical approach to selecting immunomodulating therapies for patients

As a result of new data, the treatment emphasis has become heavily weighted to treating early and aggressively. Several factors have led to this change, including the complex and progressive nature of the disease, the propensity of RRMS to transition to SPMS after several years, the finding that damaged brain early in the disease course does not recover (what is lost is gone forever), the availably of four IMTs, and the scientific and independent reviews of IMTs. No longer are neurologists waiting until the disease progresses to moderate or severe disability to initiate treatment. In fact, new diagnostic criteria encourage treatment before a second episode.

The choice of treatment is a balance between efficacy, tolerability, and convenience. Tolerability is becoming less of an issue. For example, lack of tolerability of interferon beta-1b was a major deterrent a few years ago. Now, with new techniques and protocols, only 5% of people cannot tolerate interferon beta-1b. Convenience is a relative issue. A more effective but less convenient drug may keep more people from being hospitalized for attacks or ending up in a wheelchair.

Therefore, the major factor in treatment decisions is efficacy. It is fortunate that all four IMTs are FDA approved based on scientifically valid clinical trials. These 2-year studies, however, may not tell the whole story. The goal is reducing long-term disease stability for which no treatment has any scientifically valid data. Therefore, long-term experience with the drugs becomes an important additional factor. Integrating evidence-based medicine reviews with long-term experience provides an optimal background for treating individual patients with the drug best suited for them.

Using evidenced-based medicine reviews (AAN/MS Council and Cochrane Review), interferons have demonstrated the most robust data that show that they decrease progression of disability. The two class I head-to-head trials of interferons support the AAN/MS Council recommendation that higher-dosed (and likely more frequently administered) interferons are probably more effective than lower-dose weekly interferon. In clinical practice, however, many patients seem to do well on all IMTs. Each drug has some long-term but not scientifically robust data that indicate that the people who stay on it do well after several years. In fact, each drug has responders and suboptimal responders within a population of MS patients. The factors determining response to IMT begin with dose and efficacy data but may also include the type of immunopathology, genetic factors, the underling course of MS, the patients' compliance, and yet-to-be-determined factors.

Could patients who respond to a drug with less robust efficacy data in class I trials do even better if it was switched? The data on patients who switch therapies are limited [38]. Many questions remain unanswered.

For the present, the physician is best served by understanding the conclusions of independent reviews and scientific head-to-head trials and then putting these recommendations into perspective with his or her and MS experts' experience. The practice of telling patients to make their own decisions after reviewing drug company infomercial videotapes is discouraged. The treating physician's responsibility is to educate the patient to his or her best ability and to separate marketing spin from evidence-based medicine review.

Close communication between the physician, the care team, the patient, and the families provides for the most successful long-term management of MS.

## References

[1] Compston A, Coles A. Multiple sclerosis. Lancet 2002;359:1221–31.
[2] O'Connor P. Key issues in the diagnosis and treatment of multiple sclerosis: an overview. Neurology 2002;59(Suppl 3):S1–33.

[3] Noseworthy JH, Lucchinetti G, Rodriguez G, et al. Multiple sclerosis. N Engl J Med 2000; 343(13):938–52.

[4] Sriram S, Stratton CW, Yao S, et al. Chlamydia pneumoniae infection of the central nervous system in multiple sclerosis. Proc Natl Acad Sci USA 1995;92:7440–4.

[5] Cook SD, Rohowsky-Kochan C, Bansil S, et al. Evidence for multiple sclerosis as an infectious disease. Acta Neurol Scand 1995;161(Suppl):34–42.

[6] Simon Jack H. Magnetic resonance imaging in the diagnosis of multiple sclerosis, elucidation of disease course, and determining prognosis. In: Burks JS, Johnson K, editors. Multiple sclerosis: diagnosis, medical management and rehabilitation. New York: Demos; 2000. p. 99–126.

[7] Weinshenker BG, Bass B, Rice GPA, et al. The natural history of multiple sclerosis: a geographically based study. Brain 1989;112:133–46.

[8] Weinshenker BG, Bass B, Rice GP, et al. The natural history of multiple sclerosis: a geographically based study. II. Predictive value of the early clinical course. Brain 1989;112: 1419–28.

[9] Lublin FD, Reingold SC. Defining the clinical course of multiple sclerosis: results of an international survey. National Multiple Sclerosis Society (USA) Advisory Committee on Clinical Trials of New Agents in Multiple Sclerosis. Neurology 1996;46(4):907–11.

[10] Thompson AJ, Montalban X, Barkhof F, et al. Diagnositc criteria for primary progressive multiple sclerosis: a position paper. Ann Neurol 2000;47:831–5.

[11] Hawkins SA, McDonnell GV. Benign multiple sclerosis? Clinical course, long term follow up, and assessment of prognostic factors. J Neurol Neurosurg Psychiatry 1999;67:148–52.

[12] Johnson KP, Brooks BR, Ford CC, et al. Glatiramer acetate (Copaxone): comparison of continuous versus delayed therapy in a six-year organized multiple sclerosis trial. Mult Scler 2003;9(6):585–91.

[13] Bjartmar C, Kidd G, Ransohoff RM. A real-time insight into disease progression and the role of axonal injury in multiple sclerosis. Arch Neurol 2001;58(1):37–9.

[14] Kuhlmann T, Lingfeld G, Bitsch A, et al. Acute axonal damage in multiple sclerosis is most extensive in early disease stages and decreases over time. Brain 2002;125:2202–12.

[15] Trapp BD, Peterson J, Ransohoff RM, et al. Axonal transection in the lesions of multiple sclerosis. N Engl J Med 1998;338:278–85.

[16] Ferguson B, Matyszak MK, Esiri MM, et al. Axonal damage in acute multiple sclerosis lesions. Brain 1997;120:393–9.

[17] De Stefano N, Narayanan S, Francis GS, et al. Evidence of axonal damage in the early stages of multiple sclerosis and its relevance to disability. Arch Neurol 2001;58:65–70.

[18] Arnold DL. Magnetic resonance spectroscopy: imaging axonal damage in MS. J Neuro-innunol 1999;98:2–6.

[19] Lucchinetti CF, Bruck W, et al. Heterogeneity of multiple sclerosis lesions: implications for the pathogenesis of demyelization. Ann Neurol 2000;47:707–17.

[20] Barnett MH, Prineas JW. Relapsing and remitting multiple sclerosis: pathology of the newly forming lesion. Ann Neurol 2004;55(4):458–68.

[21] Jacobs LD, Beck RW, Simon JH, et al. Intramuscular interferon beta-1a therapy initiated during a first demyelinating event in multiple sclerosis. N Engl J Med 2000;343(13): 898–904.

[22] Comi G, Filippi M, Barkhof F, et al. Early Treatment of Multiple Sclerosis Study Group. Effect of early interferon treatment on conversion to definite multiple sclerosis: a randomized study. Lancet 2001;357(9268):1576–82.

[23] McDonald W, Compston A, Edan G, et al. Recommended diagnostic material for multiple sclerosis: guidelines from the International Panel on the Diagnosis of Multiple Sclerosis. Ann Neurol 2001;50:121–7.

[24] Rice GPA, Nicolle E, Lesaux J, et al. Long term safety, compliance and evolution of neutralizing antibodies in MS patients treated with Interferon beta-1b. Mult Scler Clin Lab Res 2001;7:S54.

[25] Goodkin DE and the North American Study Group on Interferon Beta-1b in Secondary Progressive MS. Interferon beta-1b in secondary progressive MS: clinical and MRU results of a 3-year randomized controlled trial. Neurology 2000;54:2352.

[26] Burks JS. INF-beta 1b (Betaseron/Betaferon) for multiple sclerosis. Expert Rev Neurotherapeutics 2005;5(2):1–12.

[27] van den Noort S, Eidelman B, Rammohan K, et al. National Multiple Sclerosis Society (NMSS): disease management consensus statement. New York: National MS Society; 1998.

[28] Goodin DS, Frohman EM, Garmany GP Jr, et al. Disease modifying therapies in multiple sclerosis: report of the Therapeutics and Technology Assessment Subcommittee of the American Academy of Neurology and the MS Council for Clinical Practice Guidelines. Neurology 2002;22;58(2):169–78.

[29] Rice GPA, Incorvaia B, Munari L, et al. Interferon in relapsing-remitting multiple sclerosis [Cochrane review]. Cochrane Library 2001;4.

[30] Munari L, Lovati R, Boiko A. Therapy with glatiramer acetate for multiple sclerosis [Cochrane review]. Cochrane Library 2003;4.

[31] Arnon R, Sela M. Immunomodulation by the copolymer glatiramer acetate. J Mol Recognit 2003;16(6):412–21.

[32] The IFNB Multiple Sclerosis Study Group. Interferon beta-1b is effective in relapsing remitting multiple sclerosis. I. Clinical results of a multicenter, randomized, double blind, placebo controlled trial. Neurology 1993;43:655–61.

[33] The IFNB Multiple Sclerosis Study Group and the University of British Columbia MS/MRI Analysis Group. Interferon beta-1b is effective in relapsing remitting multiple sclerosis. Final outcome of the randomized controlled trial. Neurology 1995; 45:1277–85.

[34] Paty DW, Li KKB, the UBC MS/MRI Study Group and the IFNB Multiple Sclerosis Study Group. Interferon beta-1b is effective in relapsing-remitting multiple sclerosis. II. MRI analysis results of a multi-center, randomized, double-blind, placebo-controlled trial. Neurology 1993;43:662–7.

[35] European Study Group on Interferon Beta-1b in Secondary Progressive MS. Placebo-controlled multi-center randomized trial of interferon beta-1b in treatment of secondary progressive multiple sclerosis. Lancet 1998;352:1491–7.

[36] Kuhle J, Hardmeier M, Rio J, et al. Long-term follow-up of the European Study of Interferon 1b (EUSPMS) in secondary progressive MS: predictors of treatment response. Mult Scler 2004;10(2):S247.

[37] Durelli L, Verdun E, Barbero P, et al. Independent Comparison of Interferon (INCOMIN) Trial Study Group. Every other day interferon beta-1b versus once weekly interferon beta-1a for multiple sclerosis. Lancet 2002;359:1453–60.

[38] Barbero P, Verdun E, Bergui M, et al. High-dose, frequently administered interferon beta therapy for relapsing-remitting multiple sclerosis must be maintained over the long term: the interferon beta dose-reduction study. J Neurol Sci 2004;15;222(1–2):13–9.

[39] Jeffery D, Arnason B, Bigley G, et al. MRI outcomes in relapsing-remitting multiple sclerosis patients treated with 500 mcg INFB-1b versus 250 mcg every other day: first phase of the BEYOND programme. Mult Scler 2004;10(2):S244.

[40] Durelli L. Interferon beta-1b in multiple sclerosis: comparing two different doses (the OPTIMS Study). Mult Scler 2004;S248:P603.

[41] Schapiro R. Adherence to interferon β: BETA Nurse Program. Int J MS Care 2004;6:66.

[42] Jacobs L, Cookfair D, Rudick R, et al. Intramuscular interferon beta-1a for disease progression in relapsing multiple sclerosis. Ann Neurol 1996;39:285–94.

[43] Kurtzke JF. Rating neurologic impairment in multiple sclerosis: an expanded disability status scale (EDSS). Neurology 1983;33:1444–52.

[44] Cohen JA, Cutter GR, Fischer JS, et al. Benefit of interferon beta-1a on MSFC progression in secondary progressive MS. Neurology 2002;59:679–87.

[45] Sorensen PS, Ross C, Clemmesen KM, et al. Clinical importance of neutralizing antibodies against interferon beta in patients with relapsing-remitting multiple sclerosis. Lancet 2003;11;362(9391):1148–91.

[46] Panitch H, Goodin DS, et al. Randomized comparative studies of interferon β1a treatment regimens in MS: the EVIDENCE Trial. Neurology 2002;59:1496–506.

[47] PRISMS Study Group and the University of British Columbia MS/MRI Analysis Group. PRISMS-4: long-term efficacy of interferon beta-1a in relapsing MS. Neurology 2001;56: 1628–36.

[48] PRISMS Study Group. Randomized double-blind placebo-controlled study of interferon beta-1a in relapsing-remitting multiple sclerosis. Lancet 1998;352:1498–504.

[49] Secondary Progressive Efficacy Trial of Recombinant Interferon Beta-1a in MS (SPECTRIMS) Study Group. Randomized controlled trial of interferon beta-1a in secondary progressive MS. Neurology 2001;56:1496–504.

[50] Harris C, Billisberger K, Tillotson L, et al. Injection site pain: interferon beta-1b versus interferon beta-1a. J MS Care 2004;6(2):75–6.

[51] Pachner AR, Oger J, Palace J. The measurement of antibodies binding to IFN-beta in MS patients treated with IFN-beta. Neurology 2003;11;61(9 Suppl 5):S18–20.

[52] Durelli L, Ricci A. Anti interferon antibody in multiple sclerosis. Molecular basis and there impact on clinical efficacy. Frontiers Biosci 2004;9:2192–201.

[53] Coyle P. Neutralizing antibodies to Interferon beta-1b in the real world. Int J MS Care 2004; 6(2):67.

[54] Rudick RA, Simonian NA, Alam JA, et al. Incidence and significance of neutralizing antibodies to interferon beta-1a in multiple sclerosis. Multiple Sclerosis Collaborative Research Group (MSCRG). Neurology 1998;50(5):1266–72.

[55] Johnson KP, Brooks BR, Coher JA, et al. Copolymer reduces relapse rate and improves disability in RRMS. Neurology 1995;45:1268–76.

[56] Comi G, Filippi M, Wolinsky JS and the European/Canadian Glatiramer Acetate Study Group. European/Canadian multi-center, double-blinded, randomized, placebo-controlled study of the effects of glatiramer acetate on magnetic resonance imaging-measured disease activity and burden in patients with relapsing multiple sclerosis. Ann Neurol 2001;49: 290–7.

[57] Salama HH, Hong J, Zang YC, et al. Blocking effects of serum reactive antibodies induced by glatiramer acetate treatment in multiple sclerosis. Brain 2003;1269:2638–47.

[58] Teitelbaum D, Brenner T, Abramsky O, et al. Antibodies to glatiramer acetate do not interfere with its biological functions and therapeutic efficacy. Mult Scler 2004;6: 592–9.

[59] Pliskin NH, Hamer DP, Goldstein DS, et al. Improved delayed visual reproduction test performance in multiple sclerosis patients receiving interferon beta-1b. Neurology 1996; 47(6):1463–8.

[60] Fischer JS, Priore RL, Jacobs LD, et al. Neuropsychological effects of interferon beta-1a in relapsing multiple sclerosis. Multiple Sclerosis Collaborative Research Group. Ann Neurol 2000;48(6):885–92.

[61] Weinstein A, Schwid SR, Schiffer RB, et al. Neuropsychologic status in multiple sclerosis after treatment with glatiramer. Arch Neurol 1999;56(3):319–24.

[62] Wolinsky J, Coyle P, Cook S, et al. Changing therapy in relapsing multiple sclerosis: considerations and recommendations of a task force of the National Multiple Sclerosis Society. NMSS Expert Opinion Paper 2004. Available at: www.nationalmssociety.org/PRC.asp. Accessed April 4, 2005.

[63] Pirko I, Rodriguez M. Pulsed intravenous methylprednisolone therapy in progressive MS. Arch Neuro 2004;61(7):1148–9.

[64] Hartung HP, Gonsette R, Konig N, et al. Miloxantrone in progressive multiple sclerosis: a placebo-controlled, double-blind, randomized multicenter trial. Lancet 2002;360: 2018–25.

[65] Neuhaus O, Kieseier BC, Hartung HP. Mitoxantrone (Novantrone) in multiple sclerosis: new insights. Expert Rev Neurother 2004;4(1):17–26.

[66] Rudick RA, Sandrock A. Natalizumab: α4-integrin antagonist selective adhesion molecule inhibitors for MS. Neurotherapeutics 2004;4(4):571–80.

[67] Miller DH, Khan OA, Sheremata WA, et al. A controlled trial of natalizumab for relapsing multiple sclerosis. N Engl J Med 2003;348(1):15–23.

ELSEVIER
SAUNDERS

Phys Med Rehabil Clin N Am
16 (2005) 467–481

PHYSICAL MEDICINE
AND REHABILITATION
CLINICS OF
NORTH AMERICA

# Multiple Sclerosis and Spasticity

Jodie K. Haselkorn, MD, MPH[a,b,c,*],
Sharon Loomis, MD[a,b]

[a]*VA Puget Sound Health Care System, Seattle, WA*
[b]*Department of Rehabilitation Medicine, University of Washington, Seattle, WA*
[c]*Department of Epidemiology, University of Washington, Seattle, WA*

## Overview

An estimated 40% to 70% of individuals who have multiple sclerosis (MS) report impairments and disabilities that are due to spasticity [1]. In general, spasticity is characterized by increased resistance of muscle to an externally imposed stretch, often with more resistance to rapid stretch. Clinically spasticity is manifested by increased muscle tonic activity, exaggerated deep tendon reflexes, spread of activity to distant segments, and clonus with sustained stretch. Spasticity is but one symptom of the upper motoneuron syndrome, a constellation of signs that include the enhanced or positive signs of spasticity—increased responses to rapid stretch, flexor, extensor, and abductor spasms; cocontraction of antagonist muscles; hyperactive deep tendon reflexes; clonus, abnormal cutaneous reflexes; associated reactions; pain; and perceived heaviness or stiffness of muscles. Diminished or negative signs that are associated with upper motoneuron syndrome include loss of coordination, reduced speed, increased weakness, and easy fatigability.

The severity of spasticity can range widely from a minor annoyance to the initiation of a causal chain that results in severe disabilities, and ultimately, mortality. In an extreme scenario, spasticity initiates a cascade of loss of musculotendinous extensibility, limited range of motion of a single joint, multiple joint contractures, excessive pressures on skin that overlies affected joints, skin breakdown, osteomyelitis, sepsis, and death. Less extreme scenarios include secondary impairments, disabilities and reduced quality of life due to pain, reduced body image, reduced perineal hygiene, lack of sleep, and social isolation.

\* Corresponding author. RCS 117, 1660 S. Columbian Way, Seattle, WA 98108.
*E-mail address:* jodie.haselkorn@med.va.gov (J.K. Haselkorn).

Recent prevalence surveys of individuals who have MS exhibit a variability of impact among different groups. In a needs analysis that was done in Genoa, Italy, pain and spasticity were the most common symptoms that were treated with medications. Nearly 30% of the cohort was receiving treatment [2]. A much higher prevalence was reported, based on physical examination of individuals who had MS in Newcastle upon Tyne in northeast England. Forty-seven percent of individuals had spasticity on a physical examination that rated at least 2 on a Modified Ashworth Scale. Although 78% of this group was on a medication, half of these were assessed as being undertreated. The group that had moderate spasticity also did poorer on functional tasks than those who did not [3].

Spasticity is a common problem that can result in significant use of medication, yet still may be undermanaged and result in significant functional limitations. Effective management is particularly difficult in individuals who have MS for a variety of reasons [3]. Two recent systematic reviews were critical of the scientific foundation for the pharmacologic treatment of spasticity [4,5]. A recent Clinical Practice Guideline in Multiple Sclerosis by the Multiple Sclerosis Council also evaluated the evidence and provided practical strategies for management [6]. The focus of this article is to familiarize the health care provider with the management of spasticity, particularly in the context of MS, and to provide practical strategies.

## Pathophysiology of spasticity

The pathophysiology of spasticity in humans is not understood completely. Spasticity is one symptom in the condition, "upper motor neuron syndrome." The changes in muscle tone that are associated with spasticity result, in part, from alterations in the balance of inputs from reticulospinal and other descending pathways to the motor and interneuronal circuits of the spinal cord, as well as the absence of an intact corticospinal system. In the usual case when a muscle is stretched, the primary 1a afferent fibers that supply the intrafusal fibers of the muscle spindle are excited. This triggers a monosynaptic excitatory connection with the $\alpha$ motoneurons that supply the stretched muscle and results in contraction of the stretched muscle and excitatory connections with the $\alpha$ motoneuron that supplies synergistic muscles. In addition, the 1a fiber has a monosynaptic connection with a spinal interneuron that results in an inhibition of the antagonist muscle. This controlled contraction of the agonist and reciprocal inhibition of the antagonist muscles is impaired in upper motoneuron syndrome.

Lesions in the brain and the spinal cord may cause spasticity through different mechanisms and present differently. Spasticity that is caused by brain lesions is associated with a rapid response of the antigravity muscle groups (ie, flexors in the upper extremity and extensors in the lower extremity). In contrast, spasticity that is caused by spinal cord lesions is associated with slower responses and results in an increased response of flexors and extensors, including those distant from the stimulus. The hyperexcitability in the α motoneuron pool may be due to several factors, including: an imbalance in inhibitory and excitatory input, denervation supersensitivity of receptor sites to neurotransmitters, and collateral sprouting of dorsal afferents. Spasticity in MS is likely more difficulty to manage than that which is due to stroke or spinal cord injury, in part, as a result of lesions in brain and the spinal cord and the progressive nature of the disease.

Spasticity also results in changes in the periphery. Physiologic changes in the musculotendinous unit result in an increased resistance to stretch that leads to stiffness, contracture, atrophy, and fibrosis. These soft tissue changes affect normal limb movement and positioning and can exacerbate spasticity. Effective evaluation and management of spasticity depends on a determination of the abnormalities of the neural inputs and the physical properties of the soft tissues.

## Evaluation of spasticity

The clinical evaluation of spasticity requires a thorough history, functional history, and physical examination. Special studies, such as temporary nerve blocks and electromyography, can help to tease out the contribution of α motoneuron hyperexcitability versus soft tissue abnormalities and assist in treatment planning.

The presence of spasms or spasticity itself does not require treatment. The successful individualized management of spasticity depends upon inquiry into the frequency, the intensity, and the functional impacts of spasticity.

Spasticity can be increased by precipitating factors, such as increase in core body temperature that is associated with a fever or excessive exercise; infection; distended viscous, such as a full bladder or colon; noxious stimuli, such as a skin lesion; bladder or renal stone; fracture; tight clothing; menses; psychologic stress; extreme environmental temperature; hunger; an exacerbation; progression of MS; or treatment with some disease modifying or antidepressant pharmaceutical agents. If a precipitating factor is present, removal of this factor usually decreases the spasticity back to baseline levels.

Two useful measures of spasticity include the Spasm Frequency Scale [7] and the modified Ashworth Scale [8]. The Spasm Frequency Scale is obtained by history and is a 0 to 4 noninterval scale; 0 equates to no spasms and 4 equates to more than 10 spontaneous spasms per hour. The Modified Ashworth Scale also is a noninterval scale of 0 to 4 (though it includes a value for 1+) and is obtained during the physical examination [9]. Zero equates to "no increase in tone" and 4 equates to "affected part is rigid." Each joint is assigned a score. Other scales, such as an analog scale for pain or other functional interference, may be useful in addition to active and passive range of motion of the affected joints.

A functional history is essential to the decision to implement treatment, the selection of management strategies, and follow-up to determine the success of treatment. Spasticity is associated with several secondary impairments and disabilities that can be prevented. The impairments that are associated frequently with spasticity include pain, altered body image, skin breakdown, loss of sleep, fatigue, joint contractures, decubitus ulcers, and impaired sexual functioning. Spasticity also can limit the activities that are usual for an individual and his or her ability to participate socially. Limitations in this area include difficulty walking, improper positioning in a wheelchair or bed, difficult or unsafe transfers, falls, inability to drive, difficulty with self-care activities, reduced intimacy, vocational limitations, social isolation, increased care partner or attendant needs. Spasticity that interferes with desired functional status is an indication for treatment.

Physical assessment should include evaluation of tone using the Modified Ashworth Scale, strength of the agonists and antagonists, assessment of stretch reflexes, and the presence of cocontraction. Coordination and speed of active fine motor movements also may be helpful. Spasticity does vary by the time of day, positioning, availability of postural support, and effort. Therefore, what the clinician sees in passive physical examination in sitting or lying supine on an examination table may not reflect accurately the difficulties that an individual who has MS encounters throughout the course of an active day. Physical and occupational therapy can quantify strength and dexterity readily, as well as perform a thorough functional examination, including transfers, balance, mobility with and without adaptive devices, endurance, and assessment of impacts on self-care activities. Spasticity that impacts functional status should be considered for early and effective treatment.

## Treatment strategies

The Multiple Sclerosis Council for Clinical Practice Guidelines published an algorithm for management of spasticity and discussed the scientific evidence for effective treatments in individuals who have MS [6]. Although algorithms are helpful, a successful treatment strategy is one that an individual accepts and is able to incorporate his/her life over many years. Therefore, successful management of spasticity begins with thorough education of available options, an understanding of personal values and needs, and finding the most appropriate match of available options to needs.

At the outset, it is essential to identify the goals of treatment and the acceptable outcomes. Time may limit the ability to succeed with a treatment strategy, so it is important to discuss the time and effort that are involved for the person who has MS and the care partner. Potential financial barriers to any strategy also should be considered. Spasticity is dynamic throughout the day, week, month, and over the years. Therefore, successful management requires follow-up and fine tuning to meet the changing needs of the individual who has MS over the course of the disease. Commitment to a desired and feasible treatment over the long term is essential at the outset.

Based on the algorithm for management of spasticity, a helpful strategy when an individual presents with new-onset or a change in spasticity is to characterize the impact of spasticity as primarily focal or generalized. Spasticity that creates primarily focal problems often can be treated with targeted skilled rehabilitation alone or skilled rehabilitation strategies plus neuromuscular blockade. Conversely, spasticity that causes more general problems is likely to require oral or intrathecal pharmaceutical agents and skilled rehabilitation strategies.

## Skilled rehabilitation

Skilled rehabilitation is the mainstay of a treatment program for focal or generalized spasticity and was shown to improve disability and handicap [10–18]. No single particular type of rehabilitation therapy is more effective than another. The following reviews common approaches that have been associated with effective management of spasticity in individuals who have MS.

One common strategy that was shown to be effective is range of motion exercises. Range of motion exercises can reduce motoneuron excitability [18]. Range of motion exercises may decrease spasticity and is important in avoiding secondary soft tissue changes that may exacerbate spasticity and cause muscle and joint contractures. Consequently, range of motion exercise is an essential treatment for maintaining optimum joint mobility and minimizing the risk of joint contracture. Active or passive exercise through the full range of movements about a joint should be initiated as early as possible, especially for those joints that are at high risk for restriction. These joints include the vertebrae of the cervical spine, shoulder, elbow, wrist, digits of the fingers, hips, knees, and ankles.

A related strategy to range of motion exercises is stretching. Stretching can reduce secondary complication that is due to spasticity through the shortening of musculotendinous units. Stretching should be performed at least daily at the end of the available range and in a sustained fashion. Some practitioners suggest holding a stretch for more than 1 minute, whereas others suggest holding a stretch for a prolonged period of several hours.

It may be most efficient to focus stretching on those muscle groups whose shortening would cause marked functional loss, lead to medical complications, or hamper self-care. In the upper extremities, maintaining cervical extension is essential for swallowing. Loss of range about the shoulder may lead to pain and limited function for self-care activities. Limitation of elbow extension that is due to shortened elbow flexors limits effective reach and maximal use of adaptive ambulatory aides. Tight wrist extensors are associated with an inability to position the hand for optimal power and difficulty with self-care activities, writing, and all functions that involve grasp. Involvement of the finger extensors further limits grasp, and ultimately, can cause difficulty with hygiene. In the lower extremity, tight hip flexors result in limitation of full extension and difficulty with ambulation. Limited range of the knee flexors results in increased pressure over the sacrum when lying supine. Contractures in the plantarflexors are associated with toe drag and falls and place an individual who is lying supine at higher risk for skin breakdown over the calcaneus. Contractures of the plantarflexors and invertors, especially the tibialis posterior, result in an inverted plantarflexed foot that places an individual who is lying in bed at high risk for excessive skin pressure over the calcaneus and lateral malleolus.

Range of motion and stretching can be facilitated in several ways. Light pressure or stroking can decrease motoneuron excitability and facilitate an inhibitory response that may be helpful in stretching contracted tissues [14]. A splint or brace can be used to achieve prolonged stretches. Localized heating of a joint capsule with superficial heat for small joints and ultrasound for deeper structures may facilitate the ability to restore lost motion.

Although heat may facilitate stretch, local applications of cold—through cold towels or cold packs—was shown to provide temporary relief from localized spasticity, as well as improvements in strength and gait skills. Cooling garments also are helpful in reducing spasticity and enhancing an individual's ability to perform functional tasks and exercise.

The ability to exercise through a full range of motion is important to increase strength and maintain fitness. Starting and keeping up with a proper strengthening program reduces the risk of progressive weakening of the spastic muscles that results from a lack of use. Although there is no literature that suggests the need for a unique strengthening regime for individuals who have MS, a strengthening program should bring a muscle group to near fatigue without exacerbating the overall fatigue that is associated with MS. Strategies, such as exercising in a cool environment and strengthening only a few muscle groups in a session, are useful.

Although skilled rehabilitation strategies can be extremely successful, there are many instances in which these efforts are not enough. In such instances, spasticity can be treated focally with neurolytic blocks and with oral or intrathecal medications.

*Neuromuscular blocks*

Spasticity sometimes is isolated or mostly affects focal functional groups, such as the cervical extensors, elbow flexors, wrist flexors, thumb and finger flexors, hip adductors, ankle plantar flexors, and ankle invertors. Spasticity that is focal may be treated effectively using neuromuscular blockade with alcohol, phenol, or botulinum toxin that is injected through a 23 to 27 gauge needle under electromyographic, fluoroscopic, or CT guidance.

Neurolytic blockade that uses alcohol or phenol involves identification of the motor branch of a mixed nerve and injection of 2 mL to 4 mL of 100% alcohol or 2% to 5% phenol [19]. The effects are immediate. Weakness is expected. Other adverse effects are rare. This is a successful strategy in well-selected individuals and when administered by trained clinicians who manage spasticity regularly.

Besides alcohol and phenol, botulinum toxin type A (Botox in the United States and Dysport in the United Kingdom) and botulinum toxin type B (Myobloc) are used to treat spastic muscles [20]. Although the target intraneural proteins of these two subtypes differ, the mechanism of action is the same—a presynaptic inhibition of acetylcholine at the neuromuscular junction. Dosing for botulinum toxins type A and type B are different. In both cases, treatment is individualized and is dependent upon the muscles that are involved, previous response, and functional goals. For botulinum toxin type A (Botox), 400 units is the maximum dose that is given at one time, whereas for botulinum toxin type B the maximum dose in a single session is 10,000 units. For both types, sessions may be repeated after a 3-month period. The effects of the toxin become apparent within 12 hours to 7 days and the duration of effect is usually 3 to 4 months.

Injection of 400 units of botulinum type A into the thigh adductors of nine individuals who had MS resulted in significant improvement in spasticity and hygiene compared with placebo [21]. Similar improvements were found in study that evaluated Dysport in 74 individuals who had MS [22,23]. We are unaware of studies that used botulinum type B in individuals who had MS.

Adverse effects of botulinum types A or B are minimal. Gradually, muscle function returns by the regeneration or sprouting of the motor nerve to form new neuromuscular junctions. Injection with botulinum toxin types A or B can be combined with alcohol or phenol neurolysis to treat multiple muscles in a given visit and to keep the dose of either type of botulinum to less than the maximum dose.

The use of neurolytic blocks should not be considered monotherapy. Skilled rehabilitation therapies frequently are necessary to maximize function. These therapies usually are instituted or modified after injection. In addition, neurolytic blocks can be combined with various oral medications and intrathecal baclofen therapy.

Resistance to botulinum toxin results from the development of antibodies against the toxin. A lack of benefit of repeated injections suggests resistance. Antibody development occurs in less than 10% of people and can be minimized by using the smallest dose that will result in a functional effect and increasing the time interval between sessions to as long as possible (ie, ≥3 months). Several studies confirmed that people who have resistance to botulinum type A may benefit from injections with botulinum type B. The risk of antibody resistance to a single subtype may be reduced by alternating the subtypes from one session to another.

## Oral agents

Frequently, skilled rehabilitation strategies with or without neuromuscular blockade are not effective because an individual's spasticity is intense and involves multiple muscle groups. In these instances, oral agents are an effective treatment for spasticity in MS. Selection of an initial agent should be based on efficacy, side effects, cost, and personal preferences. The Multiple Sclerosis Guidelines for the management of spasticity suggest starting with baclofen or tizanidine. In all instances, it is best to start with a single agent and to increase the dosage slowly to the maximum dose or the dose that is tolerated before initiating combination therapy (many individuals who have MS cannot tolerate the maximum dosage).

*Baclofen*

Baclofen is a γ-aminobutyric acid (GABA) agonist; its primary site of action is the spinal cord, where it reduces the release of excitatory neurotransmitters and substance P by binding to the GABA-B receptor. Several studies showed that baclofen is effective in the management of spasticity by measures that assess physiology, impairment, disability, and social participation [13]. Baclofen has been shown to: (1) impact electrophysiologic measures of H-reflex modulation positively during walking [24]; (2) decrease deep tendon reflexes, clonus, resistance to stretch [13,24–32], and spasm frequency [30,33,34]; and (3) result in subjective improvements in pain, gait, and overall function [13,24,25,27,30,31,33–36]. Side effects include drowsiness, nausea, dry mouth, and dizziness [33]. Weakness and an increase in the number of falls also were reported [29,36–39].

The daily dosage of baclofen often is split up over three or four time periods. Baclofen should be started slowly, using an initial dosage of 5 mg/d and increasing every 4 to 7 days to a total recommended dosage of 80 mg/d. In community practice, dosages up to 120 mg/d and greater are not uncommon. Baclofen must be used with care in patients who have renal insufficiency because its clearance primarily is renal.

Baclofen must be tapered slowly to prevent withdrawal. Tapering may not be practical in cases of severe abdominal distress, surgery, or life-threatening conditions. Withdrawal symptoms include high fever, altered mental status, exaggerated rebound spasticity, muscle rigidity, and seizures. When baclofen has been stopped preoperatively, postoperative withdrawal can be missed and attributed to postoperative infection or other complications. In rare cases, these effects may advance to seizures, rhabdomyolysis, multiple organ-system failure, and death. Withdrawal can be prevented through early detection of symptoms and management by an informed treatment team. Despite the rare risk of withdrawal symptoms, baclofen is an effective and common agent that is used to treat spasticity.

*Tizanidine*

Tizanidine is an imidazoline derivative and a central α2-noradrenergic agonist that is effective for spasticity of cerebral and spinal origins. The spinal antispasticity effects probably are the result of inhibition of the H-reflex. In addition, tizanidine may facilitate inhibitory actions of glycine and reduce the release of excitatory amino acids and substance P. Tizanidine also may have analgesic effects.

Tizanidine was demonstrated to be an effective treatment for spasticity in several controlled clinical trials [37,38,40–43]. Tizanidine was shown to improve Ashworth Scores [44–46], cumulative limb tone, ankle dorsiflexion tone, ankle clonus, spasms, and scores on the Ambulation Index in individuals who had MS [47,48]. This agent may be particularly useful for painful spasms at night.

Tizanidine is a short-acting drug with extensive first-pass hepatic metabolism to inactive compounds following an oral dose. The half-life is 2.5 hours with peak plasma level at 1 to 2 hours. Therapeutic and side effects dissipate within 3 to 6 hours. Therefore, use must be directed to those activities and times when relief of spasticity is most important. It should be started at a low dose, 2 mg to 4 mg, usually given at bedtime. It should be titrated carefully to each patient by increasing the dosage slowly and gradually. The average maintenance dosage of tizanidine is 18 mg/d to 24 mg/d. The maximum recommended dosage is 36 mg/d. Patients who have impaired kidney function also require gradual titration and monitoring. Common side effects include dizziness, drowsiness, fatigue, and dry mouth. Rare instances of hallucinations and elevated transaminases, and an isolated instance of drug-induced hepatitis have been seen [46–48].

Tizanidine alone or in combination with baclofen plus skilled rehabilitation strategies effectively manages most generalized spasticity; however, in some circumstances, other oral agents need to be considered. These "second-line" treatments may play a useful role (see later discussion). Selection of one of these agents depends on the severity of the spasticity, associated complications, side effects, convenience, and cost.

*Dantrolene*

Dantrolene is an effective treatment for the management of spasticity in individuals who have MS [43,49–51]. This agent reduces muscle contraction at the level of the muscle fiber by affecting the release of calcium from the sarcoplasmic reticulum. Dosages are titrated from 25 mg/d to 400 mg per day, divided into 3 or 4 doses. The dose is increased slowly over a period of weeks to achieve therapeutic goals. Its peak effect is at 4 to 6 hours, with a half-life of 6 to 9 hours. Side effects in the clinical trials were common and included weakness, fatigue, nausea, diarrhea, speech difficulty, lightheadedness, dizziness, drowsiness, lack of coordination, and lethargy. Dantrolene can be hepatotoxic and regular monitoring of transaminases is essential. It should not be used with the other agents that are associated with hepatotoxicity, such as tizanidine.

*Diazepam*

Diazepam is a GABA-A agonist that binds in the brain stem within the spinal cord, and results in presynaptic inhibition and reduction of the monosynaptic and polysynaptic reflexes. Controlled clinical trials on individuals who had MS demonstrated the effectiveness of diazepam on hyperreflexia, clonus, stiffness, and cramping, as well as improving scores on a clinical scale and EMG/force recordings [51–53]. Dosages in the clinical trials ranged from 2 mg, four times per day, to 10 mg, three times per day. Dosages should be started with the lowest possible, and ideally, given at bedtime. Daytime therapy should be titrated slowly up to the maximum dosage that meets the functional objectives. The ceiling dose is 60 mg/d; however, few individuals who have MS can tolerate these dosages. Diazepam has a half-life of 20 to 80 hours and its active metabolites prolong effectiveness. Side effects include drowsiness and weakness. Muscle weakness was greater in the group that took diazepam compared with tizanidine and sedation was more common with diazepam compared with baclofen in head-to-head trials of the agents. In addition, some clinicians fear benzodiazepine dependence and addiction. Nevertheless, diazepam can be a useful agent in carefully selected individuals.

*Gabapentin*

Gabapentin is a GABA analog that modulates enzymes and results in increased glutamate. One randomized, controlled clinical trial suggests that it may have value in the treatment of spasticity. Improvements over placebo were seen in clonus, the Ashworth Scale, and subjective ratings 2 days after starting the medication. Side effects included mild drowsiness [54].

*Intrathecal management*

Intrathecal management with baclofen is a long-term spasticity management strategy for individuals who have MS who do not respond to, or cannot tolerate, oral medications. It was demonstrated to be effective in individuals who had MS in several controlled clinical trials and resulted in decreased spasm frequency, Ashworth Scores, and pain [7,55,56]. Uncontrolled studies of intrathecal management with baclofen demonstrated other benefits, including a reduction in oral medications and a decreased need for attendant care [7,57–60].

Initially, this treatment was reserved for nonambulatory individuals who had severe spasticity. More recently, however, intrathecal management with baclofen was used successfully and showed demonstrated effects on gait in ambulatory individuals who had moderate lower extremity spasticity. Evaluation of possible candidates for an implantable pump should take place at an MS Center by providers who are trained and experienced in this therapy. Before undergoing surgery, potential candidates undergo an intrathecal injection of 50 μg to 100 μg of baclofen to determine if this therapy will be effective for the individual. Candidates should be educated in advance that the "test dose" is neither individualized nor titrated and that they may experience a false perception of decrease in function from having their spasticity removed suddenly and completely. They should also be told that after pump placement, the dosage will be established individually.

The SynchroMed pump (Medtronic, Inc., Minneapolis, Minnesota) has a shape that is similar to a hockey puck. The small, circular titanium implant is approximately 3 inches in diameter and 1 inch thick. It contains a refillable reservoir for the medication, as well as a computer chip that regulates the battery-operated pump. A Synchromed II pump is smaller, more contoured, and has more reservoir capacity. Both pumps contain a programmable alarm that sounds when the reservoir needs to be refilled, the battery is low, or the pump is not delivering the baclofen.

The pump usually is placed near the waistline, avoiding the belt line. The tip of a catheter commonly is placed between the first and second lumbar vertebrae in the intrathecal space, but may be placed higher if management of trunk and upper extremity spasticity also are significant goals. The catheter is tunneled subcutaneously around the torso. The dose that is delivered by the pump is adjusted using the programmer and telemetry wand. The initial total daily dosage after implantation is approximately twice the bolus screening dose that resulted in a beneficial response, and is titrated upwards slowly to achieve desired functional goals. Maintenance dosages of baclofen for individuals who have MS range from 12 µg/d to 2000 µg/d, with average dosages ranging from 300 µg/d to 800 µg/d [7,61]. Individuals will benefit from skilled rehabilitation after pump implantation and while the dose is being titrated individually.

Early problems with pumps and catheters have become rare experiences; many individuals who have MS are approaching their third routine pump replacement because of the 5- to 7-year limit on the battery. Refills are handled routinely in the outpatient setting by a percutaneous injection using sterile technique of medication into the refill port. Frequency of refills depends on the daily dosage and the concentration of medication that is used (eg, 500 µg/mL or 2000 µg/mL) and range from monthly to every 6 months. Withdrawal symptoms should be anticipated if the pump is not refilled on time (see symptoms above).

*Surgery*

Orthopedic and neurosurgical procedures play a role in the management of MS and can be used to enhance function, restore lost function, and as palliation when rehabilitation, oral agents, and intrathecal therapy have not been completely successful [62,63]. Orthopedic procedures that are used include tenotomy, capsulotomy, osteotomy, and arthrodesis. These procedures are performed often to restore ankle and foot position, as well as hip position. They may be undertaken to facilitate ambulation in an individual who has lower extremity strength, but developed contractures after a short period of immobility (eg, after an acute prolonged hospitalization). More often, they are used to restore proper positioning in a wheel chair or bed in an individual who has long-standing spasticity and contractures to prevent further complications, such as skin breakdown. Orthopedic procedures are successful in the long run if the underlying reasons for contracture development are identified and a feasible plan for future management of spasticity is developed and agreed upon.

Neurosurgical treatments include selective dorsal rhizotomy, paravertebral or intrathecal phenol or alcohol blocks, and lumbar myelotomy [64]. With the exception of selective dorsal rhizotomy, these procedures are indicated in individuals who have no functional movement. Selection of individuals for these procedures should be done at a center that specializes in spasticity management in individuals who have MS.

## Summary

Spasticity is a common impairment in MS. It can result in significant medical complications and is associated with increased disability. Treatment strategies include skilled rehabilitation strategies, neuromuscular blocks, oral agents, intrathecal management, and surgery. Rehabilitation strategies are central, whereas other strategies are added based on the level of impairment and functional loss. Treatment strategies for spasticity management are far from optimal and are complicated in MS as a result of lesions in the brain and the spinal cord. Pharmaceutical management in MS is complicated by the numerous secondary impairments in MS and its associated polypharmacy. Head-to-head studies of the various agents are rare. The studies that exist are small and do not point to any one strategy over another. Although management is difficult, it is essential for the health, functional status, and well-being of the individual who has MS. Providers must use well-developed clinical skills to arrive at optimal individualized treatment programs and monitor them frequently. For spasticity that is unresponsive, referral to a MS Center with a spasticity program is ideal.

## Acknowledgments

The authors thank the members of the Spasticity Management Guideline Panel, the Expert Reviewers, the members of the MS Council for Clinical Practice Guidelines, the Center for Clinical Health Policy Research at Duke University, the Consortium of Multiple Sclerosis Centers, the Paralyzed Veterans of America, and United Spinal Association for their efforts to create Evidenced-Based Management Strategies for Spasticity Treatment in Multiple Sclerosis. Without the hard work of these individuals and organizations, this article would not have been possible.

## References

[1] Avourou KJ, Goldenberg E, Cleghon G. Sociodemographic and health status characteristics of persons with MS and their caregivers. Multiple Sclerosis Management 1996;3(1):6–17.

[2] Brichetto G, et al. Symptomatic medication in use in multiple sclerosis. Mult Scler 2003;9(5): 458–60.

[3] Barnes MP, et al. Spasticity in multiple sclerosis. Neurorehabil Neural Repair 2003;17(1): 66–70.

[4] Shakespeare DT, Boggild M, Young C. Anti-spasticity agents for multiple sclerosis. Cochrane Database of Syst Rev 2001(4):CD001332.

[5] Beard S, Hunn A, Wight J. Treatments for spasticity and pain in multiple sclerosis: a systematic review. Health Technol Assess 2003;7(40):1–111.

[6] Haselkorn JK, et al. Spasticity management in multiple sclerosis: evidence-based management strategies for spasticity treatment in multiple sclerosis. Multiple Sclerosis Council for Clinical Practical Guidelines. 2003: Consortium of Multiple Sclerosis Centers.

[7] Penn RD, et al. Intrathecal baclofen for severe spinal spasticity. New Engl J Med 1989; 320(23):1517–21.

[8] Ashworth B. Preliminary trial of carisoprodol in multiple sclerosis. Practitioner 1964;192: 540–2.

[9] Bohannon RW, Smith MB. Interrater reliability of a modified Ashworth scale of muscle spasticity. Phys Ther Rev 1987;67:206–7.

[10] Freeman JA, et al. The impact of inpatient rehabilitation on progressive multiple sclerosis. Ann Neurol 1997;42(2):236–44.

[11] Solari A, et al. Physical rehabilitation has a positive effect on disability in multiple sclerosis patients. Neurology 1999;52:57–62.

[12] Boynton BL, Garramone PM. Observations on the effects of cool baths for patients with multiple sclerosis. Phys Ther Rev 1959;39:297–9.

[13] Pinto OD, Polker M, Debono G. Results of international clinical trials with lioresal. Postgrad Med J 1972;48(Suppl 5):18–23.

[14] Brouwer B, Sousa de Andrade V. The effects of slow stroking on spasticity in patients with multiple sclerosis; a pilot study. Physiotherapy Theory & Practice 1995;11(1):13–21.

[15] Watson CW. Effect of lowering body temperature on the symptoms and signs of multiple sclerosis. New Engl J Med 1959;261:1253–9.

[16] Miglietta O. Evaluation of cold in spasticity. Am J Phys Med 1962;41:148–51.

[17] Kinnman J, et al. Temporary improvement of motor function in patients with multiple sclerosis after treatment with a cooling suit. J Neurol Rehabil 1997;11(2):109–14.

[18] Rosche J, et al. The effects of therapy on spasticity utilizing a motorized exercise-cycle. Spinal Cord 1997;35(3):176–8.

[19] Little J, Massagli T. Spasticity and associated abnormalities of muscle tone. In: DeLisa J, editor. Rehabilitation medicine, principles and practice, 3rd edition. Seattle: Lippincott; 2004. p. 1006–7.

[20] Bell KR, Williams F. Use of botulinum toxin type A and type B for spasticity in upper and lower limb. Am J Phys Med 2003;14(4):821–35.

[21] Snow BJ, et al. Treatment of spasticity with botulinum toxin: a double-blind study. Ann Neurol 1990;28(4):512–5.

[22] Hyman N, et al. Botulinum toxin [Dysport] treatment of hip adductor spasticity in multiple sclerosis: a prospective, randomised, double blind, placebo controlled, dose ranging study. J Neurol Neurosurg Psychiatry 2000;68(6):707–12.

[23] Francisco GE. Botulinum toxin: dosing and dilution. Am J Phys Med 2004; 83(Suppl 10):S30–7.

[24] Nielsen JF, Anderson JB, Sinkjaer T. Baclofen increases the soleus stretch reflex threshold in the early swing phase during walking in spastic multiple sclerosis patients. Mult Scler 2000; 6(2):105–14.

[25] From A, Heltberg A. A double-blind trial with baclofen (Lioresal) and diazepam in spasticity due to multiple sclerosis. Acta Neurol Scand 1975;51(2):158–66.

[26] Cendrowski W, Sobczyk W. Clonazepam, baclofen and placebo in the treatment of spasticity. Eur Neurol 1977;16(1–6):257–62.

[27] Orsnes GB, et al. Effect of baclofen on gait in spastic MS patients. Acta Neurol Scand 2000; 101(4):244–8.

[28] Nielsen JF, Sinkjaer T. Peripheral and central effect of baclofen on ankle joint stiffness in multiple sclerosis. Muscle Nerve 2000;23(1):98–105.

[29] Sawa GM, Paty DW. The use of baclofen in treatment of spasticity in multiple sclerosis. Can J Neurol Sci 1979;6(3):351–4.

[30] Basmajian JV. Lioresal (baclofen) treatment of spasticity in multiple sclerosis. Am J Phys Med 1975;54(4):175–7.

[31] Brar SP, et al. Evaluation of treatment protocols on minimal to moderate spasticity in multiple sclerosis. Arch Phys Med Rehabil 1991;72(3):186–9.

[32] Lapierre YD, Elie R, Tetreault L. The antispastic effects of Ba 34647 (B-4-p-Chlorophenyl-gamma-amino-butyric Acid) a GABA derivative. Curr Therapeutic Res Clin Exper 1974; 16(10):1059–68.

[33] Feldman RG, et al. Baclofen for spasticity in multiple sclerosis: double-blind crossover and three-year study. Neurology 1978;28(11):1094–8.

[34] Sachais BA, Logue JN, Carey MS. Baclofen, a new antispastic drug: a controlled, multicenter trial in patients with multiple sclerosis. Arch Neurol 1977;34(7):422–8.

[35] Basmajian JV, Yucel V. Effects of a GABA–derivative (BA-34647) on spasticity: preliminary report of a double-blind cross-over study. Am J Phys Med 1974;53(5):223–8.

[36] Hedley DW, Maroun JA, Espir ML. Evaluation of baclofen (Lioresal) for spasticity in multiple sclerosis. Postgrad Med J 1975;51(599):615–8.

[37] Hoogstraten MC, et al. Tizanidine versus baclofen in the treatment of spasticity in multiple sclerosis patients. Acta Neurol Scand 1988;77(3):224–30.

[38] Smolenski C, Muff S, Smolenski-Kautz S. A double-blind comparative trial of new muscle relaxant, tizanidine (DS 103–282), and baclofen in the treatment of chronic spasticity in multiple sclerosis. Curr Med Res Opin 1981;7(6):374–83.

[39] Stein R, et al. The treatment of spasticity in multiple sclerosis: a double-blind clinical trial of a new anti-spasticity drug tizanidine compared with baclofen. Acta Neurol Scand 1987;75: 190–4.

[40] Bass B, et al. Tizanidine versus baclofen in the treatment of spasticity in patients with multiple sclerosis. Can J Neurol Sci 1988;15(1):15–9.

[41] Rice GP. Tizanidine vs. baclofen in the treatment of spasticity in patients with multiple sclerosis. Can J Neurol Sci 1989;16(4):451.

[42] Eyssette M, et al. Multi-centre, double-blind trial of a novel antispastic agent, tizanidine, in spasticity associated with multiple sclerosis. Curr Med Res Opin 1988;10(10): 699–708.

[43] Sheplan L, Ishmael C. Spasmolytic properties of dantrolene sodium: clinical evaluation. Mil Med 1975;140(1):26–9.

[44] Emre M, et al. Correlations between dose, plasma concentrations, and antispastic action of tizanidine (Sirdalud). J Neurol Neurosurg Psychiatry 1994;57(11):1355–9.

[45] Nance PW, et al. Relationship of the antispasticity effect of tizanidine to plasma concentration in patients with multiple sclerosis. Arch Neurol 1997;54(6):731–6.

[46] United Kingdom Tizanidine Trial Group. A double-blind, placebo-controlled trial of tizanidine in the treatment of spasticity caused by multiple sclerosis. United Kingdom Tizanidine Trial Group. Neurology 1994;44(11 Suppl 9):S70–9.

[47] Lapierre Y, et al. Treatment of spasticity with tizanidine in multiple sclerosis. Can J Neurol Sci Suppl 1987;14(3):513–7.

[48] Smith C, et al. Tizanidine treatment of spasticity caused by multiple sclerosis: results of a double-blind, placebo-controlled trial. US Tizanidine Study Group. Neurology 1994;44 (11 Suppl 9):S34–42 [discussion S42–3].

[49] Gambi D, et al. Dantrolene sodium in the treatment of spasticity caused by multiple sclerosis or degenerative myelopathies: a double-blind, crossover study in comparison with placebo. Curr Therapeutic Res 1983;33:835–40.

[50] Gelenberg AJ, Poskanzer DC. The effect of dantrolene sodium on spasticity in multiple sclerosis. Neurology 1973;23(12):1313–5.

[51] Schmidt RT, Lee RH. Treatment of spasticity in multiple sclerosis: comparison of dantrolene sodium and diazepam. Trans Am Neurol Assoc 1975;100:235–7.

[52] Schmidt RT, Lee RH, Spehlmann R. Comparison of dantrolene sodium and diazepam in the treatment of spasticity. J Neurol Neurosurg Psychiatry 1976;39:350–6.

[53] Rinne U. Tizanidine treatment of spasticity in multiple sclerosis and chronic myelopathy. Curr Therapeutic Res 1980;28:827–36.

[54] Mueller ME, et al. Gabapentin for relief of upper motor neuron symptoms in multiple sclerosis. Arch Phys Med Rehabil 1997;78(5):521–4.

[55] Coffey JR, et al. Intrathecal baclofen for intractable spasticity of spinal origin: results of a long-term multicenter study. J Neurosurg 1993;78(2):226–32.

[56] Postma TJ, et al. Cost analysis of the treatment of severe spinal spasticity with a continuous intrathecal baclofen infusion system. Pharmacoeconomics 1999;15(4):395–404.

[57] Dressnandt J, Conrad B. Lasting reduction of severe spasticity after ending chronic treatment with intrathecal baclofen. J Neurol Neurosurg Psychiatry 1996;60(2):168–73.

[58] Lazorthes Y, et al. Chronic intrathecal baclofen administration for control of severe spasticity. J Neurosurg 1990;72(3):393–402.

[59] Ochs GA, Tonn JC. Functional outcome and clinical significance of long-term intrathecal baclofen therapy for severe spasticity. J Neurol Rehabil 1996;10(3):159–66.

[60] Siegfried J, Rea GL. Intrathecal application of drugs for muscle hypertonia. Scand J Rehabil Med 1988;17:145–8.

[61] Becker WJC, et al. Long-term intrathecal baclofen therapy in patients with intractable spasticity. Can J Neurol Sci 1995;22(3):208–17.

[62] Smyth MD, Peacock WJ. The surgical management of spasticity. Muscle Nerve 2000;23:153–63.

[63] Jarrett L, Nandi P, Thompson AJ. Managing severe lower limb spasticity in multiple sclerosis: does intrathecal phenol have a role? J Neurol Neurosurg Psychiatry 2002;73:705–9.

[64] Salome K, et al. Surgical management of spasticity by selective posterior rhizotomy: 30 years of experience. Isr Med Assoc J 2003;5(8):543–6.

ELSEVIER
SAUNDERS

Phys Med Rehabil Clin N Am
16 (2005) 483–502

PHYSICAL MEDICINE
AND REHABILITATION
CLINICS OF
NORTH AMERICA

# Multiple Sclerosis–Related Fatigue

## William S. MacAllister, PhD, Lauren B. Krupp, MD*

*National Pediatric Multiple Sclerosis Center, State University of New York at Stony Brook,*
*Stony Brook, NY 11794-8121, USA*

Fatigue is a common symptom in multiple sclerosis (MS) and often causes difficulties for both patients and health care providers. As a result of fatigue, individuals with MS experience limitations in their daily living and coping and clinicians become frustrated by management uncertainties. This article reviews current efforts to understand, measure, and treat fatigue.

## Definition

Everyone feels fatigued at some point; the problem of fatigue is not necessarily related to MS. Therefore, normal and pathologic subtypes of fatigue must be considered. Among otherwise healthy individuals, up to 20% of men and 25% of women "always feel tired" [1]. The challenge to health care providers is to determine not only when fatigue is present but also when it is different from "normal" fatigue, because fatigue associated with a disease state is more likely to have an unfavorable effect on activities of daily living, including impairment of occupational functioning, meeting responsibilities, and sustained physical functioning [2].

In 1998, the Multiple Sclerosis Council for Clinical Practice Guidelines (MS Council) published a consensus definition of MS-related fatigue. It was defined as a "subjective lack of physical or mental energy that is perceived by the individual or caregiver to interfere with usual and desired activities" [3]. Fatigue had to limit functional activities and be present more than 60% of the time. The MS Council further recognized that fatigue could be acute (newly occurring in the past 6 weeks) or chronic (lasting longer than 6 weeks). In addition, primary and secondary fatigue subtypes were distinguished. Primary fatigue is intrinsic to MS as evidenced by the observation that fatigue is worsened by heat (as are other MS symptoms), may be the first and only MS

---

\* Corresponding author. Department of Neurology, SUNY Stony Brook, HSC T-12-020, National Pediatric MS Center, Stony Brook, NY 11794-8121, USA.

*E-mail address:* lkrupp@notes.cc.sunysb.edu (L.B. Krupp).

symptom, and may precede a relapse. Secondary fatigue, in contrast, develops subsequent to other MS symptoms (eg, poor sleep, pain, and so forth).

## Characteristics of MS–related fatigue

Fatigue is a very common problem for individuals with MS. A 1984 study of 656 MS patients demonstrated that fatigue was the most commonly reported symptom [4]. In this sample, 78% of patients reported problems with fatigue. Twenty-two percent of the patients reported that fatigue caused them to reduce their level of physical activity, 14% stated that it required them to get more rest, and 10% indicated that fatigue forced them to discontinue working [4]. Subsequent research confirmed that fatigue is often the most common symptom of MS [5]. Clearly, fatigue is an MS feature that may adversely affect activities of daily living and lead to unemployment [6]. It may also have a detrimental impact on social relationships and the ability to engage in self-care activities [7] and may generally limit the ability to perform any task that necessitates physical effort [8].

Fatigue, however, is difficult to predict. This difficulty stems in part from the realization that fatigue does not correlate strongly with demographic characteristics, clinical form of MS, or other MS signs and symptoms. As an example, the relations between fatigue and age, sex, and the Expanded Disability Status Scale (EDSS) score have been low or inconsistent [9,10]. Furthermore, neuroimaging techniques such as MRI do not appear to predict fatigue reliably [11,12]. In addition, there does not appear to be a strong association between fatigue and gender in MS patients [7,13]. In contrast, general health factors and mental health have been linked to fatigue in MS [8,14]. For example, fatigue has been associated with poor overall quality of life [15] and affective disorders [16]. It is important to recognize that fatigue in MS can be independent of depression [17].

## Pathophysiology

The pathophysiology of MS-related fatigue is multifactorial and complex. Fatigue in the MS patient appears to result from dysregulation of the immune system, changes in the nervous system related to the disease process, and neuroendocrine and neurotransmitter changes. Secondary factors also contribute. It is hoped that further delineation of the patho-physiologic factors leading to fatigue will lead to improved treatments.

### Immune dysregulation

Alterations in immune system activity may underlie aspects of fatigue for MS patients. Research has suggested that immune activation may result in fatigue in the MS patient through changes in neuroendocrine function, through secretion of corticotropin-releasing hormone, corticotropin, and cortisol [18]. Thyroid function has also been implicated in the development of fatigue [19]. Attempts to correlate MS fatigue with immune system activation as assessed by circulating levels of cytokines, however, have been inconsistent, and the reported relation between fatigue and circulating markers of immune activation [17] has not been replicated [20].

Nonetheless, there are some data supporting the supposition that immune system dysregulation plays a role in fatigue, such as the fact that disease-modifying therapies (specifically, the interferon βs) produce fatigue as a side effect [21–23]. In fact, the clinical trial data that led to the approval of interferon βs demonstrated complications of fatigue [24–26]. Fatigue following interferon β injection may last several days, but often diminishes over time as the patient adjusts to these medications.

Despite the recognition that these disease-modifying therapies induce fatigue, the mechanism through which this occurs is not entirely clear. For example, one study associated interferon β administration with increase in inflammatory cytokine levels (including tumor necrosis factor α, interleukin 1, and interleukin 6) and fatigue [27]. Another study reached the opposite conclusion: interferon β administration resulted in decreases in these cytokines [28].

*Central nervous system mechanisms*

Specific central nervous system regions have been implicated in the pathophysiology of fatigue, including the premotor cortex, the limbic system, the basal ganglia, and the brainstem. Dysfunction here may be the result of immune injury, neuronal dysfunction secondary to demyelination and axonal destruction, and other changes resulting in recurrent or chronic central nervous system inflammation. Hypofunction in these areas may lead to fatigue.

Recent research has used functional neuroimaging in the study of MS-related fatigue. Although this line of research is in the preliminary stages, results have been interesting. For example, one investigation using functional MRI linked fatigue to lower levels of activation in the thalamus—possibly relevant in its role as a relay station between the motor cortex and prefrontal regions to the basal ganglia [29]. Other studies used positron emission tomography imaging to demonstrate that fatigued MS patients show decreased glucose metabolism in the prefrontal cortex and basal ganglia [30,31]. Other investigations have been less fruitful; for example, MS-related fatigue does not appear to correlate with lesion load or brain atrophy using T1- or T2-weighted MRI scans [11,32].

The destruction of the myelin sheath has been implicated in the pathophysiology of MS-related fatigue; however, as with other proposed mechanisms, its contribution remains uncertain. Some investigators have suggested that the impaired innervation of muscle groups requires a compensatory increase in central motor drive exertion, necessitating more energy depletion for a given motor function [33]. Indeed, several studies show increased central motor drive or delays in voluntary muscle activation related to impaired conduction along motor pathways [34,35]. An association between self-reported fatigue and the changes of central motor conduction or muscle activation in MS, however, has yet to be found.

*Endocrine factors*

Endocrinal abnormalities such as abnormal thyroid functioning likely play a part in the manifestation of fatigue [36]. Here, the hypothalamic-pituitary-adrenal axis is implicated, and chronic stress can lead to long-term depletion of cortisol, resulting in fatigue. Although dysregulation of the hypothalamic-pituitary-adrenal axis appears to play a role in the production of fatigue, it is not clear whether this endocrine dysfunction is a primary or secondary cause of fatigue.

*Neurotransmitter dysregulation*

Dopaminergic, histaminergic, and serotonergic pathways may also contribute to fatigue. It has been noted that disruption of serotonergic pathways can adversely affect attention and secondarily produce cognitive fatigue [37,38]. Further, adverse effects on the hypothalamus often decrease arousal and thereby produce fatigue. Modafinil, a nondopaminergic medication used to treat fatigue in MS, appears to act through mechanisms mediated by the hypothalamus [39], which suggests possible indirect evidence of hypothalamic mechanisms in fatigue.

*Secondary causes of fatigue in MS*

Several secondary factors of fatigue in MS, including deconditioning, sleep problems, depression, and medication effects, are discussed in the following sections.

*Physical deconditioning*

Deconditioning results from the failure to get adequate exercise. MS patients often experience decreased mobility, weakness, and other physical challenges. For many, this situation results in a decline in their aerobic capacity because fatigued MS patients often tend to avoid activities such as exercise. This tendency is unfortunate because it can further exacerbate fatigue in the long run. Furthermore, in severely disabled MS patients who have difficulty with mobility, respiratory muscles often become weakened, which causes an increase in the amount of energy required to breathe [40].

*Sleep dysfunction*

Problems with sleep are quite common in the general population. The estimated prevalence is approximately 12% among otherwise healthy individuals [41]. Among MS patients, however, sleep disturbances are up to three times more frequent [42]. Sleep problems in MS patients are a likely sequela of nocturnal spasms, which affect the total amount and quality of sleep. Furthermore, nocturnal incontinence may also disrupt sleep in MS patients and lead to more daytime sleepiness and fatigue. MS patients with sleep complaints may also have greater levels of depression—another potential cause of fatigue [42].

*Pain*

Sensory disturbances such as neuralgia, dysesthesia, and painful muscle spasms often play a major role in MS symptomology [43]. Physical pain and fatigue often coexist and adversely affect overall functioning for many patients [18]. Pain often contributes to physical deconditioning by further limiting activity. Likewise, pain at night often precludes restful sleep and therefore contributes to daytime sleepiness and fatigue. Further, pain often contributes to depression, which has a significant relation to overall fatigue [44].

*Depression*

Depression is a feature of MS that, when present, is intimately related to poor sleep, pain, inactivity, and fatigue. Depressive symptoms may exacerbate fatigue directly or through its psychologic consequences [45,46]. Feelings of loss of control, helplessness, and perception of illness are among the psychologic costs of MS [47]. Depression requires separate assessment and should be treated pharmacologically or through psychotherapy. Although depression is clearly a cause of fatigue that requires separate intervention, it may not be present in all MS patients experiencing fatigue.

*Medications*

It is unfortunate that many medications used to treat other symptoms in MS may contribute to fatigue. For example, several pain medications (such as opioids) have fatigue as a side effect. Antispasticity agents such as baclofen and tizanidine can also produce fatigue, as do sedatives, anticonvulsants, and antihistamines. A comprehensive list of agents known to produce fatigue as a side effect was published by the MS Council [48]; the more widely prescribed agents are shown in Table 1.

## Measurement

Measurement techniques in the assessment of fatigue can be subjective or objective. Subjective measures require patients to self-report the presence of fatigue or its severity level. In contrast, objective measures quantify the patient's level of fatigue through various parameters such as muscle force generation or cognitive/neuropsychologic testing. Because objective

Table 1
Pharmacologic agents that may contribute to fatigue in the multiple sclerosis patient

| Drug | Used for | Examples |
|------|----------|----------|
| Analgesics | Pain control | Butalbital, hydrocodone (Vicodin), oxycodone (Oxycontin) |
| Interferon therapies | Reducing MS exacerbations | Interferon beta-1a (Avonex, Rebif), interferon beta-1b (Betaseron) |
| Muscle relaxants | Spasticity, muscle strain, anxiety disorders | Tizanidine (Zanaflex), baclofen (oral or through an intrathecal pump), carisoprodal (Soma) |
| Sedatives/antihypnotics | Sleep aids, anxiety, muscle relaxation | Alprazolam (Xanax), clonazepam (Klonopin), diazepam (Valium), zolpidem (Ambien) |
| Anticonvulsants | Seizure control, pain control, depression or anxiety | Carbamazepine (Tegretol), divalproex (Depakote), gabapentin (Neurontin) |
| Antidepressants | Depression and anxiety disorders | Clomipramine (Anafranil), nefazodone (Serzone), sertraline (Zoloft) |
| Antihistamines | Allergies, hay fever | Diphenhydramine (Benadryl or other over-the-counter allergy medicines), cetirizine (Zyrtec) |
| Antipsychotics | Schizophrenia, psychoses | Clozapine (Clozaril), risperidone (Risperdal) |
| Hormone therapies | Hormone replacement, contraception | Medroxyprogesterone (Depo-Provera) |

*Data from* Multiple Sclerosis Council for Clinical Practice Guidelines. Fatigue and multiple sclerosis: evidence-based management strategies for fatigue in multiple sclerosis. Washington, DC: Paralyzed Veterans of America; 1998.

measures of fatigue have mainly been limited to research applications, the focus of this article's discussion is on subjective measures.

The advantages of subjective self-report measures of fatigue make them more practical for use in a clinical setting. For example, self-report fatigue measures are generally short, widely available, and easy for the patient to understand and complete with minimal oversight from the physician or other examiner. These measures address feelings associated with a state of fatigue, such as subjective sense of exhaustion or tiredness, attenuated motivation, and the length and frequency of such symptoms. An exhaustive review of all available self-report scales used to measure fatigue is outside the scope of this article. Table 2 lists the measures most frequently employed in the assessment of MS-related fatigue.

*Unidimensional fatigue measures in MS*

Among unidimensional measures of MS-related fatigue is the single-item visual analog scale [49] that presents patients with a single line on which to mark their fatigue severity. The far left of the line is labeled "1, Not fatigued at

Table 2
Measures of multiple sclerosis-related fatigue

| Name of scale | Author, year [ref.] | Population | Specified fatigue subscales | No. of items | Scoring |
|---|---|---|---|---|---|
| Fatigue Severity Scale | Krupp et al, 1989 [49] | MS, lupus, healthy | None | 9 | Likert Scale |
| Single-item Visual Analogue Scale of Fatigue | Krupp et al, 1989 [49] | MS, lupus, healthy | None | 1 | Visual analogue scale |
| Fatigue Assessment Instrument | Schwartz et al, 1993 [55] | Lyme, Chronic fatigue syndrome, lupus, MS, dysthymia, healthy | Fatigue severity, situation-specificity, consequences of fatigue, responds to rest/sleep | 29 | 1–7 |
| Fatigue Impact Scale | Fisk et al, 1994 [56] | MS | Physical, cognitive, psychosocial | 21 | 0–4 |
| Fatigue Descriptive Scale | Iriarte et al, 1999 [7] | MS | Spontaneous mention of fatigue, antecedent conditions, frequency, impact on life | 5 | 0–3 |
| Rochester Fatigue Diary | Schwid et al, 2002 [57] | MS | Lassitude (reduced energy) | 12 (1 item, 12 times over 24 h) | Visual analogue scale |

all," whereas the far right indicates "100, As bad as fatigue can be." Patients are to draw a mark representing their level of fatigue. Although the measure is easy to use and interpret and has been useful in studies in detecting treatment response [50], it has clear drawbacks. For example, the visual analog scale may be less reliable than other measures of fatigue and is potentially difficult to score [51]. Further, the visual analog scale measures fatigue globally but does not provide information regarding different aspects of fatigue.

Another unidimensional measure is the Fatigue Severity Scale (FSS) [49]. The FSS is a nine-item measure that uses a 7-point Likert scale response format. The FSS is typically scored by averaging the responses across items. An FSS score above 4 is indicative of severe fatigue. It is among the most widely used fatigue measure in MS, likely due to its demonstrated high validity, reliability, and internal consistency. It has also been shown to be effective in differentiating medical populations from controls and can detect treatment effects [49,52–54]. The FSS was also used by the MS Council to differentiate mild from more severe fatigue in the interest of guiding treatment.

## Multidimensional fatigue measures

To address some of the limitations inherent in unidimensional measures, multidimensional scales have been developed to measure different aspects of fatigue. The Fatigue Assessment Inventory [55], for example, assesses the severity of fatigue, situation specificity, the consequences of being fatigued, and whether or not fatigue subsides subsequent to rest or sleep.

The Fatigue Impact Scale [56] was created to assess the perceived effect of fatigue of factors such as cognitive function, physical function, and psychosocial functioning. The MS Council provides a modified version of this scale in their guidelines on fatigue [3].

The Fatigue Descriptive Scale [7] distinguishes asthenia and fatigability. It assesses spontaneous mentions of fatigue, conditions that tend to precede feelings of fatigue, the frequency at which fatigue occurs, and the adverse affect that fatigue has had on the patient's functioning. The Rochester Fatigue Diary [57] uses visual analog scales to assess different aspects of fatigue hourly over the course of a day.

Despite the obvious advantages of assessing multiple aspects of MS-related fatigue, multidimensional measures also have drawbacks. For example, multidimensional measures tend to demonstrate poorer psychometric properties (eg, lower reliability coefficients and validity coefficients and less responsiveness to fluctuation in levels of fatigue over time) [58]. Although multidimensional scales are more comprehensive, they do not provide accurate assessments of social, cognitive, or physical functioning. These assessments would require more extensive investigation (eg, confirming work attendance or assessing performance on neuropsychologic tests, and so forth), which is often difficult or impossible to achieve because it is time-consuming and may breach patient confidentiality.

## Therapy for MS–related fatigue

The treatment of fatigue in MS should first seek to eliminate or reduce factors that may contribute to it, including mood disturbance, sleep disruption, and medications that may produce fatigue as a side effect (see Table 1). If fatigue persists, more specific interventions must be considered. These interventions may include nonpharmacological interventions, medications that improve fatigue, or both.

*Nonpharmacologic approaches to the treatment of MS–related fatigue*

Nonpharmacologic interventions to improve fatigue in MS include exercise programs, nutritional improvements, cooling, and energy conservation strategies. Each has at least some empiric support, but all share common-sense features that make them palatable to patients who may be reluctant to add another medication to their regimen.

*Exercise programs*

Exercise not only serves to counteract the deconditioning that often results from inactivity (as discussed earlier) but also has the added benefits of self-esteem, improving mood, combating social isolation, decreasing the risk of cardiovascular disease, and preventing or reducing obesity [59]. Several clinical studies have examined the efficacy of exercise in improving fatigue in MS patients. Each has shown some degree of improvement. For example, a short-term study of 26 patients with moderate disability assessed exercise by way of a stationary bicycle. Those in the exercise group demonstrated significant improvement on respiratory measures and a trend toward significance on the FSS [60]. Although this study showed only trends toward reductions in fatigue, measurement issues may have precluded significant results. Further, this study was limited by poor statistical power resulting from a small sample size. Another study demonstrated that a 15-week graded exercise program resulted in improvement of fatigue on the fatigue subscale of the Profile of Mood States, but again, the FSS score did not significantly change [61].

A long-term outpatient rehabilitation program proved effective in reducing fatigue in 20 patients with progressive MS in comparison to a wait-listed control group [62]. This study used physical therapy with support services 5 h/d, 1 d/wk for a 1-year period. Fatigue was measured by the 26-item MS-Related Symptom Checklist and was significantly reduced in the treatment group compared with the control group ($P = 0.004$).

Guidelines on the implementation of exercise programs for MS patients have been more thoroughly discussed elsewhere [63]; however, the general principles are highlighted here. Clinicians must first consider the severity of neurologic impairment, the presence of other medical conditions that may affect the ability to complete an exercise program, and the need to provide a gradual, graded program. Ideally, a physical therapist knowledgeable about the unique health care needs of MS patients should be involved. As with many people, adherence to the exercise program is often an issue. Thus, it is recommended that clinicians remain positive and supportive while reinforcing adherence to the program. In the authors' experience, providing a prescription or written agenda for the exercise program helps emphasize the importance of such interventions.

*Cooling programs*

The association between heat and MS symptoms (including fatigue) has long been known. Heat adversely affects nerve impulse conduction and is often a considerable obstacle for MS patients to consider regardless of whether they participate in an exercise program [64]. Recent research demonstrates that the use of cooling garments (eg, head and vest cooling attire) may reduce fatigue for MS patients [65,66]. For patients engaging in exercise programs, cooling is essential. For exercising patients, precooling by way of water immersion and the use of cooling garments during exercise have been shown to be effective [67]. Water-based exercise programs in water less than 85°F have been suggested [68], but a more recent case study demonstrated that exercise in 94°F water did not increase fatigue [69].

*Diet*

Although there is no specific diet that combats fatigue for MS patients, developing a healthy nutrition program can be of some benefit for MS patients with significant fatigue. For example, it has been recommended that such patients avoid foods that contain refined sugars because erratic blood glucose levels can contribute to fatigue. Adequate hydration is also essential, and patients should avoid caffeine and alcohol. MS patients should eat smaller meals throughout the day rather than three large meals. The meals should be balanced and high in vitamins, minerals, protein, and complex carbohydrates. Nutrition programs for fatigued MS patients are reviewed more thoroughly elsewhere [63].

*Energy conservation*

A few studies to date have shown empiric support for the use of energy conservation techniques to reduce fatigue in MS patients. One study, for example, assessed the effectiveness of a 2-h/wk energy course led by occupational therapists. This intervention resulted in reductions in fatigue and improvements in quality of life and perceived self-efficacy [70]. Smaller investigations have found similar results. Although these results are preliminary and require replication, they suggest that referrals to an occupational therapist with expertise in this area may be helpful [71].

*Medications*

Nonpharmacologic interventions have been described as first-line therapies for the treatment of fatigue in MS patients [63]. Many patients, however, may not fully benefit from such methods or may receive incomplete relief. For such patients, the use of pharmacologic interventions may become necessary. It is unfortunate that there are no currently available Food and Drug Administration–approved medications specifically for the treatment of MS-related fatigue. Regardless, as presented in Table 3, a number of agents have been used successfully (off label) in MS patients.

*First-line medications*

Of the medications used to treat fatigue in MS, amantadine and modafinil are considered the primary agents. According to a recent consensus meeting of neurologists, amantadine is preferred for mild fatigue [72]. Mild fatigue is operationalized by an FSS score of less than 4. Amantadine is an antiviral agent used in the treatment of influenza A and the extrapyramidal symptoms in Parkinson's disease [73]. The mechanism of action is thought to involve blocking presynaptic dopamine reuptake and stimulating postsynaptic receptors. Four controlled clinical trials have evaluated the efficacy of amantadine in the treatment of MS-related fatigue. Despite different study designs, each demonstrated benefit of amantadine over placebo on self-report measures. In the first clinical trial, 62.5% of patients taking the active drug reported improved fatigue versus 21.8% on placebo ($P = 0.0005$) [10]. In another study that compared amantadine and placebo, a trend in favor of amantadine was observed in the overall fatigue score (3.18 versus 2.96; $P = 0.058$). Separate analyses of each index used in the study (ie, general energy level, concentration and memory, well-being, and the ability to solve problems) demonstrated statistically significant results; however, no significant improvement was seen in muscle strength, motivation level, or the ability to finish a task [50].

A multicenter trial that included 115 patients with a history of "chronic persistent fatigue" used a crossover analysis (controlling for changes due to time). This study involved a 2-week placebo run-in period, with two 3-week treatment periods, separated by a 2-week washout period. A general visual analog scale was used to assess daily fatigue, and participant-specific scales were also used to assess areas most often affected by each patient. Amantadine decreased daily fatigue relative to placebo, but the improvement was only statistically significant at week 1 ($P < 0.01$). Amantadine, however, was associated with a significant mean decrease in fatigue on selected activities compared with placebo at each of the 3 weeks ($P < 0.05$) [74].

Another multicenter, parallel-group, randomized trial found that amantadine significantly decreased fatigue on some but not all fatigue measures. Further, following the 2-week washout period, 79% of patients receiving amantadine versus 52% of those receiving placebo indicated that they felt better on study medication ($P = 0.03$) [52].

Modafinil is the other first-line agent used to treat MS-related fatigue recommended by the consensus meeting of neurologists; it is recommended for the treatment of severe fatigue as defined by an FSS score of 4 or above

Table 3
Drugs used to treat multiple sclerosis–related fatigue (adult doses)

| Drug | Starting dose | Usual maintenance dose | Usual maximum dose | Side effects |
|------|---------------|------------------------|--------------------|--------------|
| Amantadine (Symmetrel) | 100 mg/d in the morning | 100 mg twice per day | 300 mg/d | Insomnia, vivid dreams |
| Modafinil (Provigil) | 100 mg/d in the morning | 200 mg/d in the morning or 100 mg in the morning and 100 mg at lunchtime | 400 mg/d (some people might respond to higher doses) | Headache, insomnia |
| Pemoline (Cylert) | 18.75 mg/d in the morning | 18.75–56.25 mg/d | 93.75 mg/d | Irritability, restlessness, insomnia, potential liver problems |
| Bupropion, sustained release (Wellbutrin SR) | 150 mg/d in the morning | 150 mg twice per day | 150 tid | Agitation, anxiety, insomnia |
| Fluoxetine (Prozac) | 20 mg/d in the morning | 20–80 mg/d | 80 mg/d | Weakness, nausea, insomnia |
| Venlafaxine (Effexor-XR) | 75 mg/d in the morning | 140–180 mg/d | 375 mg | Weakness, nausea, dizziness |

[72]. Modafinil is considered a wake-promoting agent and is believed to work selectively in the central nervous system within pathways related to the hypothalamus [39,75]. Modafinil has been used in the treatment of narcolepsy [76], obstructive sleep apnea [77], and chronic fatigue syndrome [78].

Several studies have demonstrated modafinil's effectiveness in the treatment of MS-related fatigue. One study was a 9-week patient-blinded, forced-titration study of MS patients who had an average FSS score of greater than 4 [53]. Results indicated that a 200-mg dose of modafinil significantly improved fatigue in comparison to placebo on all measures of fatigue administered. Overall, 69% reported improvement on each of these self-report scales. The medication was relatively well tolerated, with the most common side effects being headache, nausea, and anxiety.

An open-label study of modafinil demonstrated a positive effect on fatigue in both relapsing remitting and secondary progressive MS patients. Significant improvement was observed on the FSS score ($P < 0.0001$) after 3 months. On global measures, 44 of 50 patients reported "clear improvement" or "some improvement." In this study, 3 patients discontinued modafinil due to nervousness or dizziness [79].

## Pemoline

The central nervous system stimulant pemoline is indicated for the treatment of attention deficit/hyperactivity disorder [80]. To date, there have been two randomized, controlled clinical trials that evaluated the effectiveness of pemoline in the treatment of MS-related fatigue. The results have been somewhat equivocal. In both studies, statistical significance was not achieved on the primary outcome measures [50,52], although a trend toward significance was evident in one study at a dosage of 75 mg/d [50]. In this study, 46.3% of patients receiving pemoline reported "good" or "excellent" relief from fatigue in comparison to 19.5% of patients in the control group ($P = 0.06$). Due to these equivocal results and the drug's association with liver problems [80], it is not generally recommended as a first-line agent. In patients who have not had favorable results with other medications, however, pemoline may be worth consideration. For patients in whom this drug is effective, it tends to work well, and some patients seem to prefer this medication to others.

## Antidepressants

Although antidepressant medications have not been systematically studied for specific treatment of fatigue in MS, given the high degree of association between fatigue and depression, antidepressants are an attractive treatment alternative, particularly in patients who show elevated depressive symptoms. There is some empiric support for the use of antidepressants in MS-related fatigue. A case study of bupropion was associated with improvements in energy and decreased irritability. These improvements were sustained over 6 months [81]. Further, a randomized trial demonstrated that treatment of depression in MS (by way of group psychotherapy, individual psychotherapy, or sertraline) was associated with improvements in fatigue [82]. In this study, changes in levels of fatigue were due to changes in mood, not other symptoms of depression such as vegetative symptoms or cognition.

*Other pharmacologic agents*

Aminopyridines (4-aminopyridines and 3,4-diaminopyridines) have been studied for the treatment of MS-related fatigue. These medications are potassium channel blockers that serve to prolong the duration of nerve action potential and improve the safety factor of nerve transmission [54]. In 1998, Sheean et al [54] conducted an open-label study on electrophysiologic parameters of motor performance in 8 patients who had a mean FSS score of 5.5. Improvements in fatigue were observed with 3,4-diaminopyridine ($P < 0.05$), but these changes were unrelated to changes in electrophysiologic tests of motor conduction and motor function. The results were attributed to a potential nonspecific central stimulant effect of the medication. Another study used a double-blind, crossover design to compare 3,4-diaminopyridine with 4-aminopyridine in 10 responders to 4-aminopyridine. Four of the patients demonstrated clinically noteworthy changes in fatigue with 3,4-diaminopyridine [83].

Although these results suggest some efficacy in the treatment of MS-related fatigue, results are preliminary and clearly require replication in larger, well-controlled studies. Furthermore, aminopyridines have high seizure risk associated with them and have been associated with hepatitis [84]. For these reasons, they are not considered first-line agents for the treatment of fatigue; safer formulations of 4-aminopyridine are being tested for symptomatic relief in MS.

A recent pilot study evaluated the efficacy of Prokarin (a transdermal blend of histamine and caffeine) [85]. In this study, a significant reduction in fatigue was seen on the Modified Fatigue Impact Scale (MFIS) of patients receiving the active medication versus placebo treatment ($P < 0.05$). This difference was evident at 4 weeks and was sustained over the 12-week duration of the study. There were some methodological concerns with this study because the patients were not properly matched at baseline: 6 of 7 patients on placebo had a progressive form of MS (primary progressive or secondary progressive), whereas only 13 of 22 patients on Prokarin had a progressive form of the disease. Thus, interpretation of these results must proceed cautiously, and larger and better-controlled trials are required to validate these results. Nonetheless, Prokarin may eventually prove to be a promising treatment for MS-related fatigue, especially considering the fact that there were no adverse reactions to the medication over the course of this study. Fig. 1 presents a suggested decision-making flowchart for the treatment of fatigue in MS.

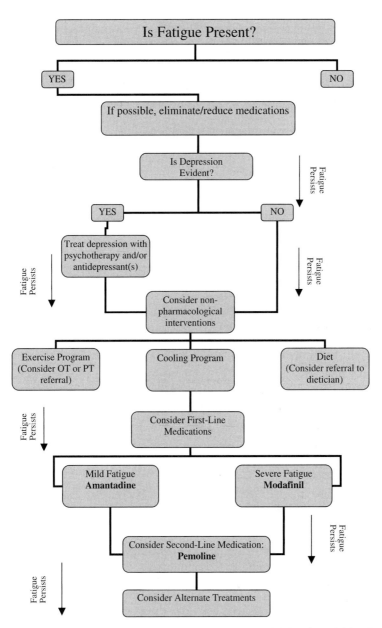

Fig. 1. Suggested decision-making flowchart for the treatment of fatigue in multiple sclerosis.

## Summary

Fatigue is a significant factor in the lives of many MS patients and the most commonly reported symptom in many studies. Fatigue is an important symptom to consider because it affects patients' social lives, occupations, and activities of daily living. Efforts to predict fatigue have been mixed, but it appears to be related to overall quality of life and mood. From a pathophysiologic perspective, fatigue in MS is multifactorial and complex, involving dysregulation of the immune system, changes in the nervous system related to the disease process, neuroendocrine and neurotransmitter changes, and other factors such as physical deconditioning, sleep disturbance, pain, and medication side effects. Various attempts to assess fatigue have been made, and many measures are now available for use in clinical practice and research. In clinical practice, these measures help guide treatment considerations. Recent research has provided valuable strategies to ameliorate fatigue in MS, and although many patients continue to experience fatigue despite interventions, many receive substantial relief. Nonpharmacologic approaches—considered the first step in treatment— include exercise programs, cooling, dietary considerations, and energy conservation strategies. For patients who continue to experience significant fatigue, several medications (although not specifically approved for use in the reduction of MS-related fatigue) have proved effective in this regard. The first-line agents include amantadine for mild fatigue and modafinil for more severe cases. Second-line agents include pemoline and antidepressant medications. Other pharmacologic agents have also shown some promise.

## Acknowledgments

The authors wish to thank Christopher Christodoulou, PhD for his helpful comments and editing and Andrew Sobel for his assistance.

## References

[1] Price RK, North CS, Wessely S, et al. Estimating the prevalence of chronic fatigue syndrome and associated symptoms in the community. Public Health Rep 1992;107(5):514–22.

[2] Krupp LB, La Rocca NG, Scheinberg LC. Fatigue in multiple sclerosis. Arch Neurol 1988; 45(4):435–7.

[3] Multiple Sclerosis Council for Clinical Practice Guidelines. Fatigue and multiple sclerosis: evidence-based management strategies for fatigue in multiple sclerosis. Washington, DC: Paralyzed Veterans of America; 1998.

[4] Freal JE, Kraft GH, Coryell JK. Symptomatic fatigue in multiple sclerosis. Arch Phys Med Rehabil 1984;65(3):135–8.

[5] Multiple Sclerosis Society of Great Britain and Northern Ireland. Symptom management survey. London: Multiple Sclerosis Society of Great Britain and Northern Ireland; 1998.

[6] Scheinberg L, Holland N, LaRocca N, et al. Multiple sclerosis; earning a living. N Y State J Med 1980;80(9):1395–400.

[7] Iriarte J, Katsamakis G, de Castro P. The Fatigue Descriptive Scale (FDS): a useful tool to evaluate fatigue in multiple sclerosis. Mult Scler 1999;5(1):10–6.

[8] Fisk JD, Pontefract A, Ritvo PG, et al. The impact of fatigue on patients with multiple sclerosis. Can J Neurol Sci 1994;21(1):9–14.

[9] Kurtzke JF. Rating neurologic impairment in multiple sclerosis: an expanded disability status scale (EDSS). Neurology 1983;33(11):1444–52.

[10] Murray TJ. Amantadine therapy for fatigue in multiple sclerosis. Can J Neurol Sci 1985; 12(3):251–4.

[11] Bakshi R, Miletich RS, Henschel K, et al. Fatigue in multiple sclerosis: cross-sectional correlation with brain MRI findings in 71 patients. Neurology 1999;53(5):1151–3.

[12] Mainero C, Faroni J, Gasperini C, et al. Fatigue and magnetic resonance imaging activity in multiple sclerosis. J Neurol 1999;246(6):454–8.

[13] Colosimo C, Millefiorini E, Grasso MG, et al. Fatigue in MS is associated with specific clinical features. Acta Neurol Scand 1995;92(5):353–5.

[14] Monks J. Experiencing symptoms in chronic illness: fatigue in multiple sclerosis. Int Disabil Stud 1989;11(2):78–83.

[15] Aronson KJ. Quality of life among persons with multiple sclerosis and their caregivers. Neurology 1997;48(1):74–80.

[16] Bakshi R, Shaikh ZA, Miletich RS, et al. Fatigue in multiple sclerosis and its relationship to depression and neurologic disability. Mult Scler 2000;6:181–5.

[17] Iriarte J, Subira ML, Castro P. Modalities of fatigue in multiple sclerosis: correlation with clinical and biological factors. Mult Scler 2000;6(2):124–30.

[18] Wessely S, Hotopf M, Sharpe M. Chronic fatigue and its syndromes. London: Oxford University Press; 1999.

[19] Jones TH, Wadler S, Hupart KH. Endocrine-mediated mechanisms of fatigue during treatment with interferon-alpha. Semin Oncol 1998;25(1 Suppl 1):54–63.

[20] Giovannoni G, Thompson AJ, Miller DH, et al. Fatigue is not associated with raised inflammatory markers in multiple sclerosis. Neurology 2001;57(4):676–81.

[21] Neilley LK, Goodin DS, Goodkin DE, et al. Side effect profile of interferon beta-1b in MS: results of an open label trial. Neurology 1996;46(2):552–4.

[22] Quesada JR, Talpaz M, Rios A, et al. Clinical toxicity of interferons in cancer patients: a review. J Clin Oncol 1986;4(2):234–43.

[23] Gottberg K, Gardulf A, Fredrikson S. Interferon-beta treatment for patients with multiple sclerosis: the patients' perceptions of the side-effects. Mult Scler 2000;6(5):349–54.

[24] Avonex (interferon beta 1a) prescribing information. Cambridge (MA): Biogen; 1996.

[25] Rebif (interferon beta-1a) prescribing information. Rockland (MA): Serono, Inc.; 2003.

[26] Betaseron (interferon beta-1b) prescribing information. Montville (NJ): Berlex Laboratories; 2003.

[27] Goebel MU, Baase J, Pithan V, et al. Acute interferon beta-1b administration alters hypothalamic-pituitary-adrenal axis activity, plasma cytokines and leukocyte distribution in healthy subjects. Psychoneuroendocrinology 2002;27(8):881–92.

[28] Rothuizen LE, Buclin T, Spertini F, et al. Influence of interferon beta-1a dose frequency on PBMC cytokine secretion and biological effect markers. J Neuroimmunol 1999;99(1): 131–41.

[29] Filippi M, Rocca MA, Colombo B, et al. Functional magnetic resonance imaging correlates of fatigue in multiple sclerosis. Neuroimage 2002;15(3):559–67.

[30] Bakshi R, Miletich RS, Kinkel PR, et al. High-resolution fluorodeoxyglucose positron emission tomography shows both global and regional cerebral hypometabolism in multiple sclerosis. J Neuroimaging 1998;8(4):228–34.

[31] Roelcke U, Kappos L, Lechner SJ, et al. Reduced glucose metabolism in the frontal cortex and basal ganglia of multiple sclerosis patients with fatigue: a 18F-fluorodeoxyglucose positron emission tomography study. Neurology 1997;48(6):1566–71.

[32] Mainero C, Faroni J, Gasperini C, et al. Fatigue and magnetic resonance imaging activity in multiple sclerosis. J Neurol 1999;246(6):454–8.

[33] Bakshi R. Fatigue associated with multiple sclerosis: diagnosis, impact and management. Mult Scler 2003;9(3):219–27.

[34] Sheean GL, Murray NM, Rothwell JC, et al. An electrophysiological study of the mechanism of fatigue in multiple sclerosis. Brain 1997;120(Pt 2):299–315.

[35] Ng AV, Kent-Braun JA. Quantitation of lower physical activity in persons with multiple sclerosis. Med Sci Sports Exerc 1997;29(4):517–23.

[36] Schwid SR, Goodman AD, Mattson DH. Autoimmune hyperthyroidism in patients with multiple sclerosis treated with interferon beta-1b. Arch Neurol 1997;54(9):1169–90.

[37] Parker AJ, Wessely S, Cleare AJ. The neuroendocrinology of chronic fatigue syndrome and fibromyalgia. Psychol Med 2001;31(8):1331–45.

[38] Heilman KM, Watson RT. Fatigue. Neurol Network Comment 1997;1:283–7.

[39] Scammell TE, Estabrooke IV, McCarthy MT, et al. Hypothalamic arousal regions are activated during modafinil-induced wakefulness. J Neurosci 2000;20(22):8620–8.

[40] Foglio K, Clini E, Facchetti D, et al. Respiratory muscle function and exercise capacity in multiple sclerosis. Eur Respir J 1994;7(1):23–8.

[41] Happe S. Excessive daytime sleepiness and sleep disturbances in patients with neurological diseases: epidemiology and management. Drugs 2003;63(24):2725–37.

[42] Clark CM, Fleming JA, Li D, et al. Sleep disturbance, depression, and lesion site in patients with multiple sclerosis. Arch Neurol 1992;49(6):641–3.

[43] Stenager E, Knudsen L, Jensen K. Acute and chronic pain syndromes in multiple sclerosis. Acta Neurol Scand 1991;84(3):197–200.

[44] Flachenecker P, Kumpfel T, Kallmann B, et al. Fatigue in multiple sclerosis: a comparison of different rating scales and correlation to clinical parameters. Mult Scler 2002;8(6):523–6.

[45] Friedberg F, Krupp LB. A comparison of cognitive behavioral treatment of chronic fatigue syndrome and primary depression. Clin Infect Dis 1994;18:S105–10.

[46] Schwartz CE, Coulthard-Morris L, Zeng Q. Psychosocial correlates of fatigue in multiple sclerosis. Arch Phys Med Rehabil 1996;77(2):165–70.

[47] Zonana-Nacach A, Roseman JM, McGwin G Jr, et al. Systemic lupus erythematosus in three ethnic groups. VI: factors associated with fatigue within 5 years of criteria diagnosis. LUMINA Study Group. LUpus in MInority populations: NAture vs Nurture. Lupus 2000;9(2):101–9.

[48] Multiple Sclerosis Council for Clinical Practice Guidelines. Washington, DC: Paralyzed Veterans Association; 1998.

[49] Krupp LB, LaRocca NG, Muir-Nash J, et al. The fatigue severity scale. Application to patients with multiple sclerosis and systemic lupus erythematosus. Arch Neurol 1989;46(10):1121–3.

[50] Weinshenker BG, Penman M, Bass B, et al. A double-blind, randomized, crossover trial of pemoline in fatigue associated with multiple sclerosis. Neurology 1992;42(8):1468–71.

[51] Krupp LB, Soefer MH, Pollina DA, et al. Fatigue measures for clinical trials in multiple sclerosis. Neurology 1998;50:A126.

[52] Krupp LB, Coyle PK, Doscher C, et al. Fatigue therapy in multiple sclerosis: results of a double blind, randomized, parallel trial of amantadine, pemoline, and placebo. Neurology 1995;45:1956–61.

[53] Rammohan KW, Rosenberg JH, Lynn DJ, et al. Efficacy and safety of modafinil (Provigil) for the treatment of fatigue in multiple sclerosis: a two-centre phase 2 study. J Neurol Neurosurg Psychiatry 2002;72(2):179–83.

[54] Sheean GL, Murray NM, Rothwell JC, et al. An open-labelled clinical and electrophysiological study of 3,4 diaminopyridine in the treatment of fatigue in multiple sclerosis. Brain 1998;121(Pt 5):967–75.

[55] Schwartz JE, Jandorf L, Krupp LB. The measurement of fatigue: a new scale. J Psychosom Res 1993;37(7):753–62.

[56] Fisk JD, Ritvo PG, Ross L, et al. Measuring the functional impact of fatigue: initial validation of the fatigue impact scale. Clin Infect Dis 1994;18(Suppl 1):S79–83.

[57] Schwid SR, Covington M, Segal BM, et al. Fatigue in multiple sclerosis: current understanding and future directions. J Rehabil Res Dev 2002;39(2):211–24.

[58] Meek PM, Nail LM, Barsevik A, et al. Psychometric testing of fatigue instruments for use with cancer patients. Nurs Res 2000;49:181–90.

[59] Sutherland G, Anderson MB. Exercise and multiple sclerosis: physiological, psychological, and quality of life stress. Journal of Sports Medicine & Physical Fitness 2002;41:421–32.

[60] Mostert S, Kesselring J. Effects of a short-term exercise training program on aerobic fitness, fatigue, health perception and activity level of subjects with multiple sclerosis. Mult Scler 2002;8(2):161–8.

[61] Petajan JH, Gappmaier E, White AT, et al. Impact of aerobic training on fitness and quality of life in multiple sclerosis. Ann Neurol 1996;39(4):432–41.

[62] Di Fabio RP, Soderberg J, Choi T, et al. Extended outpatient rehabilitation: it's influence on symptom frequency, fatigue and functional status for persons with progressive multiple sclerosis. Arch Phys Med Rehabil 1998;79:141–6.

[63] Krupp LB. Fatigue in multiple sclerosis: a guide to diagnosis and management. New York: Demos Medical Publishing, Inc.; 2004.

[64] Guthrie TC, Nelson DA. Influence of temperature changes on multiple sclerosis: critical review of mechanisms and research potential. J Neurol Sci 1995;129(1):1–8.

[65] Flesner G, Lindencrona C. The cooling-suit: case studies of its influence on fatigue among eight individuals with multiple sclerosis [abstract]. J Adv Nurs 2002;37(6):541–50.

[66] Beenakker EA, Oparina TI, Hartgring A, et al. Cooling garment treatment in MS: clinical improvement and decrease in leukocyte NO production. Neurology 2001;57(5):892–4.

[67] White AT, Wilson TE, Davis SL, et al. Effect of precooling on physical performance in multiple sclerosis. Mult Scler 2000;6(3):176–80.

[68] Woods DA. Aquatic exercise programs for patients with multiple sclerosis. Clin Kinesiol 1992;46(3):14–20.

[69] Peterson C. Exercise in 94°F water for a patient with multiple sclerosis. Phys Ther 2001;81(4): 1049–58.

[70] Mathiowetz V, Matuska KM, Murphy ME. Efficacy of an energy conservation course for persons with multiple sclerosis. Arch Phys Med Rehabil 2001;82(4):449–56.

[71] Vanage SM, Gilbertson KK, Mathiowetz V. Effects of an energy conservation course on fatigue impact for persons with progressive multiple sclerosis. Am J Occup Ther 2003;57(3): 315–23.

[72] Schapiro RT for the Working Group for Pharmacologic Therapy in Multiple Sclerosis-Related Fatigue. MS-related fatigue: toward a consensus for pharmacologic therapy. Int J MS Care 2002;4(Suppl):1–16.

[73] Symmetrel (Amantadine) package insert. Chadds Ford (PA): Endo Pharmaceuticals; 2000.

[74] Canadian MS Research Group. A randomized controlled trial of amantadine in fatigue associated with multiple sclerosis. Can J Neural Sci 1987;14:273–8.

[75] Lin JS, Hou Y, Jouvet M. Potential brain neuronal targets for amphetamine-, methylphenidate-, and modafinil-induced wakefulness, evidenced by c-fos immunocyto-chemistry in the cat. Proc Natl Acad Sci USA 1996;93:14128–33.

[76] Randomized trial of modafinil as a treatment for the excessive daytime somnolence of narcolepsy: US Modafinil in Narcolepsy Multicenter Study Group. Neurology 2000;54(5): 1166–75.

[77] Arnulf I, Homeyer P, Garma L, et al. Modafinil in obstructive sleep apnea-hypopnea syndrome: a pilot study in 6 patients. Respiration (Herrlisheim) 1997;64(2):159–61.

[78] Cochran JW. Effect of modafinil on fatigue associated with neurological illnesses. J Chronic Fatigue Syndr 2001;8:65–70.

[79] Zifko UA, Rupp M, Schwarz S, et al. Modafinil in treatment of fatigue in multiple sclerosis. Results of an open-label study. J Neurol 2002;249(8):983–7.

[80] Cylert (pemoline) package insert. Chicago: Abbott Laboratories; 2004.

[81] Duffy JD, Campbell J. Bupropion for the treatment of fatigue associated with multiple sclerosis. Psychosomatics 1994;35(2):170–1.

[82] Mohr DC, Hart SL, Goldberg A. Effects of treatment for depression on fatigue in multiple sclerosis. Psychosom Med 2003;65(4):542–7.

[83] Polman CH, Bertelsmann FW, de Waal R, et al. 4-Aminopyridine is superior to 3,4-diaminopyridine in the treatment of patients with multiple sclerosis. Arch Neurol 1994;51: 1136–9.

[84] Polman CH, Bertelsmann FW, Van Loenen AC, et al. 4-Aminopyridine in the treatment of patients with multiple sclerosis. Long term efficacy and safety. Arch Neurol 1994;51:292–6.

[85] Gillson G, Tichard TL, Smith RB, et al. A double blind pilot study of the effect of Prokarin on fatigue in multiple sclerosis [abstract]. Mult Scler 2002;8(1):30–5.

ELSEVIER
SAUNDERS

Phys Med Rehabil Clin N Am
16 (2005) 503–512

PHYSICAL MEDICINE
AND REHABILITATION
CLINICS OF
NORTH AMERICA

# Chronic Pain in Persons with Multiple Sclerosis

Dawn M. Ehde, PhD[a,*], Travis L. Osborne, PhD[a],
Mark P. Jensen, PhD[a,b]

[a]Department of Rehabilitation Medicine, Box 356490, University of Washington School of
Medicine, Seattle, WA 98195-6490, USA
[b]Multidisciplinary Pain Center, University of Washington Medical Center—Roosevelt,
4245 Roosevelt Way Northeast, Seattle, WA 98105-6920, USA

Although multiple sclerosis (MS) was once thought to be a "painless" disease [1], research in the last decade has shown that chronic pain is a common condition among persons with MS and can be severe [2–8]. The purpose of this article is to provide a summary of what is currently known concerning the nature and scope of chronic pain as a secondary condition to MS. It begins with a summary of the research literature concerning the potential causes, prevalence, severity, and impact of pain in MS and what is known concerning the factors that contribute to or are associated with adjustment to chronic pain in persons with MS. Treatment of pain in persons with MS is also discussed. As is discussed throughout the article, there are significant gaps in our understanding of chronic pain in MS, particularly with regard to its treatment.

## Potential etiologies for chronic pain

Pain can arise from a variety of sources in persons with MS. For example, the active inflammatory process that occurs with an MS exacerbation can lead to acute pain [9]. In addition, chronic neuropathic pain can result from

Supported by grant H133B031129-04 from the National Institute of Disability and Rehabilitation Research, Department of Education, and grant "Management of Chronic Pain in Rehabilitation" PO1 HD33988 from the National Institute of Child Health and Human Development, National Center for Medical Rehabilitation Research, National Institutes of Health.
 * Corresponding author.
 *E-mail address:* ehde@u.washington.edu (D.M. Ehde).

a variety of factors associated with the MS disease process itself. For example, lesions in the dorsal horn of the spinal cord can result in unpleasant tingling paresthesias and Lhermitte's sign. For some persons with MS, lesions in the trigeminal entry zone in the brainstem can lead to trigeminal neuralgia [9]. Increased muscle tone may also result in chronic pain. For example, tonic spasms can arise from demyelination in the brain stem or spinal cord, and spasticity may develop following lesions affecting the corticospinal, corticobulbar, or bulbospinal tracts [10]. Musculoskeletal pain problems may result from postural abnormalities [11] or alterations in gait. Headaches are also thought to be a potential consequence of MS [2,12].

## Nature and scope of chronic pain in MS

Historically, pain was not believed to be a significant problem among persons with MS; however, recent research indicates that between 44% and 80% of persons with MS experience pain [2–8,13–15]. A number of factors may account for the variability in the frequency of pain problems identified in different study samples, such as variations in the source from which study samples were drawn (eg, clinic versus community) and the sampling methods used (eg, random, consecutive, convenience). In addition, how pain is defined and measured varies considerably across studies. For example, in one community-based study [8] conducted by the authors' Multiple Sclerosis Research and Training Center, 44% of persons with MS completing a mail survey (N = 442) were categorized as having chronic pain. This prevalence rate is lower than many other studies of pain in MS; however, the definition used for categorizing participants as having chronic pain was more restrictive in this study than definitions used in many other studies: it required respondents to define their pain as both persistent and bothersome for a 3-month time period. Other studies have assessed pain prevalence using shorter time points such as 1 month [2] and using different definitions such as the nonstandardized categorization of "major" and "minor" pain [3]. Surprisingly, the specific questions or measures used to assess pain prevalence were not described in several studies [5,11,14,16]. Although most studies have not differentiated between acute and chronic pain, preliminary evidence suggests that chronic pain may be more prevalent than acute pain in this population [4,6,17]. Future prevalence research on MS pain should distinguish acute pain from chronic pain and provide specific definitions for what constitutes being classified as having pain.

One recent study raised the question of whether pain is truly more frequent in persons with MS relative to the general population. In a Danish population–based postal survey, Svendsen and colleagues [14] compared the rate of pain, including acute pain and chronic pain, between persons with MS (n = 771) and a randomly selected gender- and age-stratified group without MS (n = 769) from the general population. These investigators assessed pain prevalence, intensity, impact, and treatment for the month preceding completion of the survey. The investigators found that the overall frequency of reported pain was high in both groups and not statistically significantly more prevalent in persons with MS (81%) compared with persons in the reference group (63%). After adjusting for other diseases, age, and gender, however, the MS group had a higher prevalence of pain than the reference group (odds ratio = 1.45). The investigators reported that this difference was due to a significant difference ($P < 0.01$) in the prevalence of reported muscle/joint disease between the two groups. The authors also reported that the number of pain sites, pain intensity, treatment requirement, and pain impact were statistically significantly higher in persons with MS relative to the reference group. To better understand the problem of pain in MS, more research is clearly needed on the prevalence and severity of pain problems in persons with MS relative to normative reference groups.

Persons with chronic pain and MS tend to report experiencing pain in a number of different body locations and report pain from a number of sources. For example, pain in the legs, hands, and feet, respectively, were the most commonly endorsed locations for pain in one study of sensory symptoms in persons with MS [5]. A multicenter cross-sectional study [13] looked at the frequency of various types of pain in consecutive patients with MS (N = 1672) presenting to 26 MS centers in Italy. To be counted as present, the pain symptoms had to be present at the time of an in-person structured interview. The following specific types and rates of pain were found: trigeminal neuralgia (2%), Lhermitte's sign (9%), dysethetic pain (18%), back pain (16%), and painful tonic spasms (11%). Headache, pain due to optic neuritis, and musculoskeletal pain in regions other than the back were not included in this study. In this multicenter study, 43% of the sample had some form of pain, and 23% of those with pain had it in more than one location. This is consistent with the literature on pain in other disability samples that has shown that when present, chronic pain is often found in multiple sites [18]. Given that at least some pain secondary to MS is likely to be neuropathic in origin, it is not surprising that verbal descriptors of the pain have included common neuropathic terms such as burning, itching, and electric [5].

In terms of its duration, pain in persons with MS has most frequently been described as intermittent [2,5]. Because most of the research on chronic pain in MS has used cross-sectional survey designs, little is known about the course, stability, and variability of pain problems over time in persons with MS. In the only published, longitudinal follow-up study that the authors could identify, Stenager et al [7] found that the prevalence of chronic pain problems increased dramatically over a 5-year period, doubling, for example, for low back pain (from 12% to 24%) and increasing threefold for extremity pain (from 16% to 55%). Additional knowledge on the natural history of pain in MS would be useful not only for describing the problem but also for making treatment decisions, providing prognostic information, and identifying which patients with MS and pain may most be in need of pain treatment.

When assessed, pain intensity (sometimes referred to as pain severity) is typically mild to moderate for most persons with pain and MS, although a notable subset experiences more severe pain. For example, in the recent study by Ehde et al [8], many (38%) of the survey respondents described their average pain intensity as mild (1–4 on a 0–10 numeric rating scale). Approximately a fourth of those with pain, or 12% of those in the entire sample (N = 442), however, described having a chronic pain problem characterized by pain intensity that on average, over the preceding 3 months, was severe (rated 7–10 on a 0–10 scale).

## Impact of pain

The impact of chronic pain on the lives and health of persons with MS is not well understood. The few studies that have examined the impact of pain on physical and psychosocial functioning among persons with MS indicate that its impact can be severe. For example, in one study, more persons with MS reported that pain interfered with daily life "most of the time" or "all the time" than persons without MS [14]. Moreover, nearly half of persons with MS and chronic pain report that pain interferes either moderately or severely with their daily activities [8]. Persons with MS and chronic pain are also significantly more likely than those without chronic pain to report decreased activity and household work [8]. The relationship between pain and employment in MS is less clear. Although at least one study [2] suggested that over 50% of persons with MS and pain report that pain significantly interferes with their ability to work, other studies [8,16] have found in their samples that persons with MS are equally likely to be employed regardless of whether they experience pain.

The relationship between pain and various aspects of psychosocial functioning in MS is not yet well understood. The results of several studies suggest that there may be a relationship between pain and mental health in persons with MS. For instance, individuals who endorse pain report significantly poorer overall mental health than those who do not report pain [2]. Moreover, in the Ehde et al study [8], it was found that among persons with MS, depression symptom severity was significantly higher among individuals reporting chronic pain compared with those without pain. In addition, among those with chronic pain, increased pain interference with daily activities was significantly associated with depression symptom severity. Despite these findings, several studies have not observed significant differences in scores on self-report measures of depressive symptom severity between persons with MS who report pain and those without pain [4,6].

Research examining the relationship between pain and other aspects of psychosocial functioning in MS is even more limited. The minimal data available suggest that pain can contribute to problems with social functioning. More specifically, nearly one third of a sample of MS out-patients reported that pain had a negative effect on their relationships with spouses, family members, and friends [16]. In a separate study, over a third of persons with MS who experienced pain reported that pain substantially reduced their ability to fulfill various social roles (eg, spouse/partner and parent) [2]. To the authors' knowledge, the only study [6] to examine the relationship between pain and cognitive functioning in MS found that among persons with MS who were admitted to a neurology service, there were no differences in performance on a task of auditory verbal learning between those with and those without pain.

Several studies also examined whether pain in MS is associated with various indices of health. For example, one study [8], it was found that among a large community sample of persons with MS, those with chronic pain reported poorer general health than those without chronic pain. Furthermore, among those with chronic pain, increased pain interference with daily activities was significantly associated with poorer general health and increased fatigue. Increased problems with pain among persons with MS have also been shown to be significantly associated with having been hospitalized during the prior year [19] and with higher rates of health care utilization [20].

## Biopsychosocial factors in chronic pain secondary to MS

Although an understanding of MS disease variables is important in understanding pain in MS, an exclusive focus on biomedical factors results is a very limited view of pain. A more complete understanding of pain can be achieved by using a biopsychosocial model of pain and its impact. A biopsychosocial model acknowledges that biologic factors play an important fundamental role in the experience of pain for most, if not all, individuals with chronic pain [21]. It also argues, however, that psychosocial factors such as family and others' responses to pain behaviors [22,23] and pain-related cognitions, beliefs, and coping behaviors [24,25] also influence adjustment to chronic pain, including psychologic distress, pain-related disability, and health care utilization [25–27]. In the general pain literature, the biopsy-chosocial model has significantly advanced our understanding of some of the variability in individuals' adjustment to chronic pain and provided a useful theoretic framework for treatment. The biopsychosocial model is also consistent with the rehabilitation process model (developed and adopted by the Advisory Board in Medical Rehabilitation Research [28]) and the revised International Classification of Functioning [29], both of which contend that biologic, psychologic, and social factors must be taken into account when trying to understand disability.

Research has attempted to identify demographic (eg, gender, age, marital status) and disease-related factors (eg, MS subtype, disease severity, illness duration) that might be associated with pain in MS. It is unfortunate that studies differ significantly with regard to definitions and methods of assessing pain, recruitment setting (eg, inpatient, community), and the types of pain excluded from analysis, which often makes it difficult to compare findings across studies. Given these caveats, the available evidence does not suggest a strong relationship between gender and pain in MS [2,4,6,8]. The findings related to age and pain are inconclusive. Although findings from several studies indicate that pain increases with age among persons with MS [8,14,17], other studies have not observed this relationship [2,4,6]. To the authors' knowledge, only one study has examined the relationship between income and pain in MS. In this study [30], higher income was associated with decreased problems associated with pain (as measured using the Bodily Pain scale of the Short-Form-36). Other demographic variables, such as ethnicity, education level, living status (ie, living alone or with others), and marital status do not appear in the literature to have been examined.

Regarding disease-related factors, there is minimal evidence in the literature to suggest that pain in MS is related to disease subtype [2,16,31] or severity [2,4,6,17,19,30,32]. The findings from a survey of a large sample of community-dwelling persons with MS, however, indicated that those with chronic pain reported significantly greater disease severity (as measured by the self-report version of the Expanded Disability Status Scale) than those without chronic pain [8]. More research is needed to determine whether disease severity might be related to chronic pain versus acute pain in MS. To date, cross-sectional studies have typically not observed a relationship between disease duration and pain in MS [2,17,5,6,14]; however, the results of the only longitudinal study on pain in MS indicated a significant increase in the prevalence of acute and chronic pain over a 5-year period [7], highlighting the importance of longitudinal research in this area.

The full biopsychosocial model has been largely untested in samples of persons with MS. To the authors' knowledge, no studies have examined key psychosocial components of the biopsychosocial model—including pain-related cognitions, pain-specific coping behaviors, and social support—in persons with MS and chronic pain. Studies of chronic pain that have examined a biopsyochosocial model in other disability groups, including samples of individuals with spinal cord injury [33], limb loss [34–36], and cerebral palsy [37], strongly support the viability of a biopsychosocial model of chronic pain in persons with disabilities. There is a clear need to test these models more extensively in persons with MS. The results of such research will not only provide important additional tests of a biopsychosocial model of pain in the MS population but may also lead to the development of pain interventions based on this model.

## Treatment

Perhaps the most striking gap in the literature is the deficiency of knowledge about effective treatments for chronic pain in persons with MS.

The literature contains a number of descriptions of potential pharmacologic interventions for the various types of pain associated with MS [9,38] but lacks randomized clinical trials that demonstrate the efficacy of these interventions. Given that pharmacotherapeutic interventions are likely the most commonly prescribed treatment for chronic pain in persons with MS, more research on their effectiveness is needed.

A number of studies have demonstrated that treatment approaches based on biopsychosocial models of pain (eg, cognitive–behavioral interventions, operant interventions, interdisciplinary rehabilitation programs) can be effective in improving functioning and in reducing pain, psychologic distress, and pain-related disability in persons in whom pain is the primary problem. For example, in a variety of populations in which chronic pain is the primary condition (eg, arthritis, back pain, headache), cognitive behavioral interventions have been effective in improving physical and psychosocial functioning [39–42]. Several studies have also shown that continued improvements in functioning can occur as many as 6 months after completion of the active cognitive behavioral intervention [43–45]. Such treatment approaches, although having been recommended for MS-related pain as far back as 1988 [17] and described in the MS literature [46], have not yet been adequately empirically evaluated in persons with MS and chronic pain.

Given the lack of evidenced-based clinical standards for the treatment of MS pain, clinicians may turn to the broader pain treatment literature for ideas on MS pain [47]. Although potentially useful, it is unknown whether persons with significant MS pain access and utilize existing pain treatments including pain specialists and pain multidisciplinary treatment programs. A few studies have suggested that persons with MS-related pain may not be receiving adequate treatment for their pain. Goodin [3] found that only 36% of survey respondents with "major" pain had received pain treatment.

The current treatment literature is notable for its lack of attention to factors that may influence the ability of an individual with MS to benefit from or access pain treatment in the context of having this neurologic condition. A number of reasons could hypothetically account for difficulties in accessing pain treatment. Some individuals with MS have cognitive and communication impairments that may interfere with their ability to (1) be identified by health care professionals as having a pain problem, (2) access health care for pain, and (3) participate in standard pain interventions. In addition, given the potential number of other MS-related symptoms and concerns, pain may be overlooked or prioritized as less important by the person with MS, by the health care provider, or both. There may also be environmental barriers such as lack of transportation, lack of accessible pain or MS specialists, or lack of financial resources that impede treatment of pain in persons with MS. Although not studied, pain may be inadequately treated due to such barriers.

## Summary

The MS literature clearly indicates that chronic pain is a significant problem for many, although not all, persons with MS. The rates of pain have been found to vary in different studies, from 44% to 80%, depending on the sample and the specific questions used to assess the incidence and severity of pain. What is not clear is the proportion of persons who have acute pain relative to chronic pain. Although the specific frequency of pain problems in patients with MS may not be clear, there is a subgroup of patients (about 38% of those with pain in one sample) who report experiencing severe pain [8]. Preliminary research suggests that chronic pain can have a significant negative impact on a number of aspects of functioning in persons with MS, such as the ability to engage in household work and psychologic functioning. A biopsychosocial model of chronic pain, which has proved to be useful in understanding chronic pain as a primary condition and chronic pain in persons with other physical disabilities, may also be useful for understanding pain in persons with MS. Research, however, has not yet tested the utility of this model among MS populations. Longitudinal research is needed to help us learn how MS-related pain may fluctuate over time and with changes in disease status. There also is a strong need for research that examines access to pain treatment and that evaluates the efficacy of currently available pain treatments in persons with MS. The results of such research, as it is applied to help patients with MS, should contribute to an overall increase in well-being and a decrease in suffering among persons with MS and chronic pain.

## References

[1] Aring CD. Pain in multiple sclerosis. JAMA 1973;223(5):547.
[2] Archibald CJ, McGrath PJ, Ritvo PG, et al. Pain prevalence, severity and impact in a clinic sample of multiple sclerosis patients. Pain 1994;58(1):89–93.
[3] Goodin DS. Survey of multiple sclerosis in northern California. Northern California MS Study Group. Mult Scler 1999;5(2):78–88.
[4] Indaco A, Iachetta C, Nappi C, et al. Chronic and acute pain syndromes in patients with multiple sclerosis. Acta Neurol (Napoli) 1994;16(3):97–102.
[5] Rae-Grant AD, Eckert NJ, Bartz S, et al. Sensory symptoms of multiple sclerosis: a hidden reservoir of morbidity. Mult Scler 1999;5(3):179–83.
[6] Stenager E, Knudsen L, Jensen K. Acute and chronic pain syndromes in multiple sclerosis. Acta Neurol Scand 1991;84(3):197–200.
[7] Stenager E, Knudsen L, Jensen K. Acute and chronic pain syndromes in multiple sclerosis. A 5-year follow-up study. Ital J Neurol Sci 1995;16(9):629–32.
[8] Ehde DM, Gibbons LE, Chwastiak L, et al. Chronic pain in a large community sample of persons with multiple sclerosis. Mult Scler 2003;9(6):605–11.
[9] Joy JE, Johnston RB. Multiple sclerosis: current status and strategies for the future. Washington, DC: National Academy Press; 2001.
[10] Perkins FM, Moxley RT III, Papciak AS. Pain in multiple sclerosis and the muscular dystrophies. In: Block AR, Kremer F, Fernandez E, editors. Handbook of pain syndromes: biopsychosocial perspectives. Mahwah (NJ): Erlbaum; 1999. p. 349–70.

[11] Kassirer MR, Osterberg DH. Pain in chronic multiple sclerosis. J Pain Symptom Manage 1987;2(2):95–7.

[12] Rolak LA, Brown S. Headaches and multiple sclerosis: a clinical study and review of the literature. J Neurol 1990;237:300–2.

[13] Solaro C, Brichetto G, Amato MP, et al. The prevalence of pain in multiple sclerosis: a multicenter cross-sectional study. Neurology 2004;63(5):919–21.

[14] Svendsen KB, Jensen TS, Overvad K, et al. Pain in patients with multiple sclerosis: a population-based study. Arch Neurol 2003;60(8):1089–94.

[15] Beiske AG, Pedersen ED, Czujko B, et al. Pain and sensory complaints in multiple sclerosis. Eur J Neurol 2004;11(7):479–82.

[16] Warnell P. The pain experience of a multiple sclerosis population: a descriptive study. Axone 1991;13(1):26–8.

[17] Moulin DE, Foley KM, Ebers GC. Pain syndromes in multiple sclerosis. Neurology 1988; 38(12):1830–4.

[18] Ehde DM, Jensen MP, Engel JM, et al. Chronic pain secondary to disability: a review. Clin J Pain 2003;19:3–17.

[19] Vickrey BG, Hays RD, Harooni R, et al. A health-related quality of life measure for multiple sclerosis. Qual Life Res 1995;4(3):187–206.

[20] Sullivan MJL, Edgley K, Mikail S, et al. Psychological correlates of health care utilization in chronic illness. Can J Rehabil 1992;6:13–21.

[21] Novy DM, Nelson DV, Francis DJ, et al. Perspectives of chronic pain: an evaluative comparison of restrictive and comprehensive models. Psychol Bull 1995;118(2):238–47.

[22] Fordyce WE. Behavioral methods for chronic pain and illness. St. Louis (MO): Mosby Year Book; 1976.

[23] Fordyce WE, Fowler RS Jr, Lehmann JF, et al. Operant conditioning in the treatment of chronic pain. Arch Phys Med Rehabil 1973;54(9):399–408.

[24] Jensen MP, Turner JA, Romano JM, et al. Relationship of pain-specific beliefs to chronic pain adjustment. Pain 1994;57:301–9.

[25] Jensen MP, Turner JA, Romano JM, et al. Coping with chronic pain: a critical review of the literature. Pain 1991;47(3):249–83.

[26] Jensen MP, Romano JM, Turner JA, et al. Patient beliefs predict patient functioning: further support for a cognitive-behavioural model of chronic pain. Pain 1999;81(1–2): 95–104.

[27] Jensen MP, Turner JA, Romano JM. Correlates of improvement in multidisciplinary treatment of chronic pain. J Consult Clin Psychol 1994;62(1):172–9.

[28] National Institutes of Health. Research Plan for the National Center for Medical Rehabilitation Research. Washington, DC: US Government Printing Office; 1993. Publication #NIH 93-3509.

[29] World Health Organization. International Classification of Functioning, Disability, and Health: ICF. Geneva: WHO; 2001.

[30] Brunet DG, Hopman WM, Singer MA, et al. Measurement of health-related quality of life in multiple sclerosis patients. Can J Neurol Sci 1996;23(2):99–103.

[31] Heckman-Stone C, Stone C. Pain management techniques used by patients with multiple sclerosis. J Pain 2001;2(4):205–8.

[32] Nortvedt MW, Riise T, Myhr KM, et al. Quality of life in multiple sclerosis: measuring the disease effects more broadly. Neurology 1999;53(5):1098–103.

[33] Turner JA, Jensen MP, Warms CA, et al. Catastrophizing is associated with pain intensity, psychological distress, and pain-related disability among individuals with chronic pain after spinal cord injury. Pain 2002;98(1–2):127–34.

[34] Hill A. The use of pain coping strategies by patients with phantom limb pain. Pain 1993; 55(3):347–53.

[35] Hill A, Niven CA, Knussen C. The role of coping in adjustment to phantom limb pain. Pain 1995;62(1):79–86.

[36] Jensen MP, Ehde DM, Hoffman AJ, et al. Cognitions, coping and social environment predict adjustment to phantom limb pain. Pain 2002;95(1–2):133–42.
[37] Engel JM, Schwartz L, Jensen MP, et al. Pain in cerebral palsy: the relation of coping strategies to adjustment. Pain 2000;88(3):225–30.
[38] Kassirer M. Multiple sclerosis and pain. Int J MS Care 2000;2(3):30–8.
[39] Turk DC, Okifuji A, Sinclair JD, et al. Differential responses by psychosocial subgroups of fibromyalgia syndrome patients to an interdisciplinary treatment. Arthritis Care Res 1998; 11(5):397–404.
[40] Dworkin SF, Turner JA, Wilson L, et al. Brief group cognitive-behavioral intervention for temporomandibular disorders. Pain 1994;59(2):175–87.
[41] Morley S, Eccleston C, Williams A. Systematic review and meta-analysis of randomized controlled trials of cognitive behaviour therapy and behaviour therapy for chronic pain in adults, excluding headache. Pain 1999;80(1–2):1–13.
[42] Turner JA, Jensen MP. Efficacy of cognitive therapy for chronic low back pain. Pain 1993; 52(2):169–77.
[43] Bennett RM, Burckhardt CS, Clark SR, et al. Group treatment of fibromyalgia: a 6 month outpatient program. J Rheumatol 1996;23(3):521–8.
[44] Peters J, Large RG, Elkind G. Follow-up results from a randomised controlled trial evaluating in- and outpatient pain management programmes. Pain 1992;50(1):41–50.
[45] Turk DC, Rudy TE, Kubinski JA, et al. Dysfunctional patients with temporomandibular disorders: evaluating the efficacy of a tailored treatment protocol. J Consult Clin Psychol 1996;64(1):139–46.
[46] Kerns R. Psychosocial aspects of pain. Int J MS Care 2000;2(4):35–8.
[47] Robinson J, Jensen MP. Chronic pain management in patients with a history of trauma. In: Robinson LR, editor. Trauma rehabilitation. Philadelphia: Lippincott Williams & Wilkins 2005.

ELSEVIER
SAUNDERS

Phys Med Rehabil Clin N Am
16 (2005) 513–555

PHYSICAL MEDICINE
AND REHABILITATION
CLINICS OF
NORTH AMERICA

# Exercise and Rehabilitation for Individuals with Multiple Sclerosis

Theodore R. Brown, MD, MPH[a],*,
George H. Kraft, MD, MS[b]

[a]MS Hub Medical Group, 1100 Olive Way, Suite 150, Seattle, WA 98101, USA
[b]Department of Rehabilitation Medicine, University of Washington School of Medicine,
Harborview Medical Center, 325 9th Avenue, Seattle, WA 98195-6490, USA

Diagnosis occurs only once, but management takes place over a lifetime.
—George H. Kraft

Multiple sclerosis (MS) afflicts 1 in 1000 people in western countries, where it also is the leading nontraumatic cause of neurologic disability in young adults. Untreated, from symptom onset, the median time is 20 years until a cane is required and 30 years until becoming wheelchair reliant [1]. About two thirds of people with MS are unemployed and 75% of them attribute their unemployment to disability. For the purpose of this article, *impairment* refers to the primary deficit caused by the disease, *disability* denotes functional limitations imposed by the disease, and *handicap* refers to the social disadvantages resulting from a disease.

Thompson [2], who has been involved in several of the studies described in this article, reviewed the inherent difficulties in demonstrating the evidence-based effectiveness of rehabilitation for MS. Problems include the heterogeneity of disease manifestations, the variable and unpredictable course of the disease, the difficulty of blinding and providing a valid placebo, and the inconsistent use of appropriate outcome measures. The expense of therapy and the lack of an animal model are two additional problems. Among the existing outcome measures in MS, the most commonly used is the Kurtzke Expanded Disability Status Scale (EDSS)

This work was supported in part by the United Spinal Association project 659 and the National Institute on Disability and Rehabilitation Research, Department of Education grant H133B031129-04.

* Corresponding author.
*E-mail address:* berktocm@yahoo.com (T.R. Brown).

doi:10.1016/j.pmr.2005.01.005
*pmr.theclinics.com*

[3]. The scale ranges from 0 (no impairment) to 10 (death from MS), with half-point levels along the way. It focuses more on mobility than on sensory, bowel and bladder, communicative, or cognitive impairments. Different investigators have variously described this scale as a measure of impairment or of disability [4,5]. This scale, however, contains elements of impairment (eg, loss of sensation) at the lower end of the scale and disability (loss of unaided ambulation) toward the upper range of the scale. The midrange is heavily weighted on ambulation and vulnerable to inter-rater and intrarater fluctuations. For example, the difference between EDSS scores of 5.5 and 5.0 is the difference in ability to walk unaided 100 m but not 200 m. For an individual, a change in EDSS must be at least two levels (a change in 1 point) to be considered significant because the reliability of half-point changes is poor [6]. A 10-year follow-up study done by the Mayo Clinic found that a cohort of 162 MS patients had a mean change in their EDSS of only 1 point over the decade [7], yet only 15% of the patients were on disease-modifying therapy. Given that most studies of rehabilitation last less than a year and produce subtle changes, the EDSS may be too insensitive to detect a treatment effect on disease progression, causing type 2 error.

The MS Functional Composite was created as a quantitative index of neurologic function [8]. It combines the 9-hole peg test, the timed 25-foot walk, and the Paced Auditory Serial Addition Test, used as upper limb, lower limb, and cognitive impairment measures, respectively. The MS Functional Composite is less prone to inter-rater variability and more sensitive to small changes than the EDSS. The component parts of the MS Functional Composite are all well validated, but as a composite measure, it has not gained universal acceptance as a valid outcome measure of MS impairment and disability. For better or worse, the EDSS remains the "gold standard" for intervention trials [9]. In the field of rehabilitation, more specific functional measures should be encouraged.

As a chronic disease, MS has a dramatic impact on quality of life (QOL). MS disrupts established roles in the family and in society. It threatens one's educational and vocational opportunities and reduces income. It diminishes a person's self-efficacy, that is, his or her confidence in coping with the challenges of everyday life. The first attempt to gauge QOL in MS was by Rudick et al [10] who measured and compared QOL in patients with MS and two other chronic diseases: inflammatory bowel disease and rheumatoid arthritis. Of the MS patients, half had little or no impairment (EDSS ≤5) and half had higher levels of impairment. Results were that QOL was worse in the MS group. Women had lower scores than men for all three diseases, indicating a strong gender difference in the impact of chronic disease on QOL. For the MS patients, QOL correlated with level of impairment, especially with pyramidal tract, brainstem, and visual components of the EDSS. Another study by Jonssen et al [11] did not confirm the association between QOL and EDSS, so the link may not be very strong. It has also been found that physicians base their impressions of patient QOL in terms of the physical manifestations of

MS, whereas patients feel that role limitations, cognition, and emotional problems have the most significant influences on well-being [12,13].

There are conflicting reports about the relationship between disease severity, as measured by the EDSS, and depression. A study by Harper et al [14] found that EDSS correlated with physical and social QOL indices (including unemployment and low income) but was unrelated to emotional health. Less than 2% of the variance in mental health was accounted for by the EDSS. In contrast, a more recent study by Chwastiak et al [15] reported that subjects with intermediate or high scores on a self-reported version of EDSS were, respectively, three or six times as likely as subjects with low scores to have clinically significant depressive symptoms. A staggering 42% of the survey respondents reported depressive symptoms. With depression being so common, everyone with MS (not just those with advanced disease) should be clinically assessed for psychologic difficulties.

## Effect of relapses on impairment and disability

Lublin et al [16] reviewed data from a meta-analysis of primary and secondary outcomes in existing United States clinical and historical MS data sets to test the effect of relapses on development of disability. These investigators found that each attack carries a 42% chance of adding measurable residual impairment and that the mean was an additional 0.3 EDSS score per attack. Residual deficits that persist for 3 months post exacerbation usually do not resolve. Successful clinical trials with immunomodulatory drugs have shown clear evidence of or a trend toward slowed accrual of impairment while consistently showing reduced relapse rates. These studies were all conducted in ambulatory patients who continued to have relapses. In contrast, Confavreux et al [1,17] retrospectively studied a large French MS cohort and reported that relapse rates predict accrual of impairment only up to a point at which a mild degree of permanent disability is present (EDSS = 4.0). At higher levels of disability, there is a disconnection between relapses and progression of disability (ie, the rate of worsening impairment is independent of the relapse rate). Together, these findings suggest that relapses are associated with worsening impairment at the early stages of the disease (when inflammation is prominent) but probably not after marked disability has been acquired (when neurodegenerative changes predominate). Therefore, to have an effect on disability, treatment must be started early.

A confounding factor, however, is the definition and identification of a relapse or exacerbation. Traditionally, a relapse is the development of a new symptom or sign or the worsening of existing ones. However, recent research has indicated that patients may not be aware of many relapses. Frequent gadolinium-enhanced MRI scans of the brain (every 4 to 6 weeks) have shown 5 to 10 relapses not recognized by the MS patient [18]. Although initially counterintuitive, it is likely that the disease activity in the central nervous system not directly involving visual, sensory, or motor pathways may not be appreciated as a relapse. Indeed, might such activity account for the intermittent memory loss and mood dysfunction often experienced by patients with MS? After all, most of the brain's white matter does not involve visual, motor, or sensory pathways.

## Use of rehabilitation services

An investigation of rehabilitation usage patterns in North America was conducted by Hadjimichael [19]. Using a self-selected patient registry (North American Research Committee on Multiple Sclerosis [NARCOMS] data), it was found that 66% of 21,330 active registry participants had used rehabilitation at some time and that 31% were current users. The most frequently used rehabilitation service was physical therapy (PT; 41%), followed, in decreasing order, by occupational therapy (OT), psychology, massage therapy, and social worker and speech therapy. About 13% had received care from a physiatrist MS specialist. As would be expected, older age, longer duration of disease, more reported relapses, and higher disability all correlated with increased use of rehabilitation services. The survey showed that rehabilitation users tend to have fewer years of education, less income, lower rates of employment, and consequently, less private insurance coverage.

A survey done in western Washington State and published in 1986 [20] found that the use of and need for rehabilitation services and community services (eg, visiting nurse, transportation) was primarily a function of the MS patient's level of disability. Perceived need for psychology, social, and vocational services was related to the individual's youth and the recency of her or his MS diagnosis. It is unfortunate that MS is a moving target. Unlike stroke or spinal cord injury, it is a dynamic process, especially for most of individuals who have relapsing forms of MS. Rehabilitation in MS is therefore not likely to occur over a finite period of time but is an ongoing effort, which means that more frequent visits to physiatrists, physical and occupational therapists, and other specialties may be needed for MS than for most other neurologic disorders. Because it is progressive, rehabilitation professionals need to anticipate future needs and lay the groundwork for services and equipment in advance. Taking this proactive approach to therapy has been termed *over-rehabilitation* by Kraft [21]. An example would be to encourage balance and endurance training before someone has begun to experience falls or fatigue. One should initiate a vocational rehabilitation evaluation at the first sign of work-related difficulty, not when the work situation has reached a crisis point, and should order a power wheelchair before an individual will be totally dependent on it, not after.

## Effects of inpatient rehabilitation on MS

Relative to other patients admitted to the rehabilitation service, MS patients are typically younger and less disabled. They experience shorter lengths of stay and make fewer improvements in activities of daily living (ADL) and mobility than patients with head injury, spinal cord injury, or stroke [22]. Their stays are shorter because the loss of function produced by an exacerbation is usually a smaller interval of change than for most neurorehabilitation conditions that require admission. Consequently, health insurers may be unwilling to authorize more than a few weeks of inpatient rehabilitation for MS patients.

Some health professionals have felt that inpatient rehabilitation is not appropriate for persons with MS because it is a chronic, progressive disease or because rehabilitation can also be done on an outpatient basis, in a subacute rehabilitation facility, or in an acute care hospital at equal or lower costs [23,24]. Others might advocate selecting rehabilitation only for MS individuals who are still ambulatory. To expect that rehabilitation will only have an impact on a person's mobility is to shortchange the process. The goal of rehabilitation in MS is to maximize the individual's physical, emotional, social, and vocational independence and to improve QOL for them and their caregivers. Because MS impacts many aspects of a person's life, an individualized, multidisciplinary approach is essential to rehabilitation. Inpatient rehabilitation is often the most appropriate setting in which to treat complex or extensive rehabilitation needs.

Several studies of inpatient rehabilitation have been patient series and pre/post studies that reported improvements in impairment (eg, walking distance) and disability (Functional Independence Measure [FIM] score) but provided no postdischarge follow-up. Two retrospective studies of inpatient rehabilitation with similar numbers of MS patients (N = 28 and 37) and similar average lengths of stay (28 and 32 days) found statistically significant improvements on impairment and disability measures that lasted up to 3 months post discharge [25,26]. With one exception [27], a large percentage of the patients in these studies were admitted after relapses, sometimes coming directly from acute care services. Thus, a probable confounding effect of spontaneous neurorecovery limits the interpretation of the positive results.

One of the first randomized controlled trials (RCTs) was by Francabandera et al [24] who randomized 84 MS individuals with severe disability to inpatient rehabilitation (individualized PT and OT, rehabilitation nursing, and speech therapy) averaging 3 weeks or to outpatient visiting nurse, PT, and OT services (duration not specified). Despite randomization, the two groups were significantly different in functional status at entry. At 3 months post discharge, the inpatient group showed less disability than the outpatient group but equal need for home assistance. Subsequently, the inpatient group had more rapid loss of function than the outpatient group so that there was no difference in disability and no advantage to having had inpatient versus outpatient rehabilitation over 12 months of follow-up [28]. This study did not make a convincing case in favor of either rehabilitation setting.

Freeman et al [29] did two studies of inpatient rehabilitation for individuals with progressive forms of MS. The first study was an RCT with nonambulatory MS patients who received multidisciplinary inpatient rehabilitation (average length of stay = 3.5 weeks) or wait listing. This study demonstrated differences in disability (FIM score) and handicap (London Handicap Scale) but not in impairment, in favor of the rehabilitation admission group. In the second trial, the same investigators used a similar cohort without randomization, putting all subjects through an inpatient rehabilitation program. They then provided a 1-year follow-up to see how well the benefits of inpatient rehabilitation carried over into the community [5]. FIM and handicap scores were improved at discharge and were determined to be clinically meaningful (mean improvement in FIM score = 15 on a scale from 0–100) [29]. FIM scores declined back to baseline at 6 months, which suggests that 6 months may be the duration of the treatment effect of inpatient rehabilitation, after which time rehabilitation needs should be re-examined.

The publication of the second Freeman article was accompanied by another report of inpatient rehabilitation by different investigators. Solari et al [4] did an RCT of 3 weeks of inpatient rehabilitation with 50 ambulatory MS subjects. The intervention group received passive range of motion, balance and gait training with mobility aids, and strengthening. The control group had instruction in a home-based self-administered program. Both groups were followed for 15 weeks after commencement of rehabilitation. In both groups, the final EDSS was unchanged; however, the intervention group had significantly better FIM scores at discharge. This difference persisted for 9 weeks, but was nonsignificant at 15 weeks, although FIM subcomponents of self-care and locomotion remained significantly better.

Although other studies found functional benefits of inpatient rehabilitation that gradually disappeared post discharge, there has been one negative study showing no improvement in function immediately post inpatient rehabilitation stay [30]. In this study, face-to-face therapy averaged only 38 minutes a day, which may have been insufficient to produce a measurable difference. The study showed that mobility-related stress was significantly less in the intervention group, which may have translated into improved QOL.

Four other studies demonstrated that inpatient rehabilitation has a beneficial effect on QOL in MS. Jønsson et al [11] studied QOL and depression indices before and after inpatient rehabilitation (5–8 weeks) in 21 MS individuals. Significant improvements in overall QOL and fatigue, mood, endurance, Beck Depression Inventory, and anxiety levels regarding work and stair climbing were found. Solari et al [4] and Freeman et al [5] found emotional QOL and health-related QOL improvements lasting between 9 weeks and 10 months post discharge. Mostert and Kesselring [31] reported the results of 3 to 4 weeks of bicycle ergometry in an inpatient rehabilitation setting. The intervention group (n = 13) made significant gains in a few health-related QOL indicators (sport-related activity level, vitality, social functioning) and fitness parameters (maximum work rate and oxygen consumption at aerobic threshold), whereas a nonexercised control group (n = 13) that also received inpatient rehabilitation did not. Neither group had improved fatigue levels. This is the only study to have compared different inpatient rehabilitation programs.

Recently, Craig et al [32] published an RCT comparing multidisciplinary team rehabilitation versus none in the setting of inpatient admission for MS exacerbations. Mean length of stay was equivalent in the two groups (N = 53) and both received intravenous methylprednisolone for 3 days. The therapy interventions included an average of 2.6 hours of PT, 1.5 hours of OT, and other visits by rehabilitation nurses, speech therapists, and orthotists, with teaching provided on health promotion including home stretching and bladder management. The inpatient rehabilitation was often followed up by home therapy, and the investigators could not distinguish the relative contribution of inpatient and postdischarge interventions to improved outcomes. At 3 months post discharge, no significant differences existed in EDSS or QOL. There were differences favoring the multidisciplinary group in the Guy's neurologic disability scale, amended motor club assessment, human activity profile, and Barthel index.

It has been more than 2 decades since a cost–benefit analysis of inpatient rehabilitation for MS has been performed. In 1981, Feigenson et al [33] estimated the costs of care for 20 MS patients, before and after admission, for an average of 52 days of rehabilitation. Such a long average length of rehabilitation stay would not be funded today. These investigators estimated that rehabilitation improved functional independence to such an extent that the average annual cost of home services (based on an estimated hourly rate of $5.50 for a homemaker or companion) fell from $26,909 to $10,583. Savings on home care ($34,223 in inflation-adjusted 2002 US dollars [34]) meant that inpatient rehabilitation paid for itself within 1 year. These cost estimates were guessed, not based, on actual expenditures. Patients with a poor outcome (death or admission to a nursing home) were excluded from the analysis, which skewed the results in favor of cost-effectiveness. On the other hand, if similar benefits could be squeezed out of the shorter length of stays that are now typical, then the benefits/cost could be greater.

Specialized rehabilitation spa programs have been developed in Europe and at a few centers around the United States. These differ from an inpatient hospital admission in that the mountain resort settings and lack of daily vital signs and medical check-ups promotes a more holistic, empowering, and enjoyable experience. At the Jimmie Heuga Center in Colorado, groups of people with MS proceed through a 5-day program of fitness evaluation and learn principles of stress management, nutrition, and coping mechanisms. The value of this innovative program has not been tested. Vaney et al [35] studied the effects of inpatient rehabilitation (average of 4 weeks' stay with daily PT, OT, aquatic exercise, and horseback riding) on 200 consecutive MS patients in an MS specialty center in Switzerland. Only 7.5% experienced any improvement in EDSS, but 39% improved on the Rivermead Mobility Index (RMI). Italian investigators "brought the rehabilitation center to the home" and delivered individualized, multidisciplinary rehabilitation team care, then compared this intervention with usual care [36]. After 1 year, several QOL measures and a cost benefit analysis favored home-based care, but there was no difference in functional status. Bias in selection of subjects and lack of blinding are limitations of these alternative-site rehabilitation program studies.

Most MS patients enter the rehabilitation unit expecting to gain improved strength and ambulation. The sum of research indicates that those are false hopes. Seldom does inpatient rehabilitation change patients' neurologic impairments or make wheelchair users walk again. (If the patient had not previously had rehabilitative services, however, the results could be dramatic; a bed-bound patient having an EDSS of 8.5 might be made ambulatory with an EDSS of 6.5.) The admission also does not result in return to gainful employment. It is in the areas of balance, transfers, general fitness, self-care, bladder control, and use of adaptive devices that most gains are made. Because impairments cannot be modified, compensatory strategies play an important part of rehabilitation strategies. Patients and their families need guidance to set reachable goals for admission so that they do not become disappointed and uncooperative as the discharge date approaches.

It would be nice to know which MS patients are most likely to benefit from inpatient rehabilitation, but the medical literature contains conflicting reports, at least regarding the relationship between EDSS on admission and functional gain. One study found greatest improvement among the moderately to severely disabled individuals, whereas another found a trend in the opposite direction [37,38]. A third study found that baseline EDSS did not correlate in a positive or a negative way with change in disability (FIM score) resulting from inpatient rehabilitation [39]. The baseline FIM score, verbal skills, and preserved cerebellar function were the only factors that predicted the change in disability. Other investigators have remarked on the refractory nature of cognitive and cerebellar dysfunctions [38,40].

To summarize, inpatient rehabilitation for MS yields short-term benefits in function, mobility, and several aspects of QOL. Benefits have generally been more impressive in uncontrolled, retrospective trials that have included patients recovering from exacerbations. Studies that have looked for extended carryover have found that benefits dwindled by 6 to 10 months. In some studies, this finding has been attributed to disease progression, whereas in others, disease progression was not a possible explanation because the EDSS remained stable [4,5]. Because the benefits of inpatient rehabilitation are not long-term, periodic admission for rehabilitation may be needed, which is the practice of many European countries. Updated cost-benefit analysis should be done to determine the clinical effectiveness of inpatient rehabilitation for MS. In the future, there is probably more to learn from multicenter study of the individual-component specialties that make up the rehabilitation team than there is from studying the whole multidisciplinary team effect at one center. There is also a need for RCTs of inpatient rehabilitation versus outpatient and home-based rehabilitation.

## Fatigue: the leading MS symptom

Fatigue among MS individuals is defined as "a sense of physical tiredness and lack of energy, distinct from sadness or weakness" [41]. Although it is the most common symptom of MS, with a frequency of 70% or more in patient surveys, it was under-recognized before 2 decades ago [13,20,42]. Individuals with MS report many symptoms, but fatigue is usually among the most troublesome. Over 80% who have fatigue report that it is exacerbated by heat, which appears to be a difference between MS fatigue and fatigue due to other chronic diseases [43]. Fatigue is the most common primary reason given for unemployment by MS individuals [44]. Fatigue has a negative influence on mental health; mental illness may also worsen fatigue [43,44]. A worsening of fatigue may herald an MS exacerbation. The relationship between cognitive function and perceived fatigue remains uncertain, but most studies have not shown a direct association [45].

In most studies, MS fatigue is more commonly reported in women than men. It correlates weakly with age and negatively with years of education [46]. Typical clinical factors such as EDSS and disease duration have little bearing on the impact of fatigue as reported by MS individuals. In fact, individuals with shorter disease duration tend to report more fatigue than those in the same age group with longer disease duration [46]. This tendency may be because in the absence of more prominent and progressive neurologic symptoms, fatigue is the most salient and functionally limiting symptom for those with mild MS. Recent research in learning raises the question as to whether sleep is necessary for effective brain plasticity and may be a reparative mechanism in persons with MS [47].

Muscular fatigue, defined as the loss of maximal capacity to generate force during exercise, is also observed in MS [48]. Muscular fatigue correlates poorly ($r = 0.2$) with the perceived fatigue that is so commonly reported on patient questionnaires [49,50]. People with MS generally have less power and less muscle endurance than healthy controls [51,52]. Sheean et al [49] found that the force of a 45-second isometric contraction of the adductor pollicis muscle declined by 20% in control subjects and by 45% in MS patients. Another MS study found that even muscles that are not weak on maximum strength testing have increased muscular fatigue compared with normal muscles during sustained or repetitive contractions [48]. The excessive motor fatigue induced by exercise in MS may be analogous to the visual Uhthoff phenomenon previously described, but the pathogenic mechanism has yet to be described [53].

Muscular fatigue appears to result from combined central and peripheral mechanisms. Central factors may be most important, yet they have proved difficult to identify and understand. Colombo et al [54] found that the lesion load of MS plaques on brain MRI correlates with fatigue in MS individuals. Two studies of transcranial magnetic brain stimulation have found no evidence of decremental responses [49,55]. Electromyographic studies in MS have found decreased maximum motor unit firing rates [56], decreased motor unit recruitment [50], and increased surface electromyographic activity relative to force generation [57]. One group of investigators first implicated increased central motor drive and subsequently implicated decreased central motor drive as the central factor in MS muscle fatigue [57,58]. Peripheral factors are intramuscular. Muscle in persons with MS has less aerobic capacity (smaller metabolic response to exercise) than does muscle from healthy subjects. This deficiency may result from disuse and deconditioning subsequent to a sedentary lifestyle [57,59–61]. It has also been postulated that cardiovascular disregulation due to sympathetic dysfunction may contribute to decreased muscle endurance in MS [62,63].

Whereas perceived fatigue cannot be predicted by the severity of disease, the metabolic response to exercise is adversely affected by worsening impairment. Tantucci et al [64] tested 10 MS individuals with an EDSS of 1 or less and 10 matched controls at submaximal cycle ergometry. No difference in the metabolic cost of exercise was found. For individuals with more severe MS with weakness, spasticity, or ataxia, the metabolic cost of walking has been found to be two or three times greater than in normal subjects [27]. It is assumed that the high-energy cost of exercise contributes to the observed muscle fatigue.

Fatigue is not always the direct result of MS. It may be an adverse effect from spasmolytic, anticholinergic, antidepressant, analgesic, or anticonvulsant drugs. Clinicians should also consider concomitant diseases as a cause for fatigue, including anemia, hypothyroidism or other endocrine dysfunction, infection, malignancy, and sleep apnea. Psychiatric and social problems such as depression, alcohol and substance abuse, family strife, and excessive work or study could also underlie complaints of fatigue.

Krupp et al [43] developed the Fatigue Severity Scale, which they used to differentiate individuals with MS and lupus from normal subjects. The scale consists of nine statements about fatigue symptoms to which subjects respond using a 7-point Likert scale. Scores for each statement are summed. With a maximum score of 63, the mean for normal healthy controls is 21, the lower cut-off for fatigue is 36, and the mean for MS individuals is 43. In other words, most MS individuals (in fact, 91%) score above the cut-off for fatigue, with scores stacked at the top of the scale (ceiling effect) [43,65]. Some insurers use the Fatigue Severity Scale score as a determining factor for prescription approvals; however, the scale has also been criticized as insensitive to subtle change and therefore unsuitable for monitoring fatigue in clinical practice [65,66]. Fisk et al [44] developed the Fatigue Impact Scale as a more detailed measure that differentiates between physical, cognitive, and social aspects of fatigue. This scale is much more detailed, with 42 Likert-type questions. It is more sensitive but also more time-consuming.

There is a need to develop an objective muscle fatigue index that could be used alongside the existing subjective measures of fatigue for clinical and research purposes in MS.

## Safety of exercise in MS

The inability to sustain physical activity and greater impairment after elevation of body temperature has been reported and was once the basis of the "hot bath" diagnostic test for MS [67–69]. The Uhthoff phenomenon was originally described as transient amblyopia occurring with exercise or overheating [70]. The term has been applied more generally to encompass other symptoms, as described by Petajan and White [71]: "A test at rest may indicate normal function, although the individual later exhibits abnormal fatigue, conduction block or other symptoms such as spasticity or lack of coordination after only brief exercise or exposure to heat." It is less common for heating to produce this sort of focal neurologic sign than for it to produce general fatigue [72]. The Uhthoff phenomenon may be due to an exercise-associated rise in the core body temperature (which interferes with conduction across partly demyelinated axons), the fatigue of damaged neuronal pathways with repetitive nerve transmission [53], or a circulating/hormonal factor produced when temperature declines [47].

It is ironic that in the 1960s, heat, whirlpool, Hubbard tank, and sauna were regarded as useful preliminaries to exercise in MS, whereas the exercise itself was controversial [73]. Many physicians advised against exercise, even to the point of advocating bed rest because they worried about exercise-induced fatigue and induction of MS exacerbations. Fear that exercise would sap energy for ADL has also led many individuals with MS to forego exercise and recreation. In fact, there has been no evidence that exercise influences the primary pathologic processes in MS and, beyond anecdotal reports, no study of exercise in MS has ever shown a detrimental effect of training.

Ponichtera-Mulcare et al [74] measured core temperature rectally in nine MS individuals during exercise on land and in water. The mean change over the test period was 0.1°C on land and −0.1°C in water. Subjects reported no symptoms except general fatigue with the exercises. This and the cumulative results of other research reassure us that routine exercise is unlikely to raise core temperatures significantly. Even though the Uhthoff phenomenon might occur with exercise, it is usually reversible and it should not be regarded as a contraindication to exercise.

There are three reviews of the literature on exercise physiology and MS up to the year 2001 [28,72,75]. These reviews have drawn several conclusions:

1. For mild cases of MS, muscle function is close to normal.
2. MS individuals with minimal to moderate neurologic impairment usually have preserved cardiovascular responses during exercise. An exception is that some individuals with MS have a blunted heart-rate

response to increased exercise stress. These individuals tend to be more highly impaired.

3. Maximal aerobic capacity in persons with MS is influenced by the degree of physical impairment. Individuals with more impairment are able to exercise for a shorter period and achieve a lower maximal exercise intensity and lower maximal oxygen uptake.

4. Respiratory muscle dysfunction and deconditioning limit aerobic capacity.

5. Regular exercise has a positive affect on fitness as it does for healthy individuals, but improvements may be less impressive when there is more neurologic impairment.

Metabolic and physiologic studies of exercise with paraplegia have demonstrated that the small muscle mass in the upper limbs imposes an upper limit to aerobic performance [76,77]. This finding implies that people with MS who have limited use of the lower limbs due to weakness, spasticity, or cerebellar dysfunction may not be able to increase their metabolic rate sufficiently to improve aerobic fitness. Research by Schapiro et al [78] has borne this out. These investigators studied 50 MS subjects who were divided into a treatment group and a control group and stratified according to their impairment levels as measured by the EDSS. The treatment group received lectures on exercise, nutrition, and stress management and individualized, written prescriptions for 15 to 30 minutes of exercise four to five times per week. They had follow-up sessions spread over a 16-week period. The control group received no lectures or follow-up with the therapists. At baseline and week 16, all subjects underwent exercise tolerance testing with a combined arm/leg ergometer measuring heart rate, blood pressure, graded exercise time, and achieved workload. The exercise group had a small improvement in workload achievement, representing a 10% training effect. This effect was less than half the effect that would be expected for normal, sedentary individuals put through the same regimen. The investigators also found that the subjects with high degrees of disability received no significant training effect from the program. The investigators hypothesized that the highly impaired subjects' functional muscle mass was too small to take up enough oxygen to get a cardiovascular workout.

Acute exercise has an array of endocrine and immunologic effects that are somewhat dependent on the type (eccentric or concentric) and intensity of exercise. Heesen et al [79] studied serologic parameters pre and post exercise testing in three groups: MS subjects who had completed an 8-week aerobic program (n = 15), nonexercised MS subjects (n = 13), and healthy controls (n = 20). These investigators found that all groups had similar hormonal responses (increased levels of epinephrine, norepinephrine, corticotropin, cortisol, and β-endorphin), an increase in the proinflammatory cytokine interferon-γ, and unclear effects on other cytokines (tumor necrosis factor α and interleukin-10). These effects can be expected to increase blood pressure and provide mild analgesia. The relationship between exercise and inflammation in MS remains poorly understood.

In summary, exercise is safe and should be encouraged for all people with MS. Relative to healthy people, MS patients with mild impairment may need a longer training program to achieve aerobic cardiovascular benefits. More severely impaired MS patients should look to aerobics as a means to maintain rather than improve cardiovascular fitness, unless their exercise protocols are highly structured and supervised.

## Cooling and exercise tolerance

There is broad consensus that heating makes symptoms worse for some people with MS and that cooling relieves the symptoms for those individuals [80]. There is less certainty about the effects of cooling on exercise tolerance in people with MS. In healthy people, thermoregulatory reflexes (eg, sweating and vasodilatation) maintain steady core temperatures during routine exercise [81]. These reflexes, however, may be impaired in people with MS, and a rise in core temperature of even $<1°C$ may be enough to make some people experience heat symptoms. Two studies done in the 1950s reported improvements in neurologic performances using cooling baths [82,83]. Subsequently, Chiari et al [84] conducted an RCT of a cold bath (24°C) on ambulation parameters (oxygen uptake, heart rate, perceived exertion) and spasticity in 14 MS subjects in outpatient PT. The treatment resulted in paradoxically increased spasticity and no reduction in oxygen consumption or rating of perceived exertion. Cooling baths may have only a limited effect on core body temperature because of cutaneous vasoconstriction and shunting of blood elsewhere.

Wearing a cooling garment is a portable method of reducing body temperature. Depending on the apparatus, such equipment can drop body temperature by 0.5°C to 1°C over a period of 30 to 40 minutes. Capello et al [85] used a head-vest liquid cooling garment in twice-daily, 45-minute sessions to treat six thermosensitive MS subjects for 1 month. Average oral temperature reduction per session was 0.7°C. These investigators observed a "slight but definite improvement in pyramidal and cerebellar function" (based on examination by a physician). Motor and visual evoked potentials were not altered by the treatments. The subjects' subjective reports were not given. Somatosensory evoked potentials to the lower extremities were improved by a small amount, but these findings were not confirmed in a later study [86].

Kraft and Alquist [87] also showed significant benefits from a head-vest liquid cooling garment. This study was a double-blind, pre/post study with sham comparisons. The subjects were 17 persons with MS who complained of heat sensitivity. Each subject wore the garment for 60 minutes under each of two settings: garment temperature at 7°C and at 26.5°C. Significantly positive correlations between heat exchange and performance change occurred in seven of nine motor tests with the treatment condition and only in one of nine tests with the sham conditions. A treatment effect was evident for strength, dynamic coordination, and endurance capacity. The greater the heat loss, the greater the motor function gain. Syndulko et al [88] used a similar design, testing MS subjects pre and post wear of either of two different cooling systems for 90 minutes. Equal amounts of cooling (0.6°C) were achieved with an ice-pack suit and with the liquid cooling system. No significant difference was found in clinical neuroperformance and QOL measures. The same investigators gave 12 heat-sensitive MS subjects ice-pack suits for 6 weeks of twice-daily home use. Eight of the 12 subjects reported reduced fatigue and improved ambulation for up to 3 hours post cooling. A placebo effect could not be ruled out.

Woyciechowska et al [89] compared the effects of four different cooling methods in exercise on 10 MS subjects. The four measures used were wearing a cooling suit, wearing wet clothing and using a fan, drinking an ice slurry (500–1000 mL), and using sham cooling with a cooling suit. Ice ingestion before 15 minutes of exercise caused the greatest decrease in rectal temperature (−0.4°C). During an exercise protocol, there was almost no rise in rectal temperature with any of the scenarios.

The National Aeronautics and Space Administration (NASA)/MS Cooling Group conducted a well-designed cooling study on MS subjects who were not selected for heat sensitivity [90]. These investigators examined acute and chronic effects of cooling in an RTC. In the acute setting, they used high-flow and low-flow (sham) cooling garments applied for 1 hour. Body temperature reductions from baseline were mild: −0.44°C and −0.28°C for high and low flow, respectively. Each dose produced improved performance versus baseline on the MS Functional Composite, but only the high flow was significant. Significant changes occurred in the 25-foot timed walk and two measures of visual acuity, but not in measures of upper extremity or cognitive function. A month of daily cooling compared with a month of observation produced improvements on self-reported fatigue, energy, strength, and cognitive function. Because the low-dose cooling resulted in a small change in body temperature, it is difficult to determine whether the results were due to the cooling or to a placebo effect. The magnitude of the observed treatment effects was described as "very modest" and perhaps not clinically relevant. Probably the most important result of this study was showing that the benefits of cooling did not wane over a 1-month trial—the longest to date.

Most studies on cooling devices have included only subjects who complained of heat sensitivity. This practice has created a selection bias for a subset of people with MS. The magnitude of temperature increase necessary to precipitate the onset of symptoms in heat-sensitive individuals is unique to each person. Therefore, results from heat-sensitive patients should not be interpreted as applying to all individuals with MS [72].

Cooling vests with ice-pack pockets and evaporation, phase change, and external liquid cooling attachments are commercially available. The prices range from less than 50 to thousands of dollars and it is difficult to get insurers to cover these expenses. The National Multiple Sclerosis Society and the Multiple Sclerosis Association of America have programs to provide cooling vests to members. Recently, a number of low-cost cooling vests, neck wraps, arm and ankle wraps, and pillows have come on the market [91]. Drinking ice slurries is another option. Given the lack of side effects and modest benefits, some type of cooling device or environmental modification is recommended for all MS patients with heat sensitivity.

## Effects of exercise and outpatient physical therapy on MS–related impairment, disability, aerobic fitness, fatigue, and quality of life

Compared with healthy controls, people with MS have up to 30% lower aerobic capacity and even greater deficits in maximum work rate at aerobic threshold [31], which suggests a very low training level and marked deconditioning. It is obvious that effective methods of improving the fitness of people with MS need to be developed. The first investigations of exercise training in MS were uncontrolled trials with mixed quality and mixed results. In 1984, Gehlsen et al [92] did an open trial of an aquatic exercise program (freestyle swimming and shallow-water calisthenics for 1 hour, three times per week for 10 weeks) with a cohort of 10 subjects with MS. Using a dynamometer, they found muscular strength (peak torque values), power, and total work capacity improvements. The pool temperature was kept less than 27.5°C to avoid overheating. Muscle fatigue, defined as the percentage decrement in peak torque, was also improved. De Souza and Worthington [93] enrolled 40 MS subjects with moderate disability (mean EDSS = 6.0) in a study of outpatient exercise classes (frequency unspecified) and home-based PT. After 1.5 years, 50% were believed to have improved ADL and balance. These investigators found a dose-response relationship between therapy and ADL improvement and determined that functionally oriented movement exercises were more beneficial than balance exercises; however, there was a wearing-off of positive effect after the first 6 months and active range of motion (a clinical measure of strength) declined significantly in 75% of the subjects. The most common reason for poor attendance at outpatient PT was lack of transportation.

In 1994, Svensson et al [94] published an unblinded, uncontrolled study of five MS subjects who were trained for 4 to 6 weeks using an endurance program for the lower extremities (three sets of 10 repetitions of low-load strengthening with weights or exercise machine over 40–90 minutes) three times per week. Findings were reduced ratings of fatigue and improved well-being on visual analog scales.

The University of Utah established a 15-week aerobic exercise protocol (40-minute sessions of combined arm and leg ergometry three times per week) and published an uncontrolled study of 13 MS subjects [95,96]. A 21% improvement in maximum exercise capacity ($VO_2max$), no evidence of exercise-induced symptomatology, and no effect on functional performance of gait, balance, dexterity, and grip strength were found. Subsequently, Petajan et al [66] performed a second study using the same exercise protocol. This study has probably been the most influential trial of exercise in MS to date for several reasons: it was one of the first RCTs, one of the largest studies, and one of the first to show highly positive results. The investigators randomized 54 ambulatory subjects with MS to 15 weeks of aerobic training (40-minute sessions of combined arm and leg ergometry three times per week) or to nonexercise. Compared with baseline, the exercise group demonstrated significant increases in $VO_2$max (increased 22%) and upper and lower extremity strength, significant decreases in skin folds and lipid profiles (indicating reduced fat in body composition), and decreased scores on a depression/anger scale. All components of physical dimension improved on the Sickness Impact Profile, and total Sickness Impact Profile scores and measures of social interaction, emotional behavior, home management, recreation, and bowel and bladder function improved on the EDSS. Although the study did not show a beneficial effect on MS fatigue, the lack of a harmful effect on fatigue is worth noting. Four exacerbations occurred in the exercise group and three in the nonexercise group.

The main limitation of this study was that there was no follow-up assessment to determine whether there was any carryover after the program ended. Indeed, the Sickness Impact Profile scores were at their best two thirds of the way through the intervention and then worsened somewhat at the end, suggesting a wearing off of benefit and possible short-lived treatment effect.

Improvements of $VO_2$max of 21% and 22% in the first and second Utah studies, respectively, were based on the mean values for the whole treatment group. Two other studies, both involving 6-month programs of arm/leg cycle ergometry, found improvements in $VO_2$max of 15% to 19% [97,98]. One of the studies stratified the MS subjects by ambulatory status and found that those with some gait impairment (EDSS = 5–6) had only a 7% mean increase in $VO_2$max. Their improvement, however, was better than the control subjects who avoided exercise for 6 months and experienced a 12% decline in $VO_2$max [97]. Another study using intensive bicycle ergometry for 3 to 4 weeks found no significant change in $VO_2$max, but trends were more positive for the MS subjects with higher impairment [31]. Different exercise protocols and durations may explain these conflicting findings.

Precautions about progressive resistive exercises (PRE) in MS date back to the classic rehabilitation books by Howard Rusk [73]. The chief concern has always been that PRE could exacerbate fatigue [99]. Consequently, little research has been done on this topic. Only one trial of PRE in MS addressed the issue of fatigue. Kraft et al [100,101] reported the results of PRE on eight MS subjects. Three times per week for 3 months, the subjects performed PRE on bilateral quadriceps, hamstrings, triceps, and biceps. At the end of the intervention, strength had improved in all muscle groups, with more of an effect on mildly impaired subjects than on severely impaired subjects. The subjects had improved mobility and reduced self-reported disability (Sickness Impact Profile). All subjects experienced acute fatigue that lessened within 48 hours. This was a small, uncontrolled trial with no postintervention follow-up to see whether gains were maintained. In addition, it was an efficacy trial in which the subjects were exercising under constant supervision; results may be less impressive in a standard outpatient PT setting or with unsupervised PRE done at home. The importance of the study is in demonstrating that paretic muscles can be strengthened and that this may improve function. The benefits of PRE relative to more aerobic endurance exercises in MS is unknown, but they are likely to be complementary.

The concept of maintenance rehabilitation through sustained outpatient programs has been promoted by Dr. Randall Schapiro at the Fairview MS Achievement Center in Minnesota [102]. Di Fabio et al [103] reported the results of this extended outpatient program of integrated PT (balance, coordination, gait, transfer, endurance training, range of motion) and OT (ADL training) for 5 hours, 1d/wk for 1 year in persons with progressive MS. This was the first exercise study to focus on more severely disabled people with MS (EDSS = 5–8). These investigators used a longitudinal design with pre- and post-testing of the unblinded intervention group (n = 20) and wait-listed control group (n = 26). Significant effects of the rehabilitation program were reduced symptom frequency and reduced fatigue on a 6-point Likert scale (Fatigue Severity Scale was not used). No effect was found regarding functional status (Rehabilitation Institute of Chicago Functional Assessment Scale) and the EDSS was not monitored. The same investigators did an earlier, smaller study with same design using different measurements (self-administered questionnaire and functional assessment by a physical therapist) [104]. All subjects had significant disability (EDSS = 5–8) and may have been included in the study described previously. After 1 year, both groups showed a decrease in physical function (measured by Rehabilitation Institute of Chicago Functional Assessment Scale), with worse decline in the wait-listed group. The treatment group showed improvements in six areas of the Rand 36-Item Health Survey (SF-36) in which the wait-listed group did not. The differences were in physical health, bodily pain, energy/fatigue, social support, cognitive ability, and overall positive change in general health. There were negligible changes in overall QOL for both groups. Role limitations due to emotional problems increased in the treatment group, but declined in the control group. No explanation was given. The small subject number, lack of blinded and objective assessment, and lack of postintervention follow-up results are this study's weaknesses.

Recently, another RCT of outpatient therapy for progressive forms of MS was reported. Patti et al [105,106] studied 111 MS subjects with moderate to severe impairment (EDSS = 4.0–8.0; primary progressive MS, 21%; secondary progressive, 79%). This RCT excluded anyone with a minimental status score of ≤24 and anyone taking any disease-modifying therapy. The treatment group (n = 58) received 6 weeks of individualized outpatient rehabilitation (total 50–90 min/d, 6 d/wk, including PT, OT, speech pathologist, nurse, psychologist, and neurologist), followed by 6 weeks of home-based exercise program training. The control group (n = 53) received only instructions in a home exercise program. At the end of the intervention, the treatment group showed significantly improved level of disability (measured by the FIM) compared with the control group, particularly in locomotion, transfers, and self-care, which all had moderate to large effect size statistics. In the treatment group, 55% improved their FIM motor domain scores. The functional benefits lasted in the range of 4 to 6 months. Sphincter function improved to a lesser degree. The treatment group improved significantly on all eight subscales of the SF-36 QOL measure and showed 17% improvement on the Fatigue Impact Scale and 20% improvement on the Beck Depression Inventory. Cognitive subscales of the FIM and impairment (measured by the EDSS) were not changed by the intervention. At 6 months, the home exercise group had not improved or worsened across measures of impairment, disability, QOL, fatigue, depression, or social functioning. This result should not be construed as negative because worsening of these parameters might have occurred without any exercise (nonexercise controls in the study by Petajan et al [66] had worsening of fatigue and QOL outcomes). This result implies a potential benefit from a single training session on home exercises.

A systematic review conducted in 2002 by Boggild and Ford [107] found no study showing definitive proof that exercise improves MS fatigue; however, this review was conducted before Patti et al [105,106] showed mild improvement with a 6-week outpatient program. Many investigators provide anecdotal behavioral advice on fatigue management, including conserving energy, maintaining a cool environment, ceasing smoking, improving sleep habits, taking naps, and avoiding coffee and alcohol. Energy conservation studies are discussed later.

In conclusion, exercise has a beneficial effect on MS disability and QOL but not on impairment, except that strength may be improved. There is robust evidence that aerobic training improves maximum exercise capacity ($VO_2max$) for ambulatory MS individuals, whereas inactivity makes it worse. Less is known about exercise effects in semiambulatory and nonambulatory MS individuals. These individuals may receive less benefit from exercise than those who are fully ambulatory, because they cannot activate enough muscle mass to get a training effect, because exercise programs are not designed properly for them or because their adherence is poor. For more disabled people, multidisciplinary outpatient programs may provide better results than exercise alone, but these are not widely available. If people with MS follow established precautions, they will not experience exercise-associated worsening of fatigue or other symptoms lasting beyond 1 or 2 days. Adherence to exercise may yield a partial reduction of MS fatigue. Future research should compare different exercise protocols (eg, resistive exercises versus aerobics), investigate new exercise treatments for moderate to severely disabled MS individuals, and further evaluate the effects of behavioral modification and exercise on MS fatigue.

## Outpatient physical therapy effects on mobility and balance in MS

Gait impairment in MS may be caused by weakness, spasticity, fatigue, proprioceptive loss, cerebellar or vestibular nuclear dysfunction, or visual loss. Overall, about three fourths of MS individuals have some degree of ambulatory impairment [20,108]. The need for assistance in mobility is associated with older age, increasing disease duration, and divorced or separated marital status [109].

The time from symptom onset until ambulation is limited to 500 m averages 8 years and the time until a cane is required averages 20 years [1]. Compared with healthy people, MS individuals show decreased stride length; increased steps per minute (cadence); slower free speed-walking rates; less rotation at the hips, knees, and ankles (stiffer gait); increased trunk flexion; and reduced vertical lift in center of gravity. In short, they take short quick steps and lack full range of motion [110]. A survey conducted in 1983 indicated that 60% of people with MS needed assistance with ambulation [109]. Most relied on a wheelchair or physical assistance from another person. This survey indicated that orthotics are underused.

In terms of morbidity, falls are the most important sequelae of gait and balance disturbances. In one cross-sectional study of ambulatory MS individuals, 54% reported at least one fall over the previous 2 months and 32% were recurrent fallers. Impaired balance was the best predictor of falls, followed by use of an assistive device and impaired ambulation [111]. For these reasons, recommendations for mobility aids should focus on enhancing gait stability, rather than the ease and convenience of walking.

The EDSS is a gross measure of impairment and disability that should not be used to determine whether an intervention has an impact on mobility. The RMI, developed in the United Kingdom, has been used in stroke and brain injury studies and has been validated in MS [35]. This scale spans from 0 (unable to turn over in bed) to 15 (able to run 10 m in 4 seconds); a change of more than 1 point is considered reliable [112]. With the RMI, MS individuals tend to distribute out evenly, unlike the EDSS on which moderately impaired walkers bunch up at a few midpoints [35]. Timed walks (10 m, 2 minutes, and so forth) are highly quantifiable, can be compared with age-stratified normative data, and have good inter-rater reliability, but there is high individual variability of gait speed (up to 20%) [35,113]. Timing should be measured during continuous walking, not measured from start to finish [114]. In one study, the RMI was more sensitive to change over time than timed walks or the EDSS [35]. Videotape versus "live" assessment of mobility in MS was recently compared by Wiles et al [115]. They concluded that although the videotapes had higher inter-rater reliability, live assessment was more sensitive to perceived changes in gait.

Unlike mobility, balance may not be significantly altered by MS fatigue [116]. Balance assessments that have been used in MS research include the Berg Balance Test and the Timed Get-Up-and-Go, although the latter could also be considered a mobility test [117,118]. Balance platforms consist of dual plates symmetrically positioned on force transducers. Under computer control, the support surfaces are moved beneath the subject's feet. These devices can be used for balance training and balance assessment, and preliminary evidence supports their utility in MS [119]. The cost of the equipment is a limiting factor in their use. In the future, investigators might consider using the Short Physical Performance Battery that was developed by the National Institute on Aging to assess mobility, transfers, and balance. This test is well studied and validated in geriatric populations but has not been used in MS research.

In conclusion, the RMI has been used most widely as a marker of mobility in MS and is useful in most interventions when the need is to measure minor changes. Quantitative tests such as the 25-foot walk and the Timed Get-Up-and-Go are gaining popularity and useful for clinical practice. The most severely impaired individuals should be assessed with the Barthel Index or the FIM. For research purposes, it is good practice to take the average of two scores on mobility and balance tests done at different times of day or on separate days because people with MS are apt to have fluctuating performances.

Wiles et al [120] in the United Kingdom conducted a three-arm RCT of home-based PT (45 minutes with a therapist, twice weekly for 8 weeks), outpatient PT (45 minutes twice weekly for 8 weeks), or no therapy. On the primary outcome, the RMI, there was a highly significant ($P < 0.001$) treatment effect favoring either form of PT over no therapy. Significant differences were also found for global mobility and balance. There was no difference on the nine-hole peg test and no major difference between outpatient and home-based PT. The treatment effect was largely lost at 8 weeks post intervention, which led the investigators to recommend ongoing rehabilitation for MS, much as immunomodulatory drugs must continually be used in this progressive disease. Individuals and caregivers preferred home-based PT and missed fewer therapy sessions when it was home based. Physical therapists judged that home treatment was more often beneficial, but for half of the subjects, the venue made no difference. About 10% showed no benefit in home- or outpatient-based PT over placebo.

Two mobility and balance studies assessed the relative benefits of different forms of PT. Lord et al [121] treated 23 subjects with MS who were semiambulatory or better with 6 weeks of outpatient PT. Subjects were randomized to facilitation therapy (individualized, passive and active manual assistance; postural control; component practice as in Bobath technique) or to task-oriented therapy (nonindividualized, hands-off acceptance of compensatory strategies; functional tasks such as stair climbing and treadmill walking). Both treatments resulted in improved walking time, stride length, global gait score, Berg Balance Test, and RMI score. The facilitation group had nonsignificant trends toward greater benefit in all of these categories. The investigators concluded that similar gains in mobility and balance are derived from outpatient therapy whether a facilitation or a task-oriented approach is used. Armutlu et al [122] treated 26 MS patients with ataxia with 4 weeks of proprioceptive neuromuscular facilitation combined with Frenkel coordination exercises in supine, sitting, and standing positions. Half of the patients also wore long-leg splints for 20 minutes before exercise. For both groups, significant improvements were found in anterior balance, single-limb stance time, walking speed, and ambulation index. Neither study provided post-treatment follow-up, so it is not known how long the benefits were sustained. These protocols could be performed in group therapy, which might increase cost effectiveness.

Stephens et al [123] conducted a small study of awareness through movement exercise, which is a kinesiologic approach developed by Feldenkrais. The intervention was eight classes over a span of 10 weeks. Movements progressed from weight shifting to more complex changes in posture. Relative to the nonexercise controls (n = 6), the treatment group (n = 6) made significant gains in balance testing on a computerized platform test and showed a trend toward improved self-efficacy. Johnson et al [124] performed a crossover study of Feldenkrais technique versus sham for 20 subjects with MS (EDSS = 2–6). Each subject received eight weekly, 45-minute sessions of one intervention and then the other. In the Feldenkrais technique, the instructor manually put the subject through several movement patterns while giving verbal guidance. The sham was touch therapy with relaxed breathing. At the end of the trial, all subjects reported the Feldenkrais technique was more effective than sham. There was no difference between treatments or compared with baseline for self-perceived mobility, upper extremity function (nine-hole peg test), or MS symptoms. Tai Chi, the Chinese martial art form, has also been studied in an uncontrolled trial. Nineteen subjects with MS participated in an 8-week Tai Chi course taught at a Chinese medicine center in California. Walking speed and hamstring flexibility were improved and the subjects reported several subjective benefits [125].

Gehlsen et al [110] studied the effects of a 10-week aquatic exercise program on gait on 11 subjects with MS. Using videotaped gait analysis before, during, and at the end of the training, the intervention seemed to have no effect on gait. Similarly, a 6-month program of arm/leg ergometry conducted by Rodgers et al [98] failed to produce any significant improvement in videotaped gait characteristics of individuals with MS. Recently, Debolt and McCubbin [126] conducted a study that incorporated two interesting elements: unsupervised home exercise and PRE. Thirty-seven MS subjects were randomized to a 2-week instruction/6-week home program or to no exercise. The PRE were performed using no special equipment except a weighted vest and ankle weights. The vest weight was gradually increased to 1% of body weight while the exercise group performed 25 to 30 minutes of strengthening activities (eg, chair raises) three times a week. Ninety-five percent adherence was reported. The intervention resulted in significantly increased leg extensor power but no differences in balance (force platform) and mobility (Timed Get-Up-and-Go). Subjectively, subjects liked the PRE and there were no adverse effects. More detailed mobility measures and postintervention follow-up of outcomes would have strengthened this study. These three trials suggest that nonspecific exercise programs without some ambulation component are ineffective for enhancing gait.

In conclusion, outpatient and home-based PT using various techniques result in short-term gains in mobility and balance. No study has demonstrated an effect lasting beyond 2 months. Therefore, it may be that continual programs are necessary to maintain good mobility and balance in this disease. One way to make this affordable is to provide group therapy using task-oriented or kinesiology techniques. Other promising therapies such as Tai Chi and partial weight-supported treadmill training should be further studied.

## Outpatient physical therapy effects on spasticity and range of motion in MS

Spasticity in MS is due to upper motor neuron dysfunction. It is typically worse in the lower than upper extremities and may be more noticeable when a person is fatigued, anxious, in pain, infected, or in hot or cold weather. In most cases, spasticity is an undesirable impediment to function, but it may facilitate certain activities such as a pivot transfer.

In 1964, Ashworth [127], a British physician, introduced a 5-point scale to assess tone of the limbs. The Ashworth Scale, together with its modified versions, has subsequently become the world's most frequently used clinical scale in neurorehabilitation [128]. Although evidence suggests that this scale measures hypertonicity, it is commonly used to grade spasticity for clinical and research purposes [129]. The use of the same scale to measure two different symptoms is usually not a problem because hypertonicity and spasticity go hand-in-hand in the upper motor neuron syndrome, which is a common manifestation of MS. Tone is resistance to passive limb movement, whereas spasticity is hypertonicity that increases with the velocity of joint movement [130]. Resistance to passive movement is influenced by many factors, of which only one is spasticity [131].

Variations of the Ashworth Scale—all are 6-point scales and referred to as "Modified Ashworth Scales"—were introduced in 1987, 1991, and 1992 [132–134]. Subsequent studies of inter-rater agreement of the original scale and the Modified Ashworth Scales have found less reliability at the midrange scores than at both ends of the scale by clinical testing and by comparison with isokinetic measurements [135,136]. The scales also appear less reliable for the knees and ankles than for the wrists and elbows [137–140]. This finding is unfortunate because in MS, spasticity is usually more of a problem in the legs. A score of 2 has a different meaning in each of the three common versions of the Modified Ashworth Scale. Therefore, it is sometimes difficult to know whether two clinicians are using the same scale. Alternative measures of spasticity (Tone Assessment Scale, pendulum test), however, are less reliable or require expensive equipment (Cybex® testing, Owatonna, Minnesota) [141].

Stretching to prevent spasticity was once believed to be of little value in MS [73], but stretching has subsequently assumed an essential role in spasticity treatment. Much of what is believed and done to manage spasticity is based on research done on spinal cord injury, brain injury, and stroke [142]. The MS literature on this topic has focused primarily on pharmacotherapy (oral medication, intramuscular botulinum toxin neurolysis, and intrathecal baclofen). Brar et al [143] at the Rocky Mountain Multiple Sclerosis Center evaluated the effects of baclofen and stretching on spasticity in MS. In a 10-week double-blind, placebo-controlled crossover study, each of 30 ambulatory MS subjects received stretching, baclofen (20 mg or less per day), and placebo in various combinations. They measured the Ashworth Scale, Cybex flexion scores, and timed gait. With Cybex testing and the Ashworth Scale, baclofen alone and baclofen plus stretching were superior to placebo. There was a trend toward stretching plus baclofen having an additive effect, but stretching alone did not have a significant effect. Fewer subjects had improved Ashworth Scale scores on stretching than on placebo. The stretching exercises were daily 90-second stretches of four lower limb muscle groups done unsupervised at home after a single training session. Had a more aggressive stretching program been used, it might have been more effective. Other investigators have recommended that stretching be done at least twice a day [144].

A study with more intensive supervised stretching may be necessary to demonstrate the effectiveness of stretching in reducing spasticity. A 2-year prospective trial of a home stretching program for spasticity management has been launched at the University of Washington. Currently, the widely held belief that stretching reduces spasticity in MS is based on clinical experience and inference from findings in spinal cord injury and stroke literature.

Stretching may not be the only way to improve range of motion and spasticity, but very little study of other techniques has been done in MS. Rodgers et al [98] conducted an uncontrolled 6-month program of arm/leg cycle ergometry for 18 individuals with MS. This program resulted in improved hip abduction, adduction, external rotation, and hamstring looseness; however, maximum hip flexion/extension range of motion decreased, indicating that the exercise regimen increased hip flexor tightness. A daily prone stretch of hip flexors might have improved the results. Tai Chi appears to relieve muscle stiffness, and yoga may provide similar benefits;

these alternative therapies warrant further study [145]. Most MS patients with significant spasticity take antispasticity medication, and intrathecal baclofen should be considered for the most severe cases.

## A logical exercise prescription for people with MS

Petajan and White [71,146], a neurologist and an exercise physiologist, used their experience with the Utah exercise studies to write general principles of exercise in MS. They created an exercise pyramid that used progressively complex levels to suit the needs of individuals with varying degrees of impairment. The authors have modified this pyramid into a staircase to reflect the broad suitability of integrated exercises (Fig. 1). The foundation is passive range of motion, which is useful and especially important for the most physically and cognitively disabled persons. The recommended frequency of exercise should be at least daily for passive range of motion. The next step up is active range of motion, with gravity eliminated or against gravity, as strength allows. Specific muscle training is recommended for improving focal weaknesses and has been advocated when fatigue or heat sensitivity are important issues [144]. Three sets of 10 repetitions may be an appropriate regimen. Focused muscle strengthening with PRE may be effective in motivated individuals with mild impairments. Even when weakness is diffuse, with careful selection of muscles (probably not more than two per limb), resistive exercises may still be effective in strengthening. PRE is not useful for ataxia because it can be counterproductive, and PRE may be less effective for individuals with impaired balance and mobility.

The ultimate goal is to achieve integrated exercises that provide combined training on strength, endurance, balance, coordination, and flexibility. Every exercise prescription should be tailored to meet individual circumstances. For those whose primary goal is improved gait, exercise must include standing and walking. Aquatic exercise—swimming, water aerobics, or water walking—is an excellent form of integrated exercise, especially when ataxia may create

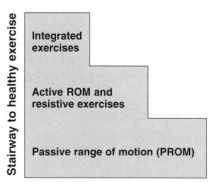

Fig. 1. An exercise "staircase" with progressively complex levels to suit the needs of individuals with varying degrees of impairment to reflect the broad suitability of integrated exercises. ROM, range of motion.

a safety concern. The hydrostatic pressure of the pool creates a low-impact environment. Even those with tetraparesis can use the water buoyancy to facilitate standing and supine swimming, with assistance and a life jacket [147]. Care should be taken to find a pool that is not too hot (above 84°F; 29°C) for those who are heat sensitive [148]. Combined arm/leg ergometry (eg, the Schwinn Airdyne [Direct Focus, Boulder, Colorado]) is useful for people with partial paralysis. Yoga may improve flexibility and reduce spasticity. Outdoor walking, aerobics, and Tai Chi are useful for balance training. Previously sedentary individuals should start aerobic exercises at a comfortable level and increase the duration and intensity of exercise at weekly or monthly intervals [146]. It is important to try to make exercise a communal/ group activity such as group aerobics. In addition to socialization, group activities may improve adherence.

To summarize, active exercise should be done at least three times a week for 20 to 30 minutes, with a 5-minute warm up and cool down. Stretching should be done for 5 to 10 minutes, with emphasis on posterior thigh, leg, and back muscles. Adherence to this regimen lowers blood pressure, decreases risk of myocardial infarction, increases bone mineralization, reduces body fat, and meets exercise requirements for weight reduction [66,78]. For the 40% of women and 44% of men with MS who are overweight, aerobic exercise is particularly important [149].

For markedly disabled MS individuals, ADL may constitute their only regular forms of physical activity. In addition to passive range of motion exercises, it is important to devise simple activities that tap underused strengths to avoid learned disuse and deconditioning. For example, keeping certain articles of daily use on a shelf above shoulder level may help to maintain a person's overhead range of motion. Frequent recreational activities also supplement the amount of exercise derived from ADL.

## Precautions: Kraft's caveats and then some

- MS rehabilitation strategies must be adapted to a progressive neurologic disease with an uncertain future prognosis. Unlike static diseases such as stroke and spinal cord injury, MS is a moving target. Individuals need to be reassessed and programs modified as appropriate. Repeated rehabilitation interventions are usually required as MS individuals acquire new impairments [150].
- Most people with MS have cognitive deficits, especially with executive function but also with memory and concentration. Some patients have problems acquiring new information; others have problems retrieving information. The therapist cannot treat MS patients like others and assume that they understand and can retrieve exercise instructions. Therefore, it is important to explain exercises to patients, have patients repeat the instructions back, and provide written copies. Over 40% of MS individuals have depression [15]. These factors hinder motivation

and adherence. Structured exercise programs with simple step-by-step instructions and multiple clinic visits may be necessary to establish and reinforce home programs.

- MS individuals' strength, balance, or coordination at rest may not reflect their ability post activity. For example, it is best to let an individual walk for a few minutes before drawing any conclusions about gait disturbances and the need for orthotics. Certain prolonged activities such as bicycle riding may be unsafe for those who experience the Uhthoff phenomenon. Neurologic symptoms that worsen with exercise, however, also resolve within 1 hour or more quickly with rapid cooling. A tepid bath for 20 to 30 minutes before and after exercise and use of an extra fan and air conditioning during exercise help minimize this problem. Individuals should wear light clothing during exercise, except for the possible addition of a cooling vest, and make use of a sport bottle filled with a cold drink [66,71,80].

- It has been recommended that all MS individuals undergo a submaximal cardiovascular stress test before starting exercise programs to determine cardiac safety and an appropriate level of exercise [142]. Others might advocate obtaining a baseline ECG before starting an exercise program. Both authors believe that such precautions are not usually necessary but should be individualized based on the individual's cardiovascular risk factors and cardiac history. A reasonable safeguard to avoid undue cardiac stress, fatigue, and the Uhthoff phenomenon is to prescribe exercise below maximal workload (a level of very strenuous exertion). To achieve an exercise intensity of 55% to 60% of $VO_2max$, the therapist may set a target heart rate using the following formulas:

Target heart rate = $(220 - \text{individual age}) \times (0.70)$
for most MS individuals

Target heart rate = $(220 - \text{individual age}) \times (0.65)$ for those with
heat sensitivity or marked deconditioning

Some individuals with MS have a blunted heart-rate response to increased exercise stress, particularly those with more severe impairment. This possibility should be taken into account when setting target heart rate and monitoring response to exercise.

- For individuals who fatigue quickly, therapeutic exercises should be divided into shorter intervals interspersed with rest periods. An individual can take a breather from walking by standing in place for a few minutes and then continuing. If a person reports an increased need for rest and a reduced tolerance for functional activity after starting a program, then the initial exercise effort was too intense and should be moderated.

- Some spasmolytic drugs (eg, baclofen and dantrolene but not tizanidine) may contribute to muscle weakness. It may be useful to have the individual exercise at different times of the day or to reduce the dose of antispasticity drug to gauge whether this improves performance.

- There is no evidence that exercise increases the exacerbation rate; however, exercise should be discontinued until the exacerbation has been stabilized and until intravenous steroids have been completed. Moreover, individuals should have medical clearance and supervision when initiating exercise programs.

## Occupational therapy for MS

People with MS tend to function in daily life below their physical capacities, and cognitive problems do not account for this discrepancy [151]. Occupational therapy (OT) can help people with MS meet their potential for independence. The principles of OT for MS have been described in various review articles [108,144]. OT has been used extensively in MS research, especially in inpatient trials in which it has been uniformly incorporated into the rehabilitation program [4,5,24,29,32,35].

A meta-analysis published in 2001 determined that OT-related treatments have a strong positive effect on MS symptomatology [152]; however, there have been few investigations of the effects of OT separate from the whole rehabilitation package. Disabling tremor is reported in nearly 30% of MS patients and is usually an action tremor [153]. Jones et al [154] conducted a nonrandomized study of inpatient OT and PT for the treatment of MS-related ataxia including tremor. Twenty-eight MS subjects with upper limb or trunkal ataxia received eight half-hour sessions of OT (postural dynamics, adaptive equipment, and damping and weighting methods) and PT (specifics not given) over 8 working days. Nine wait-listed people who received no intervention served as comparison. Baseline and immediate postintervention measurements of hand function, impairment, and ADL function were made. After completion, the intervention group had significantly improved relative to the comparison group on one ADL scale (Northwick Park Index) but not on two impairment scales (Kurtzke Functional Systems Scale and Jebsen Taylor Hand Function Scale). Intervention subjects had significantly greater improvement in visual analog scales of activity and fatigue. The conspicuous shortcomings of the study were the lack of randomization and blinding and a high drop-out rate, but the most important flaw was the lack of postdischarge measurements. Carryover to the home environment is the essence of successful rehabilitation.

Occupational therapists are frequently asked to teach the principles of "energy conservation" to MS individuals. Energy conservation means rationing activities according to one's optimum hours of function and total capacity for daily exertion and working piece-by-piece instead of trying to do too much at once [108]. Two RCTs of patient education in energy conservation (weekly 1-hour sessions for 8 weeks) found reductions in fatigue (Fatigue Impact Scale), which in one study was maintained at 6 weeks' follow-up. There were also benefits in self-efficacy and social participation [155,156]. A Cochrane review, however, cited design flaws and other weaknesses in the methodology of these two studies and concluded that the evidence was insufficient [157]. O'Hara et al [158] conducted a large RCT of individually or group-based counseling (two sessions) in self-care strategies for 268 community-dwelling individuals with MS. They found significant differences on some aspects of mental health and vitality that they used as a proxy for fatigue. Although levels of functional independence did not improve, they were maintained in the intervention group and declined in the control group. Thus, the role of OT counseling for MS symptom management is still being defined.

The priorities of therapists and their patients do not always match. It is important that occupational therapists concentrate their efforts on activities that individuals will use in practice, rather than on activities that people may not value because of environmental or behavioral circumstances.

## Assistive devices

Most MS individuals benefit from the use of some adaptive device. It may vary in size and sophistication (from cloth loops sewn onto socks to hydraulic lifts for dependent transfers). Wheelchairs and walking aids (canes, crutches, and walkers) are the most frequently prescribed devices. Leg braces are used by few people with MS [20,109]. For weakness and ataxia, a cane is an affordable and usually acceptable adaptation. Wheeled walkers with bench platforms allow an MS individual to stop for a rest while out on a walk. Scooters are useful for those whose ambulation is limited by ataxia or fatigue [159]. Ankle-foot orthoses are the most frequently prescribed orthoses. One of the authors (G.H. Kraft) recommends a nonarticulated custom-molded plastic ankle-foot orthoses for MS individuals with decreased gait stability due to dorsiflexion weakness or medial/lateral instability [150]. Weighted wrist cuffs and weighted walkers are sometimes helpful in dampening ataxic tremor [160,161].

## Rehabilitation nursing

Rehabilitation nurses are involved in MS care during inpatient admission and more commonly during outpatient care. They provide continuity and coordination of care, education, and advice on pharmacotherapy; care needs; equipment needs; bladder, bowel, and skin care; coping with disease; intimacy and advance directives; and referral for insurance and employment issues. Vital though they are, their services have been the subject of limited research, which may be because they work in a very interdisciplinary fashion and do not bill for much of what they do. The introduction of injectable therapy in 1993 was followed by an increased need for education and health care management specific to MS. This need has fostered a new MS nurse specialty with a certifying process and international organization [162]. There is also a trend toward greater involvement of nurse practitioners in MS care who can prescribe medications and bill for individual care. MS nurses and nurse practitioners are responsible for many aspects of MS individuals' primary care and rehabilitation.

One of the most common responses to MS is to restrict leisure-time activities. Physical inactivity may have multiple negative physiologic and psychologic consequences. Stuifbergen [163], an academic nurse, surveyed 37 people with MS and found that their average and maximal activity scores were much lower than the general population's and about the same as the scores of those on hemodialysis. Stuifbergen et al [164] then conducted an investigation of a nurse-directed wellness program for women with MS. Seventy-six women were randomized to eight weekly lifestyle-change classes (90 minutes' duration in groups of 8–14 women, with topics including health promotion, exercise and physical activity, healthy eating, and stress management) and twice-monthly phone calls for 3 months. Sixty-six women were randomized to the control group that had no classes or phone calls. The outcome measures were self-reported health-promoting and QOL measures. Statistically significant intervention effects were found for self-efficacy, health-promoting behaviors, mental health, and pain. The investigators believed that these results supported the following principles for nurse-directed intervention for people with MS: providing information that is specific to health promotion within the context of MS, enhancement of self-efficacy for health behaviors, and individualized goal setting and monitoring. The authors speculate that had the investigators included a measure of fatigue, this study might have also demonstrated that behavior modification improves MS fatigue.

In another study of health promotion, MS individuals were asked to identify a target area for counseling [165]. Given a list of five topics, exercise was chosen by 66%, followed by stress management (15%), improved social support (10%), fatigue management (7%), and substance abuse (1%). Then, a treatment group was given a single motivational interview and five scheduled telephone counseling sessions directed at the issue of interest to the individual. Relative to a control group, the treatment group improved significantly on measures of self-selected walking speed and health-related QOL, including physical activity, spiritual growth, and stress management. This study indicates the priorities of MS patients and suggests that even brief telephone counseling from a knowledgeable rehabilitation nurse has a positive impact.

A study done by Bourdette et al [166] investigated the effect of a multidisciplinary team clinic on MS individual care. They compared impairment (EDSS) and disability (Incapacity Status Scale) measurements at baseline and at 6 and 12 months of care at two Department of Veterans' Affairs hospitals. One clinic included a neurologist, physiatrist, psychologist, and nurse practitioner. The other clinic offered "standard medical care." There were no differences in impairment, but disability had significantly less progression with the multidisciplinary clinic. Subscores that were significantly improved with the intervention included stair climbing, dressing, mentation, and fatigue. An individual survey indicating the relative value of the components of the multidisciplinary team package would help to elucidate the contribution made by the nurse practitioner.

## Cognitive therapy

Cognitive deficits in MS may originate from either primary (neurologic) or secondary (eg, depression, drug effect) sources [167]. Slowing of information processing, abstract reasoning, and problem solving and impairment of recent memory are the most frequent problems [168]. Cognitive dysfunction is associated with MRI findings of greater brain lesion load and cerebral atrophy [169–171]. Impaired cognition does not correlate well with physical impairment (as measured by the EDSS), but it does with unemployment, social isolation, sexual dysfunction, and greater difficulty with household tasks [172,173].

Based on clinical neuropsychologic assessments, nearly 50% of all MS individuals exhibit some form of cognitive dysfunction [174]. Even in MS, individuals who do not have significant disability (EDSS ≤3.5) group scores on a range of cognitive tests fall significantly below those of healthy controls matched for age, gender, and education [172]. A World Wide Web survey conducted by the Rocky Mountain Multiple Sclerosis Center in 2003 found that 73% of respondents reported current cognitive problems. Forty-four percent had not discussed their cognitive problems with their health providers.

Neuropsychologists, speech/language pathologists, and occupational therapists are often consulted to assess and manage such problems. Four studies have shown short-term QOL benefits of inpatient and outpatient rehabilitation programs with or without cognitive therapy by psychologists, nurses, or occupational therapists [4,5,66,105]. In terms of improving cognitive function, a 1-year program including weekly PT and OT and a 6-week intensive multidisciplinary team outpatient program did not have a significant effect on cognitive function in individuals with progressive disease (EDSS = 4–8) [104,106]. Group therapy, stress management, computer-assisted retraining, and cognitive behavioral therapy, however, have been demonstrated to have substantial cognitive and emotional benefits for MS individuals [175–180]. It is still unclear how to identify individuals who would benefit from such approaches. In unselected MS patients, cognitive assessment done outside of the multidisciplinary framework and without cognitive therapy may have a counterproductive effect on QOL [181].

An important role for the neuropsychologist in MS care is helping individuals develop coping skills to deal with cognitive deficits and disease-related stress [20]. The association of emotional stress and MS exacerbations has been the subject of much research interest and debate. Until recently, the weight of evidence has indicated that stress does not have a significant effect on triggering exacerbations or on the eventual course of MS [182,183]. A study by Buljevac et al [184] published in 2003 has reignited the controversy. These investigators did a prospective cohort study (mean, 1.4 years) of 73 MS patients who kept weekly diaries with record of any stressful events. The diaries were independently evaluated by two neurologists to exclude stress directly connected to existing MS manifestations. Stressful events included occupational, financial, illness, or death in the family. There were a total of 457 stressful events and 134 exacerbations. Stress was associated with a doubling of the exacerbation rate during the subsequent 4 weeks. Infections were even more associated with exacerbation rate (threefold increase). This study has rekindled the debate as to whether stress causes relapses or may be a premonitory symptom of exacerbations [185].

Whether stress management behavior therapy can reduce exacerbations and other MS difficulties is unknown. A comparison of coping mechanisms used by MS individuals in exacerbation versus others in remission found that the former favored emotion-focused coping techniques, whereas the latter favored problem-solving and social support coping techniques [186]. Emotional preoccupation has also been identified as a marginal factor in predicting new gadolinium-positive MRI brain lesions [187]. Greater reliance on problem-focused coping and less reliance on emotion-focused coping has been associated with better psychologic adjustment to MS in a 1-year follow-up study [188]. These findings provide a rationale for teaching "better" coping mechanisms through behavioral therapy.

Neuropsychology may also help patients and their families address MS-associated behavioral problems, which are sometimes stereotyped as the "MS personality." Benedict et al [189] demonstrated that neuropsychologic counseling emphasizing insight and social skills training was more effective than standard psychologic counseling in reducing disinhibition and socially aggressive behavior in cognitively impaired MS patients.

## Speech and swallowing therapy

Charcot's [190] description of MS given in a lecture in 1877 contained a triad of symptoms including intention tremor, nystagmus, and dysarthria. Of the third symptom, he said, "The affected person speaks in a slow, drawling manner, and sometimes almost unintelligibly. It seems as if the tongue had become 'too thick' and the delivery recalls that of an individual suffering from incipient intoxication." General speech performance registers in the normal range in most individuals with MS. Problems with controlling the volume of speech (too soft or too loud) may be the most common speech problem in MS. Dysarthria is reported in 14% to 19% and it is most often found in more neurologically impaired cases [191]. It has been characterized as a mixed spastic cerebellar dysarthria, although flaccid dysarthrias are also encountered. Apraxia, anomia, and aphasia are much less common, with incidences of 3% or less [192].

MS-associated speech problems are severe enough to limit comprehensibility in about 4% of cases [193]. Evaluation by speech therapy is advised in all such cases. The immediate goal is compensated intelligibility. The ultimate result is rarely, if ever, normal speech. When oral-verbal communication is less than 50% intelligible, one should try augmentative communication devices, of which there are many kinds.

Merson and Rolnick [194] reported that the important speech pathology treatment strategies for MS dysarthria are to control speech rate, voice emphasis, and phrase shifts; to reduce phase length; and to increase voice power. These investigators gave results of inpatient and outpatient speech therapy for moderately dysarthric individuals (only some of them had MS). Individuals in both settings made similar progress (32% and 33% improvement, respectively) despite marked differences in number of treatment sessions (mean, 16.2 versus 4.7). Thus, the outpatient program appears to have been much more cost-effective. Lee Silverman Voice Therapy focuses on tasks to maximize phonatory and respiratory functions, encouraging patients to "think loud." This therapy may be useful for patients who have flaccid dysarthria and has been incorporated into two case series of MS patients, with good results [195,196].

Dysphagia is a potentially life-threatening manifestation of MS. Thomas and Wiles [197] in the United Kingdom screened 79 consecutive MS rehabilitation inpatients (mean EDSS = 6.0) with a quantitative water test for dysphagia. The test involved clinical observations during swallowing of 150 mL of water "as fast as is comfortably possible." Abnormal swallowing was found in 43%, of whom almost half had no related complaints. Calcagno et al [198] in Italy recently did a cross-sectional study of 143 MS rehabilitation inpatients (mean EDSS = 6.8). All individuals underwent clinical swallowing evaluation by a speech therapist (history taking; observation of laryngeal, tongue, and oral facial movements; and meal consumption) and trans-nasal fiberendoscopic observation of thick and liquid bolus consumption. Dysphagia was found in 34%. Both studies identified two risk factors for dysphagia: abnormal brainstem function and severity of disease. Cerebellar function was a significant risk factor in one study but not in the other. In the Italian study, dysphagia was found in 48% of the nonambulatory individuals and in 11% of the ambulatory individuals. Relative to both studies, the frequency of dysphagia would probably have been higher with videofluoroscopy and lower with a less-impaired outpatient MS population. When videofluoroscopy is used, most asymptomatic MS individuals have been found to have abnormalities [199]. The oral phase of swallowing is more frequently abnormal than the pharyngeal and esophageal phases. Fluids may be more problematic than solids, but for most dysphagic individuals, both are equally bad [200].

Questions about choking, aspiration, or swallowing difficulty should be asked as part of routine review of systems in MS. Questioning alone is not reliable, and if the risk factors previously noted are present, clinicians should have a low threshold for speech and swallowing referral. When dysphagia is reported and the individual has an EDSS of 7.5 or higher (requirement for a power wheelchair), videofluoroscopy is recommended in addition to clinical assessment [200]. Postural techniques and modification of intake volume and consistency through speech/swallowing therapy enable mildly to moderately dysphagic individuals to improve swallowing [198].

## Vocational rehabilitation

Most people with MS (71%–75%) leave the workforce [198,201]. A recent report based on in-depth guided interviews of working people with MS documented the complexity of employment issues and provided possible explanations for low employment rates in MS [202]. Health professionals, employers, legislators, and society must work together to improve the occupational activity of people with MS. Vocational rehabilitation counselors help people make practical decisions about education and occupation. They can provide advice in negotiating modifications at the workplace and terms for medical leave. As often happens, they are also consulted to assist people with MS in applying for long-term disability health insurance and benefits. Social workers should also assist in this task. In most places, government agencies offer some vocational rehabilitation services and benefits. Funding for nongovernmental vocational rehabilitation is usually only partly covered by private insurance. Organizations, including the National Multiple Sclerosis Society, can also help with vocational counseling.

## Other nonpharmacologic approaches to MS symptoms

Berg et al [203] reported a case series of spinal cord stimulation (dorsal column stimulation) in 10 MS individuals. The stimulation improved urinary hesitancy and urgency. Al-Smadi et al [145] reported nonsignificant trends toward improved pain symptoms in an RCT of transcutaneous electrical nerve stimulation applied to the backs of MS subjects. Vahtera et al [204] did an RCT of pelvic floor exercises plus electrical stimulation by way of vaginal or rectal probes. Symptoms of urinary urgency, frequency, and incontinence were significantly less in the treated group. Men responded to the treatment better than women. Another RCT of extracorporeal photopheresis in chronic progressive MS yielded negative results [205]. Danish investigators did a double-blind, placebo-controlled study of repetitive magnetic cortical stimulation on spasticity on 38 MS individuals. The protocol used twice-daily therapy for 7 days. Clinical spasticity and stretch reflex threshold were significantly improved in the treated individuals [206].

An Israeli complementary medicine clinic studied the effects of reflexology treatment on MS symptoms [207]. Seventy-one subjects with MS were randomized to 11 weeks of reflexology (manual pressure on specific points in the feet) or nonspecific massage of the calf. Paresthesias, urinary symptoms, muscle strength, and spasticity were gauged at 0, 6, 11, and 35 weeks by blinded assessors. The treatment group had significantly greater improvement in paresthesias, urinary symptoms, and spasticity. Only the difference in paresthesia improvement remained significant at 3 months' follow-up. Shortcomings of this study were the choice of sham therapy (most subjects were probably aware that reflexology involves foot and not calf massage) and the high drop-out rate (25%). Third-party coverage for massage therapy and reflexology for MS is limited. A report of an RCT of injection of local anesthesia into specific trigger points in the ankles and scalp yielded amazing effects on MS impairment (improved EDSS lasting 2–3.5 years in more than 50% of the subjects). The authors found the results unbelievable [208].

## Summary

It is the coexistence of physical and cognitive impairments, together with emotional and social issues in a disease with an uncertain course, that makes MS rehabilitation unique and challenging. Inpatient rehabilitation improves functional independence but has only limited success improving the level of neurologic impairment. Benefits are usually not long lasting. Severely disabled people derive equal or more benefit than those who are less disabled, but cognitive problems and ataxia tend to be refractory. There is now good evidence that exercise can improve fitness and function for those with mild MS and helps to maintain function for those with moderate to severe disability. Therapy can be performed over 6 to 15 weeks in outpatient or home-based settings or as a weekly day program lasting several months. Several different forms of exercise have been investigated. For most individuals, aerobic exercise that incorporates a degree of balance training and socialization is recommended. Time constraints, access, impairment level, personal preferences, motivations, and funding sources influence the prescription for exercise and other components of rehabilitation. Just as immunomodulatory drugs must be taken on a continual basis and be adjusted as the disease progresses, so should rehabilitation be viewed as an ongoing process to maintain and restore maximum function and QOL.

## References

[1] Confavreux C, Vukusic S, et al. Relapses and progression of disability in multiple sclerosis. N Engl J Med 2000;343(20):1430–8.
[2] Thompson AJ. The effectiveness of neurological rehabilitation in multiple sclerosis. J Rehabil Res Dev 2000;37(4):455–61.
[3] Kurtzke JF. Rating neurologic impairment in multiple sclerosis: an expanded disability status scale (EDSS). Neurology 1983;33(11):1444–52.
[4] Solari A, et al. Physical rehabilitation has a positive effect on disability in multiple sclerosis patients. Neurology 1999;52(1):57–62.

[5] Freeman JA, et al. Inpatient rehabilitation in multiple sclerosis: do the benefits carry over into the community? Neurology 1999;52(1):50–6.

[6] Noseworthy JH, et al. Interrater variability with the Expanded Disability Status Scale (EDSS) and Functional Systems (FS) in a multiple sclerosis clinical trial. The Canadian Cooperation MS Study Group. Neurology 1990;40(6):971–5.

[7] Pittock SJ, et al. Change in MS-related disability in a population-based cohort: a 10-year follow-up study. Neurology 2004;62(1):51–9.

[8] Cutter GR, et al. Development of a multiple sclerosis functional composite as a clinical trial outcome measure. Brain 1999;122(Pt 5):871–82.

[9] Ozakbas S, et al. Correlations between multiple sclerosis functional composite, expanded disability status scale and health-related quality of life during and after treatment of relapses in patients with multiple sclerosis. J Neurol Sci 2004;218(1–2):3–7.

[10] Rudick RA, et al. Quality of life in multiple sclerosis. Comparison with inflammatory bowel disease and rheumatoid arthritis. Arch Neurol 1992;49(12):1237–42.

[11] Jonssen A, Dock J, Ravnborg MH. Quality of life as a measure of rehabilitation outcome in patients with multiple sclerosis. Acta Neurol Scand 1996;93(4):229–35.

[12] Benito-Leon J, et al. A review about the impact of multiple sclerosis on health-related quality of life. Disabil Rehabil 2003;25(23):1291–303.

[13] Kraft GH. Health care needs of persons with multiple sclerosis in rural areas [abstract]. Arch Phys Med Rehabil 1995;76:1035.

[14] Harper AC, et al. An epidemiological description of physical, social and psychological problems in multiple sclerosis. J Chronic Dis 1986;39(4):305–10.

[15] Chwastiak L, et al. Depressive symptoms and severity of illness in multiple sclerosis: epidemiologic study of a large community sample. Am J Psychiatry 2002;159(11): 1862–8.

[16] Lublin FD, Baier M, Cutter G. Effect of relapses on development of residual deficit in multiple sclerosis. Neurology 2003;61(11):1528–32.

[17] Confavreux C, Vukusic S, Adeleine P. Early clinical predictors and progression of irreversible disability in multiple sclerosis: an amnesic process. Brain 2003;126(Pt 4): 770–82.

[18] Paty DW, McFarland H. Magnetic resonance techniques to monitor the long term evolution of multiple sclerosis pathology and to monitor definitive clinical trials. J Neurol Neurosurg Psychiatry 1998;64(Suppl 1):S47–51.

[19] Hadjimichael O. Use of rehabilitation services reported by NARCOMS registrants. Mult Scler Q Rep 2004;23(1):21–3.

[20] Kraft GH, Freal JE, Coryell JK. Disability, disease duration, and rehabilitation service needs in multiple sclerosis: patient perspectives. Arch Phys Med Rehabil 1986;67(3): 164–8.

[21] Kraft GH. Multiple sclerosis: future directions in the care and the cure. J Neuro Rehabil 1989;3(2):61–4.

[22] Carey RG, Seibert JH, Posavac EJ. Who makes the most progress in inpatient rehabilitation? An analysis of functional gain. Arch Phys Med Rehabil 1988;69(5):337–43.

[23] Reding MJ, LaRocca NG, Madonna M. Acute-hospital care versus rehabilitation hospitalization for management of nonemergent complications in multiple sclerosis. J Neuro Rehab 1987;1(1):13–7.

[24] Francabandera FL, et al. Multiple sclerosis rehabilitation: inpatient vs. outpatient. Rehabil Nurs 1988;13(5):251–3.

[25] Greenspun B, Stineman M, Agri R. Multiple sclerosis and rehabilitation outcome. Arch Phys Med Rehabil 1987;68(7):434–7.

[26] Aisen ML, Sevilla D, Fox N. Inpatient rehabilitation for multiple sclerosis. J Neuro Rehabil 1996;10(1):43–6.

[27] Olgiati R, Jacquet J, Di Prampero PE. Energy cost of walking and exertional dyspnea in multiple sclerosis. Am Rev Respir Dis 1986;134(5):1005–10.

[28] LaRocca NG, Kalb RC. Efficacy of rehabilitation in multiple sclerosis. J Neuro Rehab 1992;6:147–55.

[29] Freeman JA, et al. The impact of inpatient rehabilitation on progressive multiple sclerosis. Ann Neurol 1997;42(2):236–44.

[30] Fuller KJ, Dawson K, Wiles CM. Physiotherapy in chronic multiple sclerosis: a controlled trial. Clin Rehabil 1996;10:195–204.

[31] Mostert S, Kesselring J. Effects of a short-term exercise training program on aerobic fitness, fatigue, health perception and activity level of subjects with multiple sclerosis. Mult Scler 2002;8(2):161–8.

[32] Craig J, et al. A randomised controlled trial comparing rehabilitation against standard therapy in multiple sclerosis patients receiving intravenous steroid treatment. J Neurol Neurosurg Psychiatry 2003;74(9):1225–30.

[33] Feigenson JS, et al. The cost-effectiveness of multiple sclerosis rehabilitation: a model. Neurology 1981;31(10):1316–22.

[34] Friedman SM. The inflation calculator. Available at: www.westegg.com/inflation. Accessed February 7, 2005.

[35] Vaney C, et al. Assessing mobility in multiple sclerosis using the Rivermead Mobility Index and gait speed. Clin Rehabil 1996;10:216–26.

[36] Pozzilli C, et al. Home based management in multiple sclerosis: results of a randomised controlled trial. J Neurol Neurosurg Psychiatry 2002;73(3):250–5.

[37] Liu C, Playford ED, Thompson AJ. Does neurorehabilitation have a role in relapsing-remitting multiple sclerosis? J Neurol 2003;250(10):1214–8.

[38] Kidd D, Howard RS, Losseff N. The benefit of inpatient neurorehabilitation in multiple sclerosis. Clin Rehabil 1995;9:198–203.

[39] Langdon DW, Thompson AJ. Multiple sclerosis: a preliminary study of selected variables affecting rehabilitation outcome. Mult Scler 1999;5(2):94–100.

[40] Kraft GH. Rehabilitation still the only way to improve function in multiple sclerosis. Lancet 1999;354(9195):2016–7.

[41] Krupp LB, et al. Fatigue in multiple sclerosis. Arch Neurol 1988;45(4):435–7.

[42] Freal JE, Kraft GH, Coryell JK. Symptomatic fatigue in multiple sclerosis. Arch Phys Med Rehabil 1984;65(3):135–8.

[43] Krupp LB, et al. The fatigue severity scale. Application to patients with multiple sclerosis and systemic lupus erythematosus. Arch Neurol 1989;46(10):1121–3.

[44] Fisk JD, et al. The impact of fatigue on patients with multiple sclerosis. Can J Neurol Sci 1994;21(1):9–14.

[45] Geisler MW, et al. The effects of amantadine and pemoline on cognitive functioning in multiple sclerosis. Arch Neurol 1996;53(2):185–8.

[46] Lerdal A, Celius EG, Moum T. Fatigue and its association with sociodemographic variables among multiple sclerosis patients. Mult Scler 2003;9(5):509–14.

[47] Kraft GH, Brown T. Comprehensive management of multiple sclerosis. In: Braddom RL, editor. Physical medicine and rehabilitation. Philadelphia: Saunders; in press.

[48] Schwid SR, et al. Quantitative assessment of motor fatigue and strength in MS. Neurology 1999;53(4):743–50.

[49] Sheean GL, et al. An electrophysiological study of the mechanism of fatigue in multiple sclerosis. Brain 1997;120(Pt 2):299–315.

[50] Sharma KR, et al. Evidence of an abnormal intramuscular component of fatigue in multiple sclerosis. Muscle Nerve 1995;18(12):1403–11.

[51] Chen WY, Pierson FM, Burnett CN. Force-time measurements of knee muscle functions of subjects with multiple sclerosis. Phys Ther 1987;67(6):934–40.

[52] Armstrong LE, et al. Using isokinetic dynamometry to test ambulatory patients with multiple sclerosis. Phys Ther 1983;63(8):1274–9.

[53] van Diemen HA, et al. Increased visual impairment after exercise (Uhthoff's phenomenon) in multiple sclerosis: therapeutic possibilities. Eur Neurol 1992;32(4):231–4.

[54] Colombo B, et al. MRI and motor evoked potential findings in nondisabled multiple sclerosis patients with and without symptoms of fatigue. J Neurol 2000;247(7):506–9.

[55] Galardi L, Maderna S, et al. Assessment of central fatigue by transcranial magnetic stimulation in multiple sclerosis patients. Presented at the 1st SENIAM Workshop. Turin, Italy, September 5–6, 1996.

[56] Rice CL, Vollmer TL, Bigland-Ritchie B. Neuromuscular responses of patients with multiple sclerosis. Muscle Nerve 1992;15(10):1123–32.

[57] Ng AV, Miller RG, Kent-Braun JA. Central motor drive is increased during voluntary muscle contractions in multiple sclerosis. Muscle Nerve 1997;20(10):1213–8.

[58] Ng AV, Kent-Braun JA. Basis of muscle fatigue in multiple sclerosis. Mul Scler Q Rep 2004; 23(1):13–7.

[59] Kent-Braun JA, et al. Effects of exercise on muscle activation and metabolism in multiple sclerosis. Muscle Nerve 1994;17(10):1162–9.

[60] Kent-Braun JA, et al. Strength, skeletal muscle composition, and enzyme activity in multiple sclerosis. J Appl Physiol 1997;83(6):1998–2004.

[61] Murray TJ. Amantadine therapy for fatigue in multiple sclerosis. Can J Neurol Sci 1985; 12(3):251–4.

[62] Flachenecker P, et al. Fatigue in MS is related to sympathetic vasomotor dysfunction. Neurology 2003;61(6):851–3.

[63] Pepin EB, et al. Pressor response to isometric exercise in patients with multiple sclerosis. Med Sci Sports Exerc 1996;28(6):656–60.

[64] Tantucci C, et al. Energy cost of exercise in multiple sclerosis patients with low degree of disability. Mult Scler 1996;2(3):161–7.

[65] Horemans HL, et al. A comparison of 4 questionnaires to measure fatigue in post-poliomyelitis syndrome. Arch Phys Med Rehabil 2004;85:392–8.

[66] Petajan JH, et al. Impact of aerobic training on fitness and quality of life in multiple sclerosis. Ann Neurol 1996;39(4):432–41.

[67] Bajada S, et al. Effects of induced hyperthermia on visual evoked potentials and saccade parameters in normal subjects and multiple sclerosis patients. J Neurol Neurosurg Psychiatry 1980;43(9):849–52.

[68] Namerow NS. Temperature effect on critical flicker fusion in multiple sclerosis. Arch Neurol 1971;25(3):269–75.

[69] Davis FA, Michael JA, Tomaszewski JS. Fluctuation of motor function in multiple sclerosis related to circadian temperature variations. Dis Nerv Syst 1973;34(1):33–6.

[70] Uhthoff W. Untersuchungen über die bei der multiplen herdsklerose vorkommenden augenstörungen. Arch Psychiatr Nervenkr 1889;21:303–420.

[71] Petajan JH, White AT. Recommendations for physical activity in pati ents with multiple sclerosis. Sports Med 1999;27(3):179–91.

[72] Ponichtera-Mulcare JA. Exercise and multiple sclerosis. Med Sci Sports Exerc 1993;25(4): 451–65.

[73] Rusk HA. Rehabilitation medicine. 3rd edition. St. Louis (MO): CV Mosby; 1971.

[74] Ponichtera-Mulcare JA, et al. Maximal aerobic exercise in persons with multiple sclerosis. Clin Kinesiol 1992;46:12–21.

[75] Sutherland G, Andersen MB. Exercise and multiple sclerosis: physiological, psychological, and quality of life issues. J Sports Med Phys Fitness 2001;41(4):421–32.

[76] Astrand P, Deblom R, Messin R. Intraarterial blood pressure during exercise with different muscle groups. J Appl Physiol 1965;20:253–6.

[77] Zwiren LD, Bar-Or O. Responses to exercise of paraplegics who differ in conditioning level. Med Sci Sports 1975;7(2):94–8.

[78] Schapiro RT, et al. Role of cardiovascular fitness in multiple sclerosis: a pilot study. J Neuro Rehabil 1988;2(2):43–9.

[79] Heesen C, et al. Endocrine and cytokine responses to standardized physical stress in multiple sclerosis. Brain Behav Immun 2003;17(6):473–81.

[80] Johnson KB. Exercise, drug treatment, and the optimal care of multiple sclerosis patients. Ann Neurol 1996;39(4):422–3.

[81] Saltin B, Hermansen L. Esophageal, rectal, and muscle temperature during exercise. J Appl Physiol 1966;21(6):1757–62.

[82] Boynton BL, Garramone PM, Buca J. Cool baths as an adjunct in the treatment of patients with multiple sclerosis. Q Bull Northwest Univ Med Sch 1959;33(1):6–7.

[83] Watson CW. Effect of lowering of body temperature on the symptoms and signs of multiple sclerosis. N Engl J Med 1959;261:1253–9.

[84] Chiara T, et al. Cold effect on oxygen uptake, perceived exertion, and spasticity in patients with multiple sclerosis. Arch Phys Med Rehabil 1998;79(5):523–8.

[85] Capello E, et al. Lowering body temperature with a cooling suit as symptomatic treatment for thermosensitive multiple sclerosis patients. Ital J Neurol Sci 1995;16(8): 533–9.

[86] Robinson LR, et al. Body cooling may not improve somatosensory pathway function in multiple sclerosis. Am J Phys Med Rehabil 1997;76(3):191–6.

[87] Kraft GH, Alquist AD. Effect of microclimate cooling on physical function in multiple sclerosis [abstract]. Mult Scler Clin Lab Res 1996;2(2):114–5.

[88] Syndulko K, et al. Preliminary evaluation of lowering tympanic temperature for the symptomatic treatment of multiple sclerosis. J Neuro Rehabil 1995;9:205–15.

[89] Woyciechowska J, et al. Application of cooling techniques during exercise in MS patients. Mult Scler Manage 1995;2(2):25–9.

[90] Schwid SR, et al. A randomized controlled study of the acute and chronic effects of cooling therapy for MS. Neurology 2003;60:1955–60.

[91] Brown S. Webhead report: summer's coming: plan to cool it! Inside MS 2004;22(2):66–7.

[92] Gehlsen GM, Grigsby SA, Winant DM. Effects of an aquatic fitness program on the muscular strength and endurance of patients with multiple sclerosis. Phys Ther 1984;64(5): 653–7.

[93] De Souza LH, Worthington JA. The effect of long-term physiotherapy on disability in multiple sclerosis individuals. In: Rose FC, Edwards R, editors. Multiple sclerosis: immunological, diagnostic, and therapeutic aspects. London: John Libbey; 1987. p. 155–64.

[94] Svensson B, Gerdle B, Elert J. Endurance training in patients with multiple sclerosis: five case studies. Phys Ther 1994;74(11):1017–26.

[95] Gappmaier E, Spencer MK, White AT. Fifteen weeks of aerobic training improve fitness of multiple sclerosis individuals [abstract]. Med Sci Sports Exerc 1994;26:S29.

[96] White AT, Gappmaier E, Mino L. Response to acute exercise before and after 15 weeks of training for multiple sclerosis individuals [abstract]. Med Sci Sports Exerc 1994;26: S29.

[97] Ponichtera-Mulcare JA, Mathews T, Barrett PJ. Change in aerobic fitness of individuals with multiple sclerosis during a 6-month training program. Sports Med Train Rehabil 1997; 7:265–72.

[98] Rodgers MM, et al. Gait characteristics of individuals with multiple sclerosis before and after a 6-month aerobic training program. J Rehabil Res Dev 1999;36(3):183–8.

[99] Maloney FP. Rehabilitation of the individual with multiple sclerosis. In: Maloney FP, Burks JS, Ringel SP, editors. Interdisciplinary rehabilitation of multiple sclerosis and neuromuscular disorders. Philadelphia: JB Lippincott; 1985. p. 75.

[100] Kraft GH, Alquist AD, de Lateur BJ. Effect of resistive exercise on physical function in multiple sclerosis [abstract]. Rehabil Res Dev Rep 1995;33:328–9.

[101] Kraft GH, Alquist AD, de Lateur BJ. Effect of resistive exercise on strength in multiple sclerosis [abstract]. Rehabil Res Dev Rep 1995;33:329–30.

[102] Schapiro RT, Soderberg J, Hooley M. The multiple sclerosis achievement center: a maintenance approach toward a chronic progressive form of the disease. J Neuro Rehabil 1988;2:21–3.

[103] Di Fabio RP, et al. Extended outpatient rehabilitation: its influence on symptom frequency, fatigue, and functional status for persons with progressive multiple sclerosis. Arch Phys Med Rehabil 1998;79(2):141–6.

[104] Di Fabio RP, et al. Health-related quality of life for patients with progressive multiple sclerosis: influence of rehabilitation. Phys Ther 1997;77(12):1704–16.

[105] Patti F, et al. The impact of outpatient rehabilitation on quality of life in multiple sclerosis. J Neurol 2002;249(8):1027–33.

[106] Patti F, et al. Effects of a short outpatient rehabilitation treatment on disability of multiple sclerosis patients–a randomised controlled trial. J Neurol 2003;250(7):861–6.

[107] Boggild M, Ford H. Multiple sclerosis. Clin Evid 2002;7:1195–207.

[108] LaBan MM, et al. Physical and occupational therapy in the treatment of patients with multiple sclerosis. Phys Med Rehabil Clin N Am 1998;9(3):603–14 [vii].

[109] Baum HM, Rothschild BB. Multiple sclerosis and mobility restriction. Arch Phys Med Rehabil 1983;64(12):591–6.

[110] Gehlsen G, et al. Gait characteristics in multiple sclerosis: progressive changes and effects of exercise on parameters. Arch Phys Med Rehabil 1986;67(8):536–9.

[111] Cattaneo D, et al. Risks of falls in subjects with multiple sclerosis. Arch Phys Med Rehabil 2002;83(6):864–7.

[112] Collen FM, et al. The Rivermead Mobility Index: a further development of the Rivermead Motor Assessment. Int Disabil Stud 1991;13(2):50–4.

[113] Wade DT. Measurement in neurological rehabilitation. Oxford (UK): Oxford Medical Publications; 1992.

[114] Holden MK, et al. Clinical gait assessment in the neurologically impaired. Reliability and meaningfulness. Phys Ther 1984;64(1):35–40.

[115] Wiles CM, et al. Use of videotape to assess mobility in a controlled randomized crossover trial of physiotherapy in chronic multiple sclerosis. Clin Rehabil 2003;17(3):256–63.

[116] Frzovic D, Morris ME, Vowels L. Clinical tests of standing balance: performance of persons with multiple sclerosis. Arch Phys Med Rehabil 2000;81(2):215–21.

[117] Berg K, Wood-Dauphinee S, Williams JL. Measuring balance in the elderly. Physiother Can 1989;41:304.

[118] Mathias S, Nayak US, Isaacs B. Balance in elderly patients: the "get-up and go" test. Arch Phys Med Rehabil 1986;67(6):387–9.

[119] Kasser SL, Rose DJ, Clark S. Balance training for adults with multiple sclerosis: multiple case studies. Neurology Report 1999;23(1):5–12.

[120] Wiles CM, et al. Controlled randomised crossover trial of the effects of physiotherapy on mobility in chronic multiple sclerosis. J Neurol Neurosurg Psychiatry 2001;70(2):174–9.

[121] Lord SE, Wade DT, Halligan PW. A comparison of two physiotherapy treatment approaches to improve walking in multiple sclerosis: a pilot randomized controlled study. Clin Rehabil 1998;12(6):477–86.

[122] Armutlu K, Karabudak R, Nurlu G. Physiotherapy approaches in the treatment of ataxic multiple sclerosis: a pilot study. Neurorehabil Neural Repair 2001;15(3):203–11.

[123] Stephens J, et al. Use of awareness through movement improves balance and balance confidence in people with multiple sclerosis: a randomized controlled study. Neurology Report 2001;25(2):39–49.

[124] Johnson SK, et al. A controlled investigation of bodywork in multiple sclerosis. J Altern Complement Med 1999;5(3):237–43.

[125] Husted C, et al. Improving quality of life for people with chronic conditions: the example of t'ai chi and multiple sclerosis. Altern Ther Health Med 1999;5(5):70–4.

[126] DeBolt LS, McCubbin JA. The effects of home-based resistance exercise on balance, power, and mobility in adults with multiple sclerosis. Arch Phys Med Rehabil 2004;85(2): 290–7.

[127] Ashworth B. Preliminary trial of carisoprodol in multiple sclerosis. Practitioner 1964;192: 540–2.

[128] van Wijck FM, et al. Assessing motor deficits in neurological rehabilitation: patterns of instrument usage. Neurorehabil Neural Repair 2001;15(1):23–30.

[129] Bakheit AM, et al. The relation between Ashworth scale scores and the excitability of the alpha motor neurones in patients with post-stroke muscle spasticity. J Neurol Neurosurg Psychiatry 2003;74(5):646–8.

[130] Little JW, Massagli TL. Spasticity and associated abnormalities of muscle tone. In: DeLisa JA, editor. Rehabilitation medicine: principles and practice. Philadelphia: J.B. Lippincott; 1993. p. 666.

[131] Pandyan AD, et al. A review of the properties and limitations of the Ashworth and modified Ashworth Scales as measures of spasticity. Clin Rehabil 1999;13(5):373–83.

[132] Bohannon RW, Smith MB. Interrater reliability of a modified Ashworth scale of muscle spasticity. Phys Ther 1987;67(2):206–7.

[133] Peacock WJ, Staudt LA. Functional outcomes following selective posterior rhizotomy in children with cerebral palsy. J Neurosurg 1991;74(3):380–5.

[134] Katz RT, et al. Objective quantification of spastic hypertonia: correlation with clinical findings. Arch Phys Med Rehabil 1992;73(4):339–47.

[135] Damiano DL, et al. What does the Ashworth scale really measure and are instrumented measures more valid and precise? Dev Med Child Neurol 2002;44(2):112–8.

[136] Pandyan AD, et al. A biomechanical investigation into the validity of the modified Ashworth Scale as a measure of elbow spasticity. Clin Rehabil 2003;17(3):290–3.

[137] Sloan RL, et al. Inter-rater reliability of the modified Ashworth Scale for spasticity in hemiplegic patients. Int J Rehabil Res 1992;15(2):158–61.

[138] Bodin PG, Morris ME. Inter-rater reliability of the modified Ashworth scale for wrist flexor spasticity following stroke. Preceedings of the 11th Congress of the World Federation of Physical Therapy. London, 1991.

[139] Gregson JA. Reliability of measurements of muscle tone and muscle power in stroke individuals. Age Ageing 2000;29:223–8.

[140] Haas BM, et al. The inter rater reliability of the original and of the modified Ashworth scale for the assessment of spasticity in patients with spinal cord injury. Spinal Cord 1996;34(9): 560–4.

[141] Gregson JA, Leathley M, Moore AP. Reliability of the tone assessment scale and modified Ashworth scale as clinical tools for assessing poststroke spasticity. Arch Phys Med Rehabil 1999;80:1013–6.

[142] Taylor RS. Rehabilitation of persons with multiple sclerosis. In: Braddom RL, editor. Physical medicine and rehabilitation. Philadelphia: W.B. Saunders; 2000. p. 1177–90.

[143] Brar SP, et al. Evaluation of treatment protocols on minimal to moderate spasticity in multiple sclerosis. Arch Phys Med Rehabil 1991;72(3):186–9.

[144] Erickson RP, Lie MR, Wineinger MA. Rehabilitation in multiple sclerosis. Mayo Clin Proc 1989;64(7):818–28.

[145] Al-Smadi J, et al. A pilot investigation of the hypoalgesic effects of transcutaneous electrical nerve stimulation upon low back pain in people with multiple sclerosis. Clin Rehabil 2003; 17(7):742–9.

[146] White AT. Exercise and MS: challenges and opportunities. Mult Scler Q Rep 2004;23(1): 18–20.

[147] Woods DA. Aquatic exercise programs for individuals with multiple sclerosis. Clin Kinesiol 1992;45:14–20.

[148] Peterson JL, Bell GW. Aquatic exercise for individuals with multiple sclerosis. Clin Kinesiol 1995;49(3):69–71.

[149] Hewson DC, et al. Food intake in multiple sclerosis. Hum Nutr Appl Nutr 1984;38(5): 355–67.

[150] Kraft GH. Foreword. Phys Med Rehabil Clin N Am 1998;9(3):xi–xiii.

[151] Staples D, Lincoln NB. Intellectual impairment in multiple sclerosis and its relation to functional abilities. Rheumatol Rehabil 1979;18(3):153–60.

[152] Baker NA, Tickle-Degnen L. The effectiveness of physical, psychological, and functional interventions in treating clients with multiple sclerosis: a meta-analysis. Am J Occup Ther 2001;55(3):324–31.

[153] Alusi SH, et al. A study of tremor in multiple sclerosis. Brain 2001;124(Pt 4):720–30.

[154] Jones L, et al. The effectiveness of occupational therapy and physiotherapy in multiple sclerosis patients with ataxia of the upper limb and trunk. Clin Rehabil 1996;10:277–82.

[155] Vanage SM, Gilbertson KK, Mathiowetz V. Effects of an energy conservation course on fatigue impact for persons with progressive multiple sclerosis. Am J Occup Ther 2003;57(3): 315–23.

[156] Mathiowetz V, Matuska KM, Murphy ME. Efficacy of an energy conservation course for persons with multiple sclerosis. Arch Phys Med Rehabil 2001;82(4):449–56.

[157] Steultjens EM, et al. Occupational therapy for multiple sclerosis. Cochrane Database Syst Rev 2003;(3):CD003608.

[158] O'Hara L, et al. Evaluation of the effectiveness of professionally guided self-care for people with multiple sclerosis living in the community: a randomized controlled trial. Clin Rehabil 2002;16(2):119–28.

[159] Hutchinson B. Rehabilitation interventions for people with multiple sclerosis. Mult Scler Q Rep 2004;23(1):3–11.

[160] Kraft GH. Movement disorders. In: Basmajian JV, Kirby RL, editors. Medical rehabilitation. Baltimore (MD): Williams and Wilkins; 1984. p. 162–5.

[161] Aisen ML, et al. The effect of mechanical damping loads on disabling action tremor. Neurology 1993;43(7):1346–50.

[162] Costello K, Halper J, Harris C, et al. Multifaceted roles of the MS nurse. Int J Mult Scler Care 2003;S14.

[163] Stuifbergen AK. Physical activity and perceived health status in persons with multiple sclerosis. J Neurosci Nurs 1997;29(4):238–43.

[164] Stuifbergen AK, et al. A randomized clinical trial of a wellness intervention for women with multiple sclerosis. Arch Phys Med Rehabil 2003;84(4):467–76.

[165] Bombardier CH, Blake K, Cunniffe M. Brief counseling for health promotion among persons with multiple sclerosis (Abstract). Intl J MS Care 2004;6(2):59–64.

[166] Bourdette D, et al. Evidence that a multidisciplinary team care clinic is more effective than standard medical care in treating veterans with multiple sclerosis [abstract]. Neurology 1991;41(Suppl):353.

[167] Arnett PA, et al. Depressed mood in multiple sclerosis: relationship to capacity-demanding memory and attentional functioning. Neuropsychology 1999;13(3):434–46.

[168] Beatty WW. Cognitive and emotional disturbances in multiple sclerosis. Neurol Clin 1993; 11(1):189–204.

[169] Rao SM, et al. Correlation of magnetic resonance imaging with neuropsychological testing in multiple sclerosis. Neurology 1989;39(2 Pt 1):161–6.

[170] Rovaris M, et al. Relation between MR abnormalities and patterns of cognitive impairment in multiple sclerosis. Neurology 1998;50(6):1601–8.

[171] Comi G, et al. Brain MRI correlates of cognitive impairment in primary and secondary progressive multiple sclerosis. J Neurol Sci 1995;132(2):222–7.

[172] Ruggieri RM, et al. Cognitive impairment in patients suffering from relapsing-remitting multiple sclerosis with EDSS < or = 3.5. Acta Neurol Scand 2003;108(5):323–6.

[173] Rao SM, et al. Cognitive dysfunction in multiple sclerosis. II. Impact on employment and social functioning. Neurology 1991;41(5):692–6.

[174] Rao SM, et al. Cognitive dysfunction in multiple sclerosis. I. Frequency, patterns, and prediction. Neurology 1991;41(5):685–91.

[175] Crawford JD, McIvor GP. Group psychotherapy: benefits in multiple sclerosis. Arch Phys Med Rehabil 1985;66(12):810–3.

[176] Crawford JD, McIvor GP. Stress management for multiple sclerosis patients. Psychol Rep 1987;61(2):423–9.

[177] Foley FW, et al. Efficacy of stress-inoculation training in coping with multiple sclerosis. J Consult Clin Psychol 1987;55(6):919–22.

[178] Larcombe NA, Wilson PH. An evaluation of cognitive-behaviour therapy for depression in patients with multiple sclerosis. Br J Psychiatry 1984;145:366–71.

[179] Jonsson A, et al. Effects of neuropsychological treatment in patients with multiple sclerosis. Acta Neurol Scand 1993;88(6):394–400.

[180] Plohmann AM, et al. Computer assisted retraining of attentional impairments in patients with multiple sclerosis. J Neurol Neurosurg Psychiatry 1998;64(4):455–62.

[181] Lincoln NB, et al. Evaluation of cognitive assessment and cognitive intervention for people with multiple sclerosis. J Neurol Neurosurg Psychiatry 2002;72(1):93–8.

[182] Taylor A, Taylor RS. Neuropsychologic aspects of multiple sclerosis. Phys Med Rehabil Clin N Am 1998;9(3):643–57 [vii–viii.].

[183] Goodin DS, et al. The relationship of MS to physical trauma and psychological stress: report of the Therapeutics and Technology Assessment Subcommittee of the American Academy of Neurology. Neurology 1999;52(9):1737–45.

[184] Buljevac D, et al. Self reported stressful life events and exacerbations in multiple sclerosis: prospective study. BMJ 2003;327(7416):646.

[185] Galea I, Newman TA, Gidron Y. Stress and exacerbations in multiple sclerosis: whether stress triggers relapses remains a conundrum [author reply]. BMJ 2004;328(7434):287.

[186] Warren S, Warren KG, Cockerill R. Emotional stress and coping in multiple sclerosis (MS) exacerbations. J Psychosom Res 1991;35(1):37–47.

[187] Mohr DC, et al. Moderating effects of coping on the relationship between stress and the development of new brain lesions in multiple sclerosis. Psychosom Med 2002;64(5):803–9.

[188] Pakenham KI. Adjustment to multiple sclerosis: application of a stress and coping model. Health Psychol 1999;18(4):383–92.

[189] Benedict RH, et al. Neuropsychological counseling improves social behavior in cognitively-impaired multiple sclerosis patients. Mult Scler 2000;6(6):391–6.

[190] Charcot JM. Lectures on the diseases of the nervous system, vol. 1. London: The New Sydenham Society; 1877.

[191] Darley FL, Brown JR, Goldstein NP. Dysarthria in multiple sclerosis. J Speech Hear Res 1972;15(2):229–45.

[192] Lacour A, et al. Acute aphasia in multiple sclerosis: a multicenter study of 22 patients. Neurology 2004;62(6):974–7.

[193] Beukelman DR, Kraft GH, Freal J. Expressive communication disorders in persons with multiple sclerosis: a survey. Arch Phys Med Rehabil 1985;66(10):675–7.

[194] Merson RM, Rolnick MI. Speech-language pathology and dysphagia in multiple sclerosis. Phys Med Rehabil Clin N Am 1998;9(3):631–41.

[195] Sapir S, et al. Effects of intensive phonatory-respiratory treatment (LSVT) on voice in two individuals with multiple sclerosis. J Med Speech-Lang Pathol 2001;9(2):141–51.

[196] Hartelius L, Nord L. Speech modification in dysarthria associated with multiple sclerosis: an intervention based on vocal efficiency, contrastive stress, and verbal repair strategies. J Med Speech-Lang Pathol 1997;5(2):113–40.

[197] Thomas FJ, Wiles CM. Dysphagia and nutritional status in multiple sclerosis. J Neurol 1999;246(8):677–82.

[198] Calcagno P, et al. Dysphagia in multiple sclerosis—prevalence and prognostic factors. Acta Neurol Scand 2002;105(1):40–3.

[199] Wiesner W, et al. Swallowing abnormalities in multiple sclerosis: correlation between videofluoroscopy and subjective symptoms. Eur Radiol 2002;12(4):789–92.

[200] De Pauw A, et al. Dysphagia in multiple sclerosis. Clin Neurol Neurosurg 2002;104(4):345–51.

[201] Minden SL, Marder WD, Harrold LN. Multiple sclerosis: a statistical portrait. A compendium of data on demographics, disability, and health service utilization in the United States. New York: National Multiple Sclerosis Society; 1993.

[202] Johnson KL, et al. The cost and benefits of employment: a qualitative study of experiences of persons with multiple sclerosis. Arch Phys Med Rehabil 2004;85(2):201–9.

[203] Berg V, et al. The value of dorsal column stimulation in multiple sclerosis. Scand J Rehabil Med 1982;14(4):183–91.

[204] Vahtera T, et al. Pelvic floor rehabilitation is effective in patients with multiple sclerosis. Clin Rehabil 1997;11(3):211–9.

[205] Rostami AM, et al. A double-blind, placebo-controlled trial of extracorporeal photo-pheresis in chronic progressive multiple sclerosis. Mult Scler 1999;5(3):198–203.

[206] Nielsen JF, Sinkjaer T, Jakobsen J. Treatment of spasticity with repetitive magnetic stimulation: a double-blind placebo-controlled study. Mult Scler 1996;2(5):227–32.

[207] Siev-Ner I, et al. Reflexology treatment relieves symptoms of multiple sclerosis: a randomized controlled study. Mult Scler 2003;9(4):356–61.

[208] Gibson RG, Gibson SL. Neural therapy in the treatment of multiple sclerosis. J Altern Complement Med 1999;5(6):543–52.

ELSEVIER
SAUNDERS

Phys Med Rehabil Clin N Am
16 (2005) 557–570

PHYSICAL MEDICINE
AND REHABILITATION
CLINICS OF
NORTH AMERICA

# Health Promotion in People
# with Multiple Sclerosis

Charles H. Bombardier, PhD*, Rohini Wadhwani, BS,
Chiara LaRotonda, MSW

*Multiple Sclerosis Rehabilitation Research and Training Center,
Department of Rehabilitation Medicine, Box 359740,
University of Washington School of Medicine, Harborview
Medical Center, 325 9th Avenue, Seattle, WA 98195-6490, USA*

Health promotion is essential to effective management of chronic diseases. Health-promotion activities have the potential to improve the overall physical, emotional, and social health of persons with multiple sclerosis (MS) within reasonable bounds [1]. As illustrated in Fig. 1, health-promotion activities are unrelated to physical abilities; that is, most everyone with MS can engage in and benefit from some sort of health-promotion activity. Most important, health-promotion activities can mitigate the impact of physical disabilities on quality of life [2].

Health promotion is described in various ways: wellness promotion, disease management, lifestyle modification, and self-management. Health promotion has at least two dimensions: content and process. The content of health promotion for people with MS is the focus of this article; however, the process by which health promotion occurs also merits discussion.

## Processes of health promotion

How health promotion is accomplished varies from being entirely initiated and maintained by the person with chronic illness (eg, the use of self-help materials in the absence of professional health care) to being prescribed, organized, and delivered by health care providers (eg, comprehensive inpatient rehabilitation). Health promotion, however, usually implies more

Funded in part by the National Institute on Disability and Rehabilitation Research grant H133B980017 and the Department of Education, National Institute on Disability and Rehabilitation Research grant H133B031129-04.
  * Corresponding author.
  *E-mail address:* chb@u.washington.edu (C.H. Bombardier).

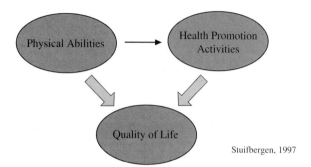

Fig. 1. Health promotion and MS. (*From* Stuifbergen AK, Roberts GJ. Health promotion practices of women with multiple sclerosis. Arch Phys Med Rehabil 1997;78:S3–9; with permission.)

responsibility on the part of the person with the chronic disease than in traditional medical care.

Lorig [3] described five core self-management skills: problem solving, decision making, resource use, forming effective partnerships with health care providers, and taking action. This model emphasizes training and empowering those with chronic diseases to proactively manage their own health in collaboration with health care providers. Self-management interventions have been shown to improve health status and lower health care costs in people with heart disease, arthritis, asthma, and diabetes [3]. The self-management model may be useful for many people with MS; however, some people may also benefit from more structure and monitoring on the part of the health care system.

Wagner's [4] model of chronic disease management is more encompassing and focuses on the provider side of the health-promotion equation. It describes how an organized, proactive care system would provide self-management education and support for patients. Equally important, a prepared system would provide (1) decision support for health care providers to develop and implement evidence-based guidelines, (2) reorganized health care teams that can provide systematic follow-up, and (3) enhanced information systems such as disease registries, tracking systems, and automatic reminders to give patients and providers feedback on performance. If Wagner's analysis is correct, the future health of people with MS depends not only on changing the behavior of individuals with MS but also on changing the behavior of health care organizations and how prepared they are to support more effective management of this chronic disease.

## Targets of health promotion

Health-promotion interventions in MS can target many different aspects of the disease and how it is managed. The authors selected domains that seemed to have the most potential for improving the lives of people with MS. Examples include remaining active or exercising, improving stress management, building social support and coping skills, enhancing compliance with disease-modifying therapies, improving diet and nutrition, and avoiding substance misuse.

*Exercise*

Exercise appears to be a safe, popular, and powerful means of improving health and functioning among people with MS. In terms of safety, people with MS have been carefully monitored in a number of research studies and shown to have very low rates of negative side effects or adverse reactions [5,6]. Exercise does not appear to increase the frequency of exacerbations [5]. General fatigue typically is the only symptom reported in response to exercise [6], and graded exercise programs result in reduced fatigue as conditioning improves [7,8]. Those with heightened thermosensitivity can significantly dampen elevation of exercise-induced body temperature through 30 minutes of precooling the lower extremities in a 16°C to 17°C bath [9]. Other strategies such as using fans, exercising in pools with colder temperatures, and using cooling vests may also be helpful. Exercise should be reduced or discontinued during an exacerbation, especially if cortico-steriod treatment is required [5].

The popularity of exercise is evident among people with MS and researchers. Somerset et al [10] reported that the single most requested type of medical information was advice about exercise, with 41% requesting such information. At the Multiple Sclerosis Rehabilitation Research and Training Center at the University of Washington, a survey of 739 community residents with MS showed that they were more interested in exercise than any other health-promotion activity [11]. Eighty-six percent of the total sample was very interested or somewhat interested in learning more about ways to exercise safely. There has also been a sharp rise in interest among researchers, as shown by the recent publication of many new studies on outpatient rehabilitation [12], aerobic training [13,14], home-based resistance exercise [15], and yoga [8].

Evidence for positive health benefits of exercise among people with MS is substantial and growing [5,6]. Beginning with the seminal work by Petajan and colleagues [7], exercise has been shown to result in widespread positive effects among people with MS. This widely cited randomized controlled study showed that three 40-minute sessions of combined arm and leg ergometry over a 15-week period resulted in diminished fatigue along with improvements in strength, aerobic conditioning, mobility, and bowel and bladder functioning compared with controls receiving no treatment. The exercise intervention also led to improvements in psychosocial variables including mood, social interactions, home management, and recreation. Other studies have confirmed the positive effects of exercise on fatigue (using yoga or a stationary bicycle) [8], strength [15], and vitality, social interaction, and activity level [13]. Respiratory muscle strength and ventilatory capacity can also be improved with a 3- to 5-week respiratory muscle training program [16]. Although most exercise research has been performed on people with mild MS-related disability (Expanded Disability Status Scale ≤6), Di Fabio et al [17] investigated the benefits exercise among people with chronic, progressive MS. He provided one group of patients with 5 hours of outpatient rehabilitation services 1 d/wk for a year. Compared with a wait-list control group, the group receiving rehabilitation demonstrated a significant reduction in fatigue and other symptoms and a trend toward less decline in functional status. This study lends credence to the claim that some form of exercise is possible for anyone with MS (from passive range of motion to an integrated strength training program) and that exercise may be beneficial for people with MS regardless of disease severity [5].

Recommendations for exercise and physical activation have been published for the physician wanting to promote this form of rehabilitation for patients with MS [5]. The more challenging task is perhaps determining the best way to approach exercise promotion in sedentary patients with MS. There is mixed evidence that physician counseling alone can improve physical activity in people without disabilities [18]; however, there are a number of strategies that may improve the effectiveness of physician counseling. These include providing a written prescription for exercise, providing intensive counseling with educational materials, scheduling follow-up visits, using telephone call reminders or interactive mail interventions, and making referrals to existing community programs for social support (eg, walking or water aerobics programs). Alternatively, referral can be made to physical or occupational therapists to initiate and monitor home- or clinic-based range of motion, conditioning, or strengthening programs. More comprehensive rehabilitation services and follow-up may be indicated for patients with multiple disabilities, comorbidities, or risk factors [17].

Patients who want to become more active may also benefit from counseling regarding the benefits of "lifestyle exercise" as illustrated by the physical activity pyramid [5]. When formal exercise programs are not feasible, patients can be encouraged to begin exercising by more fully participating in basic and advanced activities of daily living such as shopping, housework, and childcare. Those who maximize their activity at this level can be counseled to build inefficiencies into their daily life, such as parking further from the supermarket or taking stairs rather than an elevator. The next level of lifestyle exercise involves participation in active recreation such as walking, swimming, hiking, dancing, golf, or gardening. Regular lifestyle exercise is thought to preserve fitness and adaptive functioning and may be feasible for many people for whom formal exercise is not an option [5].

*Stress management*

Stress has been anecdotally linked to onset and to exacerbation of MS since the nineteenth century. Moxon's [19] 1873 case report suggested a possible association between his patient having discovered her husband involved in an extramarital affair and the onset of her MS. Charcot [20], who was the first to describe MS as we know it today, suggested that "long continued grief and vexation" may be causally linked to disease activity. More recent investigations into the relationship between stress and disease onset have proved to be inconclusive and fraught with methodological difficulties [21–23]. Although there may not be enough evidence to implicate stress as a cause of MS, several studies have found a significant relationship between stress and exacerbation of MS symptoms.

A recent study done by Buljevac et al [24] showed that the occurrence of stressful life events was associated with a doubling of the exacerbation rate during the subsequent 4 weeks. Stressful events included stress related to a holiday, illness of or problems with a close family member, job stress, financial problems, and death of a relative or friend. Another study found that 85% of MS exacerbations were associated with stressful life events in the preceding 6 weeks [25].

Data also suggest that different types of stress may have differential effects. In a prospective study done by Franklin et al [26], it appeared that the quality, as opposed to the quantity, of stressful life events was associated with acute exacerbations of MS symptoms. In this study, those who experienced qualitatively extreme stressful life events, rated by patients with respect to desirability, controllability, and impact on self-esteem, were 3.7 times more likely to suffer an exacerbation than those not exposed to such events. Those patients who experienced exacerbations, however, did not experience a greater number of stressful life events than nonexacerbating controls. Another study done retrospectively on MS patients in Israel suggested that stress may play a protective role [27]. These patients were exposed to the threat of missile attacks over a 5-week period during the Persian Gulf War and showed a significantly lower number of relapses during the 2 months following the attack compared with their frequency during the preceding 2 years. The discrepancies among these research findings typify the complex nature of stress. Further examination is necessary to elucidate the effects of different types of stress (eg, extreme versus moderate, positive versus negative, and chronic versus acute stress) on disease activity.

In addition to the potentially causal link between stress and disease activity, the disabling symptoms, unpredictable course, and lack of a cure make MS an extremely stressful condition. After adjusting for age, gender, and education, Schwartz et al [28] found that stress increased the risk of disease progression and, conversely, disease progression increased the risk of reported stress. This bidirectional relationship emphasizes the critical importance of developing stress management techniques that help patients with MS cope with the diagnosis and progression of their disease.

Stress management may be addressed as part of a total wellness approach that includes components such as exercise, recreation, meditation, relaxation, hypnosis, and cognitive restructuring. Traditionally, patients have developed these techniques on their own with input from books, tapes, lectures, and workshops. Stress management training programs may also be beneficial for those persons with MS looking for a more structured approach to learning these skills.

Stress management interventions that focus on developing the techniques of relaxation, meditation, and cognitive restructuring have been associated with positive health outcomes in persons with hypertension, heart disease, and rehabilitation patients [29–32]. In a randomized controlled trial of patients with ischemic heart disease, Ornish et al [31] found that those who received a stress management intervention significantly increased their exercise tolerance, reduced plasma lipid levels, had less frequent episodes of angina, reduced medication intake by one half, lost more weight, and were more likely to stop smoking. In a study of patients with chronic illnesses including MS, Mandel and Keller [32] found that subjects who participated in a stress management program showed a significant decrease in state anxiety and a significant decrease on a measure of somatization compared with controls. These studies suggest that stress management programs could potentially offer somatic and psychologic benefits to persons with MS. Due to the potent relationship between stress and MS, stress management interventions and methods of promoting other wellness activities must be developed further.

## Social support and coping with multiple sclerosis

Although MS is currently incurable, psychologic adjustment to its effects can be mediated by various coping strategies on the part of the individual with the disease. Two broad types of coping styles—problem-focused and emotion-focused—have been identified [33] and can be applied to the successful management of life with MS. Problem-focused coping attempts to change the effects of a potential problem by acting directly on the environment or on oneself, whereas emotion-focused coping attempts to change the internal meaning of the problem or the way in which one addresses it [34].

Problem-focused coping has been positively correlated with higher levels of psychologic adjustment and self-esteem in patients with MS [35,36], whereas several other studies [37,38] have confirmed that higher levels of psychologic distress are significantly related to emotion-focused coping. A relationship between control of the effects of the disease and coping style may be ascertained through evidence that MS patients who are currently experiencing an exacerbation tend to favor emotion-focused coping [39].

Similarly, patients with MS were found to use emotion-focused coping during times of higher uncertainty and higher perceived danger [36]. It may be that people with MS cope with the effects of their disease by using emotion-focused coping, thus allowing them to exert some perceived control over an uncontrollable disease. These emotion-focused coping strategies, such as benefit finding [40], may be especially constructive if previous attempts at problem-focused coping have proved ineffective.

Social support and the social network can be seen as integral aspects of coping from an emotion-focused and a problem-focused coping perspective. Individuals with MS may use social support to realign internal perspectives concerning the disease [41] and to address more practical concerns such as mobility and health care access. Increased social support has been shown to be correlated with increased levels of physical disability in MS patients [42,43]. In a 2004 study by Williams et al [44] that surveyed 451 veterans with MS, social support was conceptualized as constantly changing due to the influence that physical disability has on the ability to manage independently. Furthermore, social support was described as an indicator of overall health. There were some significant differences in terms of social support between married and unmarried men and women. Married men reported higher levels of all types of social support than did married women. Interestingly, low annual income (below $22,000) was related to low social support for women but not for men, with unmarried low-income women who live alone reporting the lowest levels of social support. This finding is especially relevant considering that women have been found to be more likely than men to seek social support as a proactive coping strategy [38]. These data shed light on the various circumstances that can enhance or impede social support among patients with MS and on the relative importance of social support as a coping strategy.

Given its importance to emotion-focused and problem-focused coping styles, it seems especially important to find ways to enhance social support through clinical intervention in the MS population [45]. The most useful interventions of this type feature a socially supportive environment that addresses concerns common to the experience of MS using problem-focused coping methods. Stuifbergen et al [46] described a successful wellness intervention program that used three main intervention processes: provision of accurate health knowledge within the context of MS, with an emphasis on health promotion; enhancement of self-efficacy for health behavior through performance accomplishment, vicarious experience, verbal persuasion, and emotional arousal; and individualized goal setting for health behavior change. This knowledge and goal-focused portion of the program was followed by three months of telephone support from a health care professional to encourage progress and goal attainment. The intervention resulted in improved creation and maintenance of health-promoting behaviors among women with MS. In a later randomized trial of the effectiveness of this program [47], participants agreed on the need for the combination of the educational intervention and the supportive problem-solving environment.

MS peer support groups exemplify an emotion-focused approach to social support. These groups foster mutual information sharing, sympathy, listening, and unconditional positive regard among individuals with MS. Despite the ubiquity of MS support groups, the literature is mixed regarding the helpfulness of this type of intervention. Recent research indicates that support groups are not as helpful to those who are dealing with health care access barriers or are not already in contact with health care professionals [48] and may actually be detrimental to those with better mental health functioning [49]. Intriguingly, it has been suggested that one of the main benefits of peer support groups is that of providing peer support in addition to [50,51] (or even instead of) receiving it. Schwartz and Sendor [41] found that compared with contemporaries who merely received peer support in the form of one 15-minute telephone call a month from another patient with MS, those who provided the peer support showed pronounced improvement in confidence, self-esteem, depression, and role functioning.

*Compliance with disease-modifying therapies*

Despite the consensus that disease-modifying therapies (DMTs) are effective at reducing exacerbations and disease activity, it is thought that DMTs are underused and frequently discontinued [52]. This problem presents a tremendous opportunity for health-promotion efforts that enhance compliance with DMTs. Multiple characteristics influence adherence to DMTs, including those of the patient, the disease, the treatment, and the health care provider. Important patient characteristics include injection anxiety [53], unrealistic therapeutic expectations [54], depression [54,55], and low self-efficacy [56]. Disease characteristics associated with reduced adherence are loss of feeling or numbness, perceived worsening of the disease [52,57], impaired cognition, and physical ability to perform self-injection [58].

Provider characteristics also influence adherence. Providers who demonstrate greater empathy, instill a sense of purpose, and promote less formal relationships achieve better rates of adherence to DMTs with their patients. [59]. Holland et al [60] applied the transtheoretic stages of change model [61] to the problem of nonadherence to DMTs and emphasized that different therapeutic strategies should be applied depending on whether the patient is not considering, is contemplating, or is ready to adopt the use of DMTs. Many of the principles of self-management training described previously also apply to the problem of nonadherence to DMTs, and pharmaceutical companies are offering programs that use these principles, such as training videos, toll-free help lines, and home nursing visits. Although a thorough review of the relevant adherence literature is beyond the scope of this article, it bears mentioning that specific interventions such as aggressive treatment of depression [55] and needle anxiety [53] can improve adherence.

*Diet and nutrition*

Good nutrition is among the cornerstones of health-promotion activities. Although there is no direct evidence that nutrition is involved in the etiology of MS, good nutrition can decrease the risk of developing other chronic diseases, reduce the risk of secondary conditions, and enhance quality of life [2,62]. For example, diets high in calcium and vitamin D may reduce the risk of osteoporosis, diets low in saturated fat may reduce the risk of cardiovascular disease, and maintaining an appropriate intake of calories reduces the risk of obesity. Good nutrition may also improve symptoms specific to MS such as fatigue and constipation. Furthermore, it has been suggested that certain diets may reduce the number and severity of relapses and slow down progression of the disease [63].

Examination of the relationship between nutrition and MS has focused largely on the influence of dietary fat on disease activity. In a longitudinal study of MS patients over a 34-year period, Swank and Dugan [64] found that patients who consumed a low-fat diet (<20 g/d) experienced less disability and a death rate of 31% compared with more serious disability and death rates of 79% to 81% in those who did not follow dietary recommendations. Patients in this study also appeared to be specifically intolerant to saturated animal fat. One epidemiologic study has also suggested this relationship [65] but, to date, no other trials have corroborated these findings.

Essential fatty acids (EFAs) may be an important link in our understanding of the relationship between dietary fat and MS. Poly-unsaturated fatty acids, such as those found in vegetable and fish oils, play a significant structural role in the CNS as components of brain tissue and the myelin sheath. Low levels of omega-6 and omega-3 EFAs have been demonstrated in the erythrocytes and serum of MS patients [66,67]. Furthermore, it has been shown that plasma EFA status is significantly correlated with dietary intake of EFAs in persons with MS [68]. Studies on the relationship of EFA supplements, in particular omega-3 and omega-6 polyunsaturated fatty acids, have shown mixed results. In a meta-analysis of three controlled trials, Dworkin et al [69] demonstrated that patients with minimal or no disability who received omega-6 supplements showed a smaller increase in disability than controls and that omega-6 treatment reduced the severity and duration of relapses among patients of all levels of disability. In a controlled trial by Bates et al [70], however, no significant benefit of omega-3 and omega-6 supplements was demonstrated, and only a minor trend was shown in favor of the group treated with omega-3 polyunsaturated fatty acids. Although these findings are inconclusive, a diet low in saturated fats and rich in EFAs such as those found in vegetable oils, wild game, and seafood is now recommended.

Constipation is a common MS symptom that can be successfully managed by diet. The prevalence of constipation in persons with MS ranges from 34% to 54%, which is considerably higher than the general population [71,72]. This high prevalence may be due to reduced rectal sensation, poor functioning of pelvic floor muscles, and decreased physical activity [71]. Constipation may cause considerable physical and social discomfort and can have long-term consequences such as anal fissures and hemorrhoids. Simple dietary strategies such as increasing fluid and fiber intake may effectively prevent and manage constipation and should be emphasized to those with MS.

Osteoporosis is another nutrition-related disease that is of concern for women with MS. Two studies on the eating patterns of women with MS have shown an inadequate intake of calcium [73,74]. Inadequate calcium intake and sedentary lifestyle compounded by the use of steroids among many people with MS increase the risk for osteoporosis. Supplemental calcium intake, in addition to weight-bearing exercise, is an important strategy for the prevention of osteoporosis.

A high prevalence of weight gain has been reported in persons with MS [74,75]. In a study by Hewson [75], 40% of female subjects and 44% of male subjects were considered overweight. Weight gain may have deleterious effects including increasing the risk of heart disease and decreasing mobility. Symptoms such as fatigue, muscle weakness, and balance problems make physical activity difficult for many people with MS. A decrease in physical activity reduces the amount of calories expended and caloric intake must therefore be adjusted or weight gain will occur.

Although diet therapy for the treatment of MS has shown mixed results and specific dietary guidelines for people with MS have not been established, diets lower in saturated fats and calories and high in polyunsaturated fats, fiber, and calcium are based on sound nutritional advice that is generalizable to everyone. For persons with MS, good nutritional practices may provide the added benefits of reducing disease activity and enhancing quality of life.

### Alcohol or other drug abuse

Alcohol and drug abuse should not be ignored in people with MS. In a large survey of 708 community residents with MS, 14.0% of respondents screened positive for possible alcohol abuse or dependence and 7.4% reported misusing illicit drugs or prescription medications within the previous month [76]. People who are younger and still working and those with less severe MS were more likely to report these behaviors. Alcohol and drug misuse were associated with greater depressive symptomatology. Substance abuse is particularly worrisome in this population because of the possibility that it may cause more motor and cognitive impairment in people with MS than the general population. Fortunately, most people who admitted alcohol or drug misuse were also interested in learning more about ways to stop or cut down. Health care providers should consider screening for substance abuse, especially in people with depressive symptoms, and use existing guidelines to provide brief advice to help patients stop or cut down on their use of alcohol or drugs (see http://www.niaaa.nih.gov/publications/physicn/htm for guidelines).

## Summary

Chronic diseases like MS present unique challenges and opportunities for patients and the medical care system. Patients are challenged because they are under tremendous pressure to actively engage themselves in multiple prevention, treatment, and health maintenance behaviors, often before they feel ready. Health care providers are challenged because health-promotion activities require more time, counseling skills, and organizational resources than traditional, acute medical care. Patients, clinicians, and researchers face the challenge of determining which health-promotion activities are not only supported by the evidence but also appropriate for a given patient. New models of health promotion are being developed that integrate self-help and professional help. These approaches have been applied in other chronic diseases and should be adapted and studied among people with MS.

## Acknowledgments

The authors are grateful to Chris Schwartzenberg for his editing help.

## References

[1] Holland N. Foreword. In: Kraft GH, Catanzaro M, editors. Living with multiple sclerosis: a wellness approach. New York: Demos; 1996. p. ix–x.

[2] Stuifbergen AK, Roberts GJ. Health promotion practices of women with multiple sclerosis. Arch Phys Med Rehabil 1997;78:S3–9.

[3] Lorig K. Self-management education: more than a nice extra. Med Care 2003;41:699–701.

[4] Wagner EH. Chronic disease management: what will it take to improve care for chronic illness? Eff Clin Pract 1998;1:2–4.

[5] Petajan JH, White AT. Recommendations for physical activity in patients with multiple sclerosis. Sports Med 1999;27:179–91.

[6] Sutherland G, Andersen MB. Exercise and multiple sclerosis: physiological, psychological, and quality of life issues. J Sports Med Phys Fitness 2001;41:421–32.

[7] Petajan JH, Gappmaier E, White AT, et al. Impact of aerobic training on fitness and quality of life in multiple sclerosis. Ann Neurol 1996;39:432–41.

[8] Oken BS, Kishiyama S, Zajdel D, et al. Randomized controlled trial of yoga and exercise in multiple sclerosis. Neurology 2004;62:2058–64.

[9] White AT, Wilson TE, Davis SL, et al. Effect of precooling on physical performance in multiple sclerosis. Mult Scler 2000;6:176–80.

[10] Somerset M, Campbell R, Sharp DJ, et al. What do people with MS want and expect from health-care services? Health Expect 2001;4:29–37.

[11] Blake KD, Bombardier CH, Cunniffe M, et al. Health promotion in multiple sclerosis: problems and desire for help. Paper presented at the Consortium of Multiple Sclerosis Centers. Chicago, June 6, 2002.

[12] Patti F, Ciancio MR, Cacopardo M, et al. Effects of a short outpatient rehabilitation treatment on disability of multiple sclerosis patients–a randomized controlled trial. J Neurol 2003;250:861–6.

[13] Mostert S, Kesselring J. Effects of a short-term exercise training program on aerobic fitness, fatigue, health perception and activity level of subjects with multiple sclerosis. Mult Scler 2002;8:161–8.

[14] Schulz KH, Gold SM, Witte J, et al. Impact of aerobic training on immune-endocrine parameters, neurotrophic factors, quality of life and coordinative function in multiple sclerosis. J Neurol Sci 2004;225:11–8.

[15] DeBolt LS, McCubbin JA. The effects of home-based resistance exercise on balance, power, and mobility in adults with multiple sclerosis. Arch Phys Med Rehabil 2004;85:290–7.

[16] Olgiati R, Girr A, Hugi L, et al. Respiratory muscle training in multiple sclerosis: a pilot study. Schweiz Arch Neurol Psychiatr 1989;140:46–50.

[17] Di Fabio RP, Choi T, Soderberg J, et al. Health-related quality of life for patients with progressive multiple sclerosis: influence of rehabilitation. Phys Ther 1997;77:1704–16.

[18] Eden KB, Orleans CT, Mulrow CD, et al. Does counseling by clinicians improve physical activity? A summary of the evidence for the US Preventive Services Task Force. Ann Intern Med 2002;137:208–15.

[19] Moxon W. Case of insular sclerosis of brain and spinal cord. Lancet 1873;5:261–2.

[20] Charcot J. Lectures on the diseases of the nervous system delivered at La Salpetriere [lecture delivered 1868]. London, 1877.

[21] LaRocca NG. Psychosocial factors in multiple sclerosis and the role of stress. Ann N Y Acad Sci 1984;436:435–42.

[22] Mohr DC, Goodkin DE, Bacchetti P, et al. Psychological stress and the subsequent appearance of new brain MRI lesions in MS. Neurology 2000;55:55–61.

[23] Li J, Johansen C, Bronnum-Hansen H, et al. The risk of multiple sclerosis in bereaved parents: a nationwide cohort study in Denmark. Neurology 2004;62:726–9.

[24] Buljevac D, Hop WC, Reedeker W, et al. Self reported stressful life events and exacerbations in multiple sclerosis: prospective study. BMJ 2003;327:646.

[25] Ackerman KD, Heyman R, Rabin BS, et al. Stressful life events precede exacerbations of multiple sclerosis. Psychosom Med 2002;64:916–20.

[26] Franklin GM, Nelson LM, Heaton RKB, et al. Stress and its relationships to acute exacerbations in multiple sclerosis. J Neurol Rehabil 1988;2:7–11.

[27] Nisipeanu P, Korczyn AD. Psychological stress as risk factor for exacerbations in multiple sclerosis. Neurology 1993;43:1311–2.

[28] Schwartz CE, Foley FW, Rao SM, et al. Stress and course of disease in multiple sclerosis. Behav Med 1999;25:110–6.

[29] Crowther H. Stress management training and relaxation imagery in treatment of essential hypertension. J Behav Med 1983;6:169–87.

[30] Langosch W, Seer P, Brodner G, et al. Behavior therapy with coronary heart disease patients: results of a comparative study. J Psychosom Res 1982;26:475–84.

[31] Ornish D, Scherwitz LW, Doody RS, et al. Effects of stress management training and dietary changes in treating ischemic heart disease. JAMA 1983;249:54–9.

[32] Mandel AR, Keller SM. Stress management in rehabilitation. Arch Phys Med Rehabil 1986; 67:375–9.

[33] Lazarus R, Folkmna S. Stress, appraisal, and coping. New York: Springer; 1984.

[34] Fontana A, McLaughlin M. Coping and appraisal of daily stressors predict heart rate and blood pressure levels in young women. Behav Med 1998;4:5–16.

[35] Pakenham KI. Adjustment to multiple sclerosis: application of a stress and coping model. Health Psychol 1999;18:383–92.

[36] Wineman NM, Durand EJ, Steiner RP. A comparative analysis of coping behaviors in persons with multiple sclerosis or a spinal cord injury. Res Nurs Health 1994;17: 185–94.

[37] Jean VM, Paul RH, Beatty WW. Psychological and neuropsychological predictors of coping patterns by patients with multiple sclerosis. J Clin Psychol 1999;55:21–6.

[38] McCabe MP, McKern S, McDonald E. Coping and psychological adjustment among people with multiple sclerosis. J Psychosom Res 2004;56:355–61.

[39] Warren S, Warren KG, Cockerill R. Emotional stress and coping in multiple sclerosis (MS) exacerbations. J Psychosom Res 1991;35:37–47.

[40] Mohr DC, Dick LP, Russo D, et al. The psychosocial impact of multiple sclerosis: exploring the patient's perspective. Health Psychol 1999;18:376–82.

[41] Schwartz CE, Sendor M. Helping others helps oneself: response shift effects in peer support. Soc Sci Med 1999;48:1563–75.

[42] O'Brien MT. Multiple sclerosis: the role of social support and disability. Clin Nurs Res 1993; 2:67–85.

[43] Gulick EE. Social support among persons with multiple sclerosis. Res Nurs Health 1994;17: 195–206.

[44] Williams R, Turner A, Hatzakis M, et al. Social support among veterans with multiple sclerosis. Rehabil Psychol 2004;49:106–13.

[45] Stuifbergen AK, Seraphine A, Roberts G. An explanatory model of health promotion and quality of life in chronic disabling conditions. Nurs Res 2000;49:122–9.

[46] Stuifbergen AK, Becker H, Rogers S, et al. Promoting wellness for women with multiple sclerosis. J Neurosci Nurs 1999;31:73–9.

[47] Stuifbergen AK, Becker H, Blozis S, et al. A randomized clinical trial of a wellness intervention for women with multiple sclerosis. Arch Phys Med Rehabil 2003;84:467–76.

[48] Peters TJ, Somerset M, Campbell R, et al. Variables associated with attendance at, and the perceived helpfulness of, meetings for people with multiple sclerosis. Health Soc Care Community 2003;11:19–26.

[49] Uccelli MM, Mohr LM, Battaglia MA, et al. Peer support groups in multiple sclerosis: current effectiveness and future directions. Mult Scler 2004;10:80–4.

[50] Reynolds F, Prior S. Sticking jewels in your life: exploring women's strategies for negotiating an acceptable quality of life with multiple sclerosis. Qual Health Res 2003;13:1225–51.

[51] Maton KI. Social support, organizational characteristics, psychological well-being, and group appraisal in three self-help group populations. Am J Community Psychol 1988;16: 53–77.

[52] Hadjimichael O, Vollmer T. Adherence to injection therapy in MS: patients survey. Neurology 1999;52(Suppl 2):A549.

[53] Mohr DC, Cox D, Epstein L, et al. Teaching patients to self-inject: pilot study of a treatment for injection anxiety and phobia in multiple sclerosis patients prescribed injectable medications. J Behav Ther Exp Psychiatry 2002;33:39–47.

[54] Mohr DC, Goodkin DE, Likosky W, et al. Therapeutic expectations of patients with multiple sclerosis upon initiating interferon beta-1b: relationship to adherence to treatment. Mult Scler 1996;2:222–6.

[55] Mohr DC, Goodkin DE, Likosky W, et al. Treatment of depression improves adherence to interferon beta-1b therapy for multiple sclerosis. Arch Neurol 1997;54:531–3.

[56] Fraser C, Morgante L, Hadjimichael O, et al. A prospective study of adherence to glatiramer acetate in individuals with multiple sclerosis. J Neurosci Nurs 2004;36:120–9.

[57] Mohr DC, Likosky W, Boudewyn AC, et al. Side effect profile and adherence to in the treatment of multiple sclerosis with interferon beta-1a. Mult Scler 1998;4:487–9.

[58] Holland N, Wiesel P, Cavallo P, et al. Adherence to disease-modifying therapy in multiple sclerosis: part I. Rehabil Nurs 2001;26:172–6.

[59] Mohr DC, Goodkin DE, Masuoka L, et al. Treatment adherence and patient retention in the first year of a phase-III clinical trial for the treatment of multiple sclerosis. Mult Scler 1999;5: 192–7.

[60] Holland N, Wiesel P, Cavallo P, et al. Adherence to disease-modifying therapy in multiple sclerosis: part II. Rehabil Nurs 2001;26:221–6.

[61] Prochaska JO, DiClemente CC, Norcross JC. In search of how people change. Applications to addictive behaviors. Am Psychol 1992;47:1102–14.

[62] Marge M. Health promotion for persons with disabilities: moving beyond rehabilitation. Am J Health Prom 1988;2:29–35.

[63] Swank RL. Multiple sclerosis: fat-oil relationship. Nutrition 1991;7:368–76.

[64] Swank RL, Dugan BB. Effect of low saturated fat diet in early and late cases of multiple sclerosis. Lancet 1990;336:37–9.

[65] Alter M, Yamoor M, Harshe M. Multiple sclerosis and nutrition. Arch Neurol 1974;31: 267–72.

[66] Crawford MA, Budowski P, Hassam AG. Dietary management in multiple sclerosis. Proc Nutr Soc 1979;38:373–89.

[67] Thompson RH. A biochemical approach to the problem of multiple sclerosis. Proc R Soc Med 1966;59:269–76.

[68] Fitzgerald G, Harbige LS, Forti A, et al. The effect of nutritional counseling on diet and plasma EFA status in multiple sclerosis patients over 3 years. Hum Nutr Appl Nutr 1987;41: 297–310.

[69] Dworkin RH, Bates D, Millar JH, et al. Linoleic acid and multiple sclerosis: a reanalysis of three double-blind trials. Neurology 1984;34:1441–5.

[70] Bates D, Cartlidge NEF, French JM. A double blind controlled trial of long chain n-3 polyunsaturated fatty acids in the treatment of multiple sclerosis. J Neurol Neurosurg Psychiatry 1989;52:18–22.

[71] Chia YW, Fowler CJ, Kamm MA, et al. Prevalence of bowel dysfunction in patients with multiple sclerosis and bladder dysfunction. J Neurol 1995;242:105–8.

[72] Sullivan SN, Ebers GC. Gastrointestinal dysfunction in multiple sclerosis. Gastroenterology 1983;84:1640.

[73] Stuifbergen AK, Becker H. Health promotion practices in women with multiple sclerosis: increasing quality and years of healthy life. Phys Med Rehabil Clin N Am 2001;12:9–22.

[74] Timmerman GM, Stuifbergin AK. Eating patterns in women with multiple sclerosis. J Neurosci Nurs 1999;31:152–8.

[75] Hewson DC. Is there a role for gluten-free diets in multiple sclerosis? Hum Nutr Appl Nutr 1984;38:417–20.

[76] Bombardier CH, Blake KD, Ehde DM, et al. Alcohol and drug abuse among persons with multiple sclerosis. Mult Scler 2004;10:35–40.

ELSEVIER
SAUNDERS

Phys Med Rehabil Clin N Am
16 (2005) 571–582

PHYSICAL MEDICINE
AND REHABILITATION
CLINICS OF
NORTH AMERICA

# Mitigating the Impact of Multiple Sclerosis on Employment

## Kurt L. Johnson, PhD, CRC[a,*], Robert T. Fraser, PhD[a,b]

[a]Department of Rehabilitation Medicine, Box 356490,
University of Washington School of Medicine, Seattle, WA 98195-6490, USA
[b]Department of Neurology, University of Washington School of Medicine, Seattle,
WA 98195-6490, USA

The diagnosis of multiple sclerosis (MS) is often made when people are in their mid-20s and early in their careers. At least 90% of people with MS report a history of employment [1]. According to a recent survey of 736 subjects with MS, 66% had at least a community college degree and only 2 failed to complete high school (University of Washington Rehabilitation Research and Training Center on Multiple Sclerosis, unpublished data, 2003). In contrast to what might be expected based on higher educational levels and advances in disease-modifying therapies, people with MS are unemployed at a rate of 70% to 80% 5 years after diagnosis [2]. Of those who are unemployed, approximately 40% would like to return to work [3]. Many people with MS may retire prematurely or move from higher- to lower-demand positions. These changes can have adverse economic consequences for individuals and society [4,5]. Even when compared with people who have disabilities in general or epilepsy, people with MS progress at a higher frequency and more quickly toward long-term disability and Social Security Disability Insurance (SSDI) benefits [6]. Premature retirement and unemployment for people with MS cannot be explained solely by physical disability factors. There is an interaction between physical/psychosocial disability and social program factors (health insurance, disability subsidy, social services) that contributes to employment status [7].

Physical factors that may serve as barriers to employment include limitations in mobility and dexterity, bowel and bladder dysfunction,

The authors gratefully acknowledge support from the National Institute on Disability and Rehabilitation Research grant H133B031129-4 for their work as part of the National Rehabilitation Research and Training Center on Multiple Sclerosis.

* Corresponding author.
*E-mail address:* kjohnson@u.washington.edu (K.L. Johnson).

spasticity, vision changes [7,8], and temperature intolerance [9]. Changes in cognitive status, however, appear to be salient in understanding employment status. The prevalence of cognitive changes based on neuropsychologic assessment has been estimated to range from 50% to 70% [10,11]. Cognitive deficits have been found to present more disability in the workplace for people with MS than physical disability, and people with cognitive deficits are employed at a much lower rate than those without cognitive deficits [12,13].

Fatigue, pain, and depression may also contribute to overall work-related disability. People with MS are more likely to experience depression and psychologic distress, which is often underdiagnosed and undertreated [14–16]. Similarly, most people with MS experience MS-related chronic or acute pain at some point during the course of their disease [17]. Fatigue is one of the major barriers to employment faced by people with MS. Fatigue may be acute or chronic and may exacerbate other symptoms [18,19]. Fatigue may result from sustained cognitive effort and ultimately results in reduced cognitive performance [20].

Johnson et al [21] and Yorkston et al [22] conducted qualitative interviews with 16 subjects who were employed or recently employed to understand their perspectives on the value of employment and barriers to continuing employment. Respondents indicated that there were costs and benefits to working. On the plus side, respondents highly valued employment. Working contributed to self-esteem and identity, financial security, and social interaction and helped them to focus on work activity rather than on symptoms such as pain. On the negative side, work often detracted from the energy available for activities outside of employment such as leisure and family time, and particularly in the presence of cognitive changes, work could be stressful. Several respondents indicated that they had been advised to discontinue employment by their physician to "avoid stress," but the respondents declined, observing that unemployment and poverty would also be stressful.

Johnson et al [21] found that fatigue, cognitive changes, and stress served as significant barriers and were often intertwined. Respondents reported that fatigue reduced cognitive efficiency, that thinking was fatiguing, and that dealing with cognitive changes in the workplace was very stressful. Many reported that multitasking, maintaining attention in the face of distractions and interruptions, thinking quickly, remembering, and learning new material were all difficult, and the compensatory strategies that they employed required effort and could be stressful. A significant factor in their experience of stress was related to concerns about the perspectives of coworkers and supervisors. In many instances, respondents reported that others in the workplace would overestimate the impact of cognitive and physical symptoms of MS on their ability to work and underestimate the efficacy of compensatory strategies. Respondents were very cautious about disclosing their MS status because of concerns about potential discrimination. Of equal concern was a lack of appreciation for well-intended but poorly received attempts by employers to mitigate stress or protect the employee by making unilateral decisions about the conditions of employment, such as not offering promotional opportunities.

Structured interventions to preserve employment have not been as effective as might have been anticipated. Although elements of the interventions themselves (which have included clinic-based counseling, community-based counseling and planning for disclosure and accommodation, and workplace-based accommodations) were effective, many people with MS declined to participate due to concerns about the consequences of disclosure, lack of time or energy, or other reasons [23–25]. Johnson et al [21] recommended that health care workers may be in an excellent position to provide limited advice and referral information to assist people with MS to preserve employment or to leave when continuing employment is no longer feasible or desirable.

### Accommodations for employment

Not only do many people with MS prefer to work but they also have legal protection against discrimination in employment under federal law and, in many states, local law. Under the Americans with Disabilities Act [26], if a qualified individual with a disability (ie, MS must affect one or more major life area) can perform the essential functions of the job (ie, functions that are clearly central to job) with or without accommodation and if the employer is a covered entity (ie, 15 or more employees under federal law; as few as 8 employees under some state laws), then the employer may not discriminate based on disability status and is required to provide or pay for reasonable accommodations necessary for the employee to perform the job. "Reasonable" is not defined in the law but is based on administrative regulations and case law. What is reasonable depends on the size of the employer, amount of revenue, and other factors, and reasonable accommodations cannot impose an undue hardship on the employer. From a practical perspective, large employers, including governmental agencies, have a much higher threshold for what is "reasonable" than smaller employers. It is important to note, however, that many accommodations cost nothing or are inexpensive. People with MS can seek consultation about their legal rights under the Americans with Disabilities Act from their local Disability Technical Assistance Center (http://www.adata.org/dbtac.html) or the US Department of Justice (http://www.usdoj.gov/). The following sections describe examples of workplace accommodations derived from the authors' clinical experience, reports by their research subjects and patients, and the literature. These examples are meant only to illustrate the range of potential accommodations that may be useful. Additional information on accommodations may be found at http://www.jan.wvu.edu/, and information about assistive technology accommodations may be found at http://www.abledata.com.

*Fatigue*

Severe fatigue may represent an exacerbation and require limited or extended time off from work until the exacerbation is resolved. More frequently, however, fatigue may occur spontaneously or as the workday progresses. It is useful to help patients establish patterns of their fatigue, if possible. For example, many individuals with MS report that their fatigue increases as the day progresses. In this case, an accommodation strategy might include modifying the order in which work tasks are engaged so that tasks requiring more concentration are completed earlier in the day and routine tasks are completed later on. Other accommodations might include combining the lunch and afternoon breaks and napping in the office or any other private place where a cot or floor mat could be set. Some of the authors' clients are able to refresh themselves with a 15-minute "power nap" in the office, whereas others split their day to allow them to go home for a 2-hour rest.

*Cognitive changes*

The primary objective for accommodating cognitive changes is to build into the work structure strategies and tools to compensate for cognitive deficits including memory impairment, inability to multitask, and other variations in cognitive function. Seemingly simple interventions such as reducing the clutter on the desktop or computer screen and minimizing distractions by providing a private office or privacy screen may help. Developing clear organizational routines can also be useful. People who previously had thrived on working on multiple tasks simultaneously may need to rethink their approach to work and sequence tasks instead.

Many workers make extensive use of electronic mail and other computer-related tools. One subject described being overwhelmed by "inbox chaos." Electronic mail programs can be configured to sort incoming mail into folders, color code various messages, or both, allowing the employee to increase efficiency. Calendars ranging from hardcopy day-timers to computer calendars can be very useful, allowing the employee to keep track of appointments, tasks, and to-do lists, reducing the demands on working memory. These features are also available on personal digital assistants and newer cell phones. Text pagers may be linked to computer-based calendars so that reminders are automatically sent to the text pager.

Learning new material may be difficult. For example, reviewing a legal brief, marketing plan, or operations manual may seem overwhelming. Developing strategies that employ classic study skills such as repetition, outlining the content, and highlighting key points for further review may be helpful. Some of our clients and subjects have also noted that they make voice notes using digital recorders for review before meetings.

## Heat sensitivity

People with MS can mitigate the impact of heat sensitivity on employment by limiting their trips outdoors during hotter parts of the day, by requesting control over the temperature in their work environment, and by using portable, personal air conditioning units or fans in their work areas. Some employees benefit from cooling jackets or heat extraction systems.

## Mobility

For people with mobility limitations, strategies to limit mobility demands may be useful. For example, an employee may request that the workstation be located to minimize the distance to key contact points such as other work groups, the restroom, the cafeteria, and so forth. It is also useful to reduce mobility demands associated with coming to and from work to preserve energy. For example, an individual may benefit from using a personal vehicle rather than public transportation and requesting preferential parking. For individuals who have limited endurance for walking, a powered mobility device such as a scooter or wheelchair may be used in the workplace. One of the authors' subjects was independent in mobility at home and in the community but was required to travel significant distances around a large building at work. As an accommodation, she received a powered wheel chair, which she used only at work.

## Vision

Changes in vision may be accommodated by modifying the overhead lighting or providing task lighting. Closed-circuit television devices can be used to magnify and manage print contrast to permit reading of hard-copy material. For individuals who have difficulty seeing the content on the computer screen, various screen magnification programs exist that can be enabled within the operating system or purchased separately.

## Requesting accommodations

As noted earlier, many individuals with MS are reluctant to request accommodations from their employers. They may be reluctant to acknowledge to themselves the need for accommodations or they may be concerned, perhaps legitimately, about potential changes in attitudes toward them by their employer and coworkers if they disclose their MS status. Johnson et al [21] found that respondents in their study were particularly concerned about disclosing their cognitive deficits. Many individuals with MS are able to make accommodations on their own by employing compensatory strategies; however, for some, it is necessary to make a formal request to the employer for accommodations. These requests should be made to the human resources specialist or, in larger organizations, the disability management unit.

## Disability benefits

The patient with MS, particularly the newly diagnosed, can be overwhelmed with barriers and challenges within the workplace. Some well-paid, midcareer individuals simply want to give up. The decision-making process is enhanced when patients have a clear grasp of issues surrounding disability benefits, insurance, and other variables.

### Family Medical Leave Act

The Family Medical Leave Act (FMLA) is a federal law that enables the patient to use up to 12 weeks of nonpaid medical leave over 12 months due to the disability. It can be used at one time, but this is often not the best utilization of the act. For some individuals, taking a few weeks off, then beginning to work half-time, and then increasing to three-fourths time best uses the unpaid medical leave that this act provides. Some individuals may choose to use only an hour per day of FMLA time and spread this "off work" time over a protracted period to enable them to keep their jobs. Strategies for using FMLA time depend on the unique needs of each individual. Often in larger companies, a specialist deals with FMLA. In smaller companies, the human resources personnel department representative can act as a resource.

The FMLA applies to private and public companies with 50 or more workers. It is necessary to have worked 1250 hours during the year to be eligible for FMLA, and the highest paid 10% of employees in an organization are excluded. More information can be found at http://www.dol.gov/esa/whd/fmla/.

### Short- and long-term disability insurance

Many employees have short-term and long-term disability insurance coverage. The terms of these policies vary, and it is critical that the employee understand his or her policy. Often, short-term disability policies can be invoked after sick leave has been exhausted that pay the covered employee 60% to 80% of the salary for 3 months to 2 years. If the employee has a long-term disability policy, then it would typically begin after the short-term disability benefit ended. Generally, to qualify for long-term disability, the employee must not be able to perform the functions of his or her job or a similar job due to disability. Many long-term disability policies include a vocational rehabilitation benefit that pays for services necessary to return the beneficiary to work if that is feasible.

Employees who have paid Social Security taxes for the required number of quarters may be eligible for SSDI, a federal long-term disability program. To be eligible for SSDI, the individual must be "totally disabled," which is defined as unable to perform any job in the national economy at a level that would generate "substantial and gainful activity," defined as earning more than $860 per month.

*Receiving subsidy and working*

If the patient proceeds to the point of receiving long-term medical disability, it does not necessarily mean that work is no longer an option. An existing long-term disability plan needs to be reviewed with regard to new work-attempt efforts, potential financial penalties, and so forth. Many long-term disability policies allow the recipient to earn some supplementary income without jeopardizing the benefit.

Patients on SSDI can earn up to $860 per month without having a reduction in their benefit, which can significantly improve economic well-being. Individuals on SSDI considering a return to full-time employment can use the 9-month trial work period available with SSDI to test the waters without the risk of losing their benefits. The Social Security Administration also has several work incentive programs that allow recipients to deduct the cost of various disability-related employment expenses from their total gainful earnings (eg, personal assistance or special technology such as computers and voice recognition systems). This allowable deduction permits individuals who earn more than $860 and incur disability-related expenses to remain below the income threshold and continue their benefits. Under this scenario, the beneficiary not only has increased earnings but also has access to technology and services otherwise unavailable. After 2 years, SSDI recipients are eligible for Medicare.

People with MS who are not eligible for SSDI may be eligible for supplemental security insurance (SSI), a federal welfare program. SSI has similar requirements with respect to disability status to SSDI but also requires that the recipient be poor. Generally, people seeking SSI will not have a significant employment history. SSI payments are markedly less than a person would receive under SSDI, and the provisions for earning additional income are much more restrictive, although disability-related employment expenses can be used to reduce income as described previously. Because the SSI benefit is reduced dollar for dollar by earned income, there may be significant advantages for an individual to work and yet retain eligibility for SSI. With SSI, the patient is immediately eligible for Medicaid, and after 2 years, the patient is eligible for Medicare. In addition, there is no work trial.

**Resources and programs for employment**

*State vocational rehabilitation agencies*

The federal-state vocational rehabilitation program funds vocational rehabilitation agencies in each state. These offices, divisions, or departments of vocational rehabilitation (DVR) provide services to individuals with disabilities seeking to enter or return to employment. In some states, there is a separate agency to serve people who are blind; in other states, the agencies are combined. The goal is not simply to provide the participant with employment but to maximize the fit between the individual and the job and to consider potential career development. To be eligible for DVR services, the individual must have a significant disability that interferes with employment. In some states where there is not adequate funding to serve all applicants, an order of selection has been invoked whereby applicants with the most severe disabilities receive priority for services. Many individuals with MS would fall into this highest priority because of the combination of cognitive and physical limitations. Although there is no financial-means test for eligibility, participants who have financial resources may be asked to pay for or cost-share some components of service. DVR can provide or pay for services necessary to achieve employment, including counseling, vocational assessment, assistive technology, education and training, medical services (including neuropsychologic assessment), tools and uniforms, job development and placement, job retention services, and case management. An individual who is currently employed may be eligible for DVR services if their employment status is at risk due to disability. DVR can assist the individual and employer in designing and implementing accommodations to preserve employment.

Because many people with MS are at the midcareer level, returning to formal education may not be realistic. Rather, they may find it useful to participate in a series of community job tryouts authorized under the 1993 US Department of Labor waiver. This waiver provides an individual with a disability up to 215 hours for unpaid job tryouts for vocational exploration, establishing task proficiency, training or skill building, or all of these options. DVR may pay a community rehabilitation provider to establish a tryout under this waiver, and patients with MS can determine whether they can function in a new job, what specific accommodations or additional training they may need, and most important, determine whether working is a viable option. The job site tryout time can vary from as little as 2 hours a day to a full days' work. In some cases, the time may be protracted (eg, the individual works less than a full-time day) because patients are receiving medical treatment or have other commitments. Employment liability insurance costs are typically paid by DVR or the specific providers with whom they have contracted to establish the tryout. Referral information to local vocational rehabilitation agencies may be found at http://www.jan.wvu.edu/sbses/vocrehab.htm.

*A new option: Ticket to Work*

The Social Security Administration developed the national Ticket to Work program through which an individual on Social Security subsidy is assigned a voucher that can be used by any certified employment network within a state to provide a person with job placement assistance. These employment networks can be diverse vocational service agencies or private sector businesses. All state DVR are members of employment networks.

If a patient uses Ticket to Work, he or she should make certain that the job accepted will be permanent and has adequate medical coverage. One advantage to this program is that the patient may get back onto SSDI or SSI with accompanying medical coverage if the position does not work out. Employability is then re-evaluated while subsidy and medical coverage are provided. Although this program represents a major effort on the part of the Social Security Administration to help people on subsidy re-enter employment, this voucher system of employment assistance seems to have been poorly conceptualized. The staggered payment system to reimburse the provider is particularly unattractive to community agencies, and given the economic conditions confronting states, the buy-in mechanism relative to Medicaid may not always be available, putting a prospective employee at risk if the employer does not provide health care insurance. In addition, part-time employment is not considered an outcome in this program, making it of limited value to many patients with MS, and the employment networks will not accept the cases of people seeking less than full-time work. More information on the Ticket to Work program can be found at http://www.yourtickettowork.com/program_info.

### WorkSource: a state employment agency

WorkSource state employment agencies are located in each state. They offer employers the necessary services for recruiting potential employees. Work-Source centers are often "one-stop" centers that bring together many of the services and resources needed by job seekers. These resources may include a DVR counselor, an employment specialist, a veterans specialist, and access to the Internet and electronic job boards. Job-seeking skill modules are usually available to help a patient organize a job search, develop knowledge of the job market, and so forth. Many WorkSource centers also have linkages to short-term training monies or provide individuals with computer training in Word, Excel, and other software programs that may make them more employable.

### Projects with Industry

Across the United States, there are approximately 100 Projects with Industry programs that are funded by the Rehabilitation Services Administration to meet critical job placement indices relating to the needs of people with disabilities seeking employment. Many of these programs arrange for the patient to meet with a liaison state vocational rehabilitation counselor, which in some cases, may be housed within a WorkSource center. A local provider (if available) can be identified by contacting the International Association of Business, Industry, and Rehabilitation at http://www.inabir@paltech.com.

### Internet resources

The National Multiple Sclerosis Society Web site (http://www.nationalmssociety.org/) has online programs that can be helpful for individuals dealing with employment decisions such as disclosure or accommodations. The National Epilepsy Foundation Web site (http://efa.org) has a "career search" workstation on their Web site, which is a useful tool because in addition to basic information on items such as cover letters, resumes, disclosure of disability, and so forth, it has direct links to effective job search engines for individuals with and without disability. It is literally a "one stop" shopping center for individuals conducting Web-based job searches and organizing their job search.

## Making decisions about employment

A number of costs and benefits need to be weighed by people with MS choosing to continue or discontinue employment or to pursue a new job path. Individuals who are well informed about the process and the resources available to them are more likely to make successful decisions. Vocational success takes planning and consistency. Through observing thousands of individuals work their way through vocational programs over the years, it is evident that the qualities of planning, consistently engaging with rehabilitation services, and willingness to meet with employers are a winning combination.

Health care providers and rehabilitation counselors can contribute to a successful outcome. The rehabilitation counselor is part counselor, information broker, evaluator, coach, and partner in vocational planning with the patient (to include financial considerations). In cases of greater degree of impairment (particularly cognitive), the rehabilitation counselor is required to take an increasingly active role in brokering the client to the employment community, including arranging of job-site supports.

The health care provider's role is not only to optimize medical treatment but also to consider the whole patient. Employment issues are critical to people with MS and may represent a myriad of patient strengths and limitations. It takes just a few minutes to ask about the work picture and whether patients have tried some of the strategies and resources identified in this article. When issues are identified, referrals can be made. Should a referral be made to a rehabilitation counselor or rehabilitation psychologist? Can a social worker help clarify the financial picture? Can a brief letter from the physician to the DVR clarify the extent of disability across physical and cognitive domains and improve eligibility for services? Will a letter to an employer endorsing accommodations consideration provide a patient the time to put together a plan to preserve employment? Above all, health providers should be optimistic and encouraging about the patient's vocational efforts whenever possible. Even part-time work can help maintain economic security, emotional equilibrium, and quality of life.

As Johnson et al [21] have noted, decisions to leave employment should be made deliberately. Health care workers can be particularly helpful by encouraging early and ongoing discussions about employment status. During exacerbations when patients are frightened and sick, patients should be encouraged by their health care worker to bide their time until the exacerbation has resolved before making important decisions, especially with regard to employment. Employment serves as a proxy for issues critical to patients' perceived quality of life and well-being, and MS clearly has an impact on employment. Physicians and others providing health care to people with MS should routinely ask about employment and support thoughtful decision making about employment status.

## References

[1] LaRocca NG, Hall HL. Multiple sclerosis program: a model for neuropsychiatric disorders. New Dir Ment Health Serv 1990(45):49–64.

[2] Kornblith AB, La Rocca NG, Baum HM. Employment in individuals with multiple sclerosis. Int J Rehabil Res 1986;9(2):155–65.

[3] LaRocca N, Kalb R, Scheinberg L, et al. Factors associated with unemployment of patients with multiple sclerosis. J Chronic Dis 1985;38(2):203–10.

[4] Jackson MF, Quaal C, Reeves MA. Effects of multiple sclerosis on occupational and career patterns. Axone 1991;13(1):16–27.

[5] Hassink G, Manegold U, Poser S. Early retirement and occupational rehabilitation of patients with multiple sclerosis. Rehabilitation (Stuttg) 1993;32(2):139–45.

[6] Fraser R, McMahon B, Danczy-Hawley C. Progression of disability benefits: a perspective on multiple sclerosis. J Voc Rehabil 2003;19(3):173–9.

[7] Johnson K, Amtmann D, Yorkston K, et al. Medical, psychological, social, and pro-grammatic barriers to employment for people with multiple sclerosis. J Rehabil 2004(70): 38–50.

[8] Joy JE, Johnston RB Jr. Characteristics and management of major symptoms. In: Joy JE, Johnston RB Jr, editors. Multiple sclerosis: current status and strategies for the future. Washington, DC: National Academy Press; 2001. p. 115–75.

[9] Gulick EE, Yam M, Touw MM. Work performance by persons with multiple sclerosis: conditions that impede or enable the performance of work. Int J Nurs Stud 1989;26(4): 301–11.

[10] Heaton RK, Nelson LM, Thompson DS, et al. Neuropsychological findings in relapsing-remitting and chronic-progressive multiple sclerosis. J Consult Clin Psychol 1985;53(1): 103–10.

[11] Rao SM, Leo GJ, Bernardin L, et al. Cognitive dysfunction in multiple sclerosis. I. Frequency, patterns, and prediction. Neurology 1991;41(5):685–91.

[12] Beatty WW, Blanco CR, Wilbanks SL, et al. Demographic, clinical, and cognitive characteristics of multiple sclerosis patients who continue to work. J Neurol Rehabil 1995; 9(3):167–73.

[13] Rao SM, Leo GJ, Ellington L, et al. Cognitive dysfunction in multiple sclerosis. II. Impact on employment and social functioning. Neurology 1991;41(5):692–6.

[14] Fassbender K, Schmidt R, Mossner R, et al. Mood disorders and dysfunction of the hypothalamic-pituitary-adrenal axis in multiple sclerosis: association with cerebral in-flammation. Arch Neurol 1998;55(1):66–72.

[15] Mohr DC, Goodkin DE, Likosky W, et al. Identification of Beck Depression Inventory items related to multiple sclerosis. J Behav Med 1997;20(4):407–14.

[16] Patten SB, Metz LM. Depression in multiple sclerosis. Psychother Psychosom 1997;66(6): 286–92.

[17] Maloni HW. Pain in multiple sclerosis: an overview of its nature and management. J Neurosci Nurs 2000;32(3):139–44.

[18] Hubsky EP, Sears JH. Fatigue in multiple sclerosis: guidelines for nursing care. Rehabil Nurs 1992;17(4):176–80.

[19] Krupp LB, Alvarez LA, LaRocca NG, et al. Fatigue in multiple sclerosis. Arch Neurol 1988; 45(4):435–7.
[20] Krupp LB, Elkins LE. Fatigue and declines in cognitive functioning in multiple sclerosis. Neurology 2000;55(7):934–9.
[21] Johnson KL, Yorkston KM, Klasner ER, et al. The cost and benefits of employment: a qualitative study of experiences of persons with multiple sclerosis. Arch Phys Med Rehabil 2004;85(2):201–9.
[22] Yorkston KM, Johnson K, Klasner ER, et al. Getting the work done: a qualitative study of individuals with multiple sclerosis. Disabil Rehabil 2003;25(8):369–79.
[23] Rumrill PD Jr, Steffen JM, Kaleta DA, et al. Job placement interventions for people with multiple sclerosis. Work 1996;6(3):167–75.
[24] Rumrill PD. Project alliance final performance report. New York: National Multiple Sclerosis Society; 1996.
[25] LaRocca NG, Kalb RC, Gregg K. A program to facilitate retention of employment among persons with multiple sclerosis. Work 1996;7(1):37–46.
[26] Americans with Disabilities Act. Vol 42; 1990.

ELSEVIER
SAUNDERS

Phys Med Rehabil Clin N Am
16 (2005) 583–594

PHYSICAL MEDICINE
AND REHABILITATION
CLINICS OF
NORTH AMERICA

# Taking Part in Life: Enhancing Participation in Multiple Sclerosis

Kathryn M. Yorkston, PhD, BC-NCD[a],*,
Kurt L. Johnson, PhD, CRC[b], Estelle R. Klasner, PhD[c]

[a]Division of Speech Pathology, Department of Rehabilitation Medicine, Box 356490,
University of Washington School of Medicine, Seattle, WA 98195-6490, USA
[b]Division of Rehabilitation Counseling, Department of Rehabilitation Medicine, Box 356490,
University of Washington School of Medicine, Seattle, WA 98195-6490, USA
[c]Department of Rehabilitation Medicine, University of Washington School of Medicine,
Seattle, WA 98195-6490, USA

Multiple sclerosis (MS) is a multifaceted condition that can be viewed from many perspectives. The physician may view it in terms of management of a complex and interacting set of symptoms, with the goal of reducing or eliminating these symptoms. The physical therapist or occupational therapist may view it in terms of changes in functional status, with the goal of improving function in activities of daily living (ADL). Although these perspectives are legitimate, it is clear that the individual living with MS, the insider, has a somewhat different perspective. A growing body of research focusing on the lived experience of MS suggests that goals of individuals with MS are global and personal. They include such objectives as "to fashion a life" [1] or "to craft a life" by incorporating MS into one's personal, family, and work life [2]. From the perspective of individuals living with chronic disease, focusing on symptoms or functional status alone does not adequately reflect the meaning of their experience [3]. Taking part in meaningful activities can be viewed as a common goal that is important to health care providers and to individuals living with MS.

The purpose of this article is to (1) review the literature related to the insider's experience of MS, focusing especially on taking part in valued activities; (2) suggest a model for understanding/measuring the adequacy of participation, including factors that may influence it and domains such as

---

This work was support by the National Institute of Disability and Rehabilitation Research grant H133BO31129.

* Corresponding author.

*E-mail address:* yorkston@u.washington.edu (K.M. Yorkston).

employment that are key to the construct; and (3) suggest strategies that health care providers can employ as mentors or partners in achieving the goal of full participation.

## The insider's experience

The following example illustrates the importance of recognizing various perspectives on MS. A 40-year-old woman with MS stumbles and falls at her place of work. The physician may view this scenario from the perspective of symptom management and seek information about leg strength and coordination along with complicating factors such as heat sensitivity or fatigue. The physical therapist may view this from the perspective of functional status and question whether mobility aids are needed to maintain independence. The individual with MS, on the other hand, may view this scenario from a more global and personal perspective and ask questions like What do my coworkers think of me? Should I really be working? How can I manage financially if I can no longer work? What will I do if I can no longer work? Failure to appreciate these differences in perspective may be frustrating to all involved.

The research community is beginning to appreciate the need to understand the perspective of individuals with MS who are the only true "experts" in the lived experience of MS. Qualitative studies are well suited to the study of complex phenomena that cannot easily be separated from the context in which they occur. Living with MS is certainly one of these phenomena. A number of qualitative research studies are available to examine the insider perspective [4–12].

Several themes emerged repeatedly after interviewing individuals with MS. The first was the issue of control. For many individuals, MS was viewed as a major loss of control [3]. Coping with MS involved maintaining control over the condition [13] or over certain aspects of it such as mobility [5]. The notion of control was also reflected in the desire to take charge of their lives. Participants suggested that picking and choosing activities allowed them to alter their lifestyles while maintaining control [7]. Although control was universally important, it was manifest in different ways for different individuals. For some, control meant maintaining independence, whereas for others it meant having prompt access to medical services [4]. The value of maintaining control that emerged from the qualitative research literature is consistent with quantitative studies using regression models that point toward the value of enabling autonomy and self-reliance [14]. A second theme identified by individuals living with MS was the value of participation, including taking part in meaningful social, recreational, and work activities [15]. Work is considered vital for self-esteem and self-worth [8,16]. Engaging in meaningful occupations or activities is central to achieving good quality of life and a positive self-image [6].

One of the important challenges for the field of rehabilitation in MS is capturing the perspective of the insider when measuring outcomes. Dijkers[17] makes a strong argument that the field needs to go beyond the traditional measures of function and health status that were developed in the 1970s and 1980s to capture outcomes that are meaningful to the individual living with MS. The following section defines the term *participation* and suggests that this construct may be useful in measuring client-centered outcomes in MS.

## Participation

### *Definition*

Participation, a major component of the International Classification of Function, Disability, and Health, is defined by the World Health Organization as involvement in life situations [18]. Recently, "optimal social participation" has been characterized as the absence of disruption in the accomplishment of life habits [19]. The presence of disability has been found to lead to participation that is less diverse, is restricted more to the home setting, involves fewer social relationships, and includes less active recreation [20]. Because participation reflects the consequences of all aspects of life experience of people with MS, the construct of participation is multifaceted and can only be understood if it is placed within a broad biopsychosocial framework.

For individuals with MS, participation is an outcome that reflects the influence and interaction of many factors, including the pattern and level of function and disability along with environmental and personal factors. Fig. 1 depicts a model of participation. Function and disability, environmental factors, and personal factors contribute to the level of participation. Function and disability is a domain that includes different types and levels of impairment and limitations in activity. Impairment reflects problems in body function, including physical, sensory, and cognitive changes and depression, fatigue, and pain. Limitations in activities include difficulties that an individual may have in ADL related to basic personal care (bathing, dressing, eating, grooming) or to personal business (using the telephone, shopping, food preparation, transportation). The latter activities are considered instrumental ADL [21]. Environmental factors include factors that make up the physical, social, and attitudinal environment in which people live and conduct their lives. Personal factors include the internal influences or attributes of the person, including self-efficacy and positive adaptation.

### *Factors influencing participation*

Participation is a multidimensional global construct that comprises many domains including personal and household management, leisure or

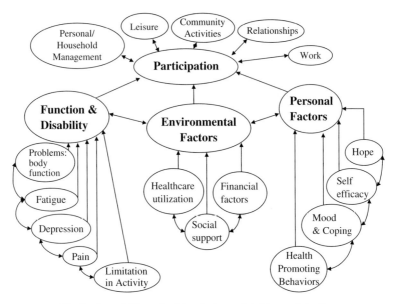

Fig. 1. A model hypothesizing factors related to participation.

recreations activities, community involvement, relationships, and work. Table 1 contains definitions and example of activities in each of these domains. These domains reflect many activities performed within the context of their social environment. Some of these activities, such as personal or household management, are not open to choice but still serve the goal of independence and survival [22]. Other activities are chosen to promote a personally important goal, such as when an individual decides to sing in the church choir or continue to work in a valued job.

*Measuring participation*

Traditionally, participation has been measured using time-use surveys or prevalence rates for certain activities [23,24]. The difficulty with these approaches is that they do not provide information about value, activity preferences, meaning, and enjoyment [20,25,26]. For example, knowing how many times per week an individual travels outside the home does not indicate whether this level of activity is acceptable to the individual. When viewed from the perspective of the individual with MS, participation can be measured by asking the question, how satisfied are you with your ability to take part in this activity? When measured in this way, participation may fall under the category of *activity-related quality of life* [27], a term referring to an assessment of quality of everyday life that includes what a person does (functional activities, community participation, and behaviors) and that individual's feelings about or appraisal of the level of participation in those activities.

Table 1
Domains related to participation

| Domain | Definition | Example |
|---|---|---|
| Personal management | Involvement in situations related to self-care or medical care | Tending to medical routines (eg, taking medicine, making appointments with doctors) |
| | | Arranging personal services (eg, making an appointment for a haircut) |
| Household management | Involvement in situations related to managing a household and those living together in it | Helping others in the household (eg, driving others, doing their laundry) |
| | | Managing finances (eg, budgeting, paying bills, doing taxes) |
| Leisure | Involvement in situations related to discretionary activities not related work or other duties (quiet or active activities) | Taking part in quiet leisure activities (eg, reading a book, watching TV, browsing the Web, playing computer games) |
| | | Taking part in active leisure activities (eg, playing sports, going to a movie or play, visiting a museum) |
| Community involvement | Situations related to community involvement (eg, civil roles, activities in the community, and moving from one place to another within the community) | Engaging in civic/community activities (eg, voting, attending Parent-Teacher Association or garden club) |
| | | Getting around the community |
| Relationships | Involvement is situations related to social roles that connect or bind participants (family, friends and romantic relationships) | Staying connected with family (eg, phoning one's parents, corresponding by written or electronic mail) |
| | | Interacting/maintaining relationships with one's children |
| Work | Involvement in situations related to paid or unpaid (volunteer) employment or school work | Working (paid employment) |
| | | Taking part in volunteer work |

## Benefits of enhanced participation

Participation is important from the perspectives of the health care provider and the individual living with MS. For the health care provider, participation represents the convergence of many factors and may be considered a "metaoutcome" of rehabilitation. Participation may be enhanced in many ways: by minimizing the impairment, by increasing performance on important activities, by providing adequate environmental support, by reducing social and environmental barriers, and by enhancing personal coping strategies. For many different groups, enhancing participation has substantial benefits. Social participation has been associated with enhanced cognition and perceived quality of life in middle-aged [28] and aging populations [29–31]. The social impact of MS on the individuals living with the condition and on the family has also been examined [32]. The ability to continue in gainful employment or to maintain social contacts and leisure activities correlates with the course and severity of MS and cognitive function. Withdrawal from social activities and a shrinking circle of friends is common among individuals with MS, especially those with severe disability. Approximately one fourth of those studied reported that they stopped visiting friends and family members because of poor mobility associated with MS, which reflects significant reduction in participation in preferred activities.

If maximizing participation is central to the field of rehabilitation and captures issues important to health care providers and to individuals living with MS, then measuring the levels of participation accurately and comprehensively is essential for setting goals, selecting and prioritizing interventions, and examining efficacy. In other words, the concept of participation should be central to the management of MS. The following section describes some strategies that may assist health care providers in maximizing participation.

## Strategies for intervention: what the physician needs to know

Thus far, this article has highlighted the importance of enhanced participation as an essential measure of outcomes in MS. Participation is critical from the perspectives of the health care provider and the individual living with MS. Developing strategies to enhance participation is a complex process that requires excellent communication between the health care provider and the client. Because the quality of this communication influences treatment outcomes, the final section of this article reviews the literature related to health care communication in MS and offers some strategies for facilitating the communication and enhancing participation.

### The insider perspective

Qualitative studies have provided insights into the preferences of individuals with MS with respect to health care decisions. It is clear from interviewing individuals with MS about health care communication that many prefer "to take charge" of their own health care. One of the primary factors contributing to this preference is that individuals with MS believe they, rather than health care providers, have the "big picture." One individual with MS summed up this attitude by saying, "The medical profession knows so little...it's been clear to me since the very beginning that [the ball] was in my court" [2]. Individuals with MS believe that health care providers have an incomplete picture of their experience. They indicate that MS is only one dimension of their existence and that managing MS health care services is only one aspect of the multiple resources that they access to help them deal with the disease itself [2].

Differences in perspective between individuals living with MS and health care providers may lead to the appearance of disagreement and may cause frustration. Studies suggest that individuals with MS and their health care providers differ in their assessment of the relative importance of different elements of quality of life [33]. For example, health care providers may focus primarily on physical disability, but those functional limitations are often not the main determinant of life satisfaction for individuals living with MS. Differences in viewpoints between health care workers and patients can lead to the notion expressed by some individuals with MS that "nobody listened" and to the failure of health care providers to inquire about experiences related to MS that are salient to the individual [7].

## Trajectory and changes over time

Health care communication related to MS is further complicated by the fact that management strategies and styles may need to change over time in response to changing severity of the condition. Critical periods include the time around the diagnosis of MS, the period of mild disability when the individual with MS is crafting a life in the context of MS, the time during acute exacerbation of symptoms, and a later period when progression is constant and the disability is increasingly severe. The literature contains studies reflecting best practices for health care communication around the time of diagnosis. During this early phase, the role of the health care provider is to listen, to believe the patients' perspective, and to provide appropriate information [34]. Health care providers need to take the patient's accounts of symptoms seriously, to provide reassurance, and to be thoughtful in presenting the "bad news" related to diagnosis.

The middle phase of management may be characterized as "taking part in life in the context of MS." Here, a partnership in decision making may be most appropriate. Thorne and colleagues [2] suggested a shift from the mentorship that was appropriate during the early phases of management to a relationship that is better described as a partnership in managing the unique manifestations of this particular disease, in this particular body, and in this particular life. During this phase, individuals with MS continue to need information. Survey data from large groups of individuals with MS reveal that information or advice about exercise is the single most requested area, followed by information about course-altering drugs. Other significant areas include sexuality, fatigue, changes in cognition, and pain [35]. Information and advice must be tailored to an individual's unique circumstances and symptoms so that they can develop strategies for living as well as possible in the context of their disease [36].

During periods of acute exacerbation of symptoms, needs shift to information about drugs, including side effects, long-term effects, and new drugs [37]. Again, individuals with MS express the preference for information that is up-to-date and personally relevant. During the advanced stages of MS, management strategies shift once more. Qualitative interviews of individuals with MS and severe disability suggest that MS becomes an all-encompassing illness resulting in substantial limitations in independence and participation [38]. The relationship with health care providers involves supportive action to enhance control over the life course and to address existential issues.

## Strategies for health care communication

Appropriate strategies for health care communication are critical for good management of any condition. These strategies are particularly important in a complex condition such as MS whereby symptoms vary across individuals and over time and environmental, social, and personal factors influence an individual's experience. The following strategies may be helpful in assisting an individual with MS to construct a life within the context of that complex condition.

### Listen to the perspective of individuals living with multiple sclerosis

Throughout this article, the perspective of the individuals living with MS has been highlighted. Respecting this perspective and acknowledging that it might be different from that of the health care provider is a major factor in establishing good health care communication. Individuals with MS are the experts in living with MS. Their past experience has taught them how to manage the condition [39]. They have set the global priorities of how they wish to craft their lives within the context of MS. Health care professionals, on the other hand, are the experts in a number of components of management of MS. They are skilled in the identification and management of symptoms. They have information about the latest developments in course-altering medication and specific techniques to improve or maintain function. Management of MS is most effective when various perspectives are identified, acknowledged, and respected as legitimate viewpoints. The role of the health care provider is to form a partnership to enhance the ability of the individual with MS to take part in activities that have personal value and meaning.

At times, it is difficult for the health care provider to relinquish the role as expert. Health care providers are often trained to accept responsibility for the complete care of the person with MS, thereby taking charge of the situation. Establishing a partnership between the individual with MS and the care provider allows them to manage difficulties together and share information on an ongoing basis and provides learning opportunities for the person with MS and the health care provider [40]. To facilitate a successful partnership, each partner needs to become aware of communication styles, boundaries, and needs. Health care providers should understand how the person with MS communicates and what style makes the person feel most comfortable. For example, some individuals overstate their symptoms and consider each one to be a crisis, whereas other individuals understate how they are feeling and often do not report serious symptoms. Health care providers need to gauge individual communication styles so that they can communicate the needed information. The individual who treats each symptom as serious requires a different communication style than the person who understates how he or she feels. The information needs of individuals with MS vary from person to person and are dictated by stage of illness. The next section addresses information needs of individuals with MS.

*Need for individualized information—more is better than less*

To make good decisions, individuals with MS must have good information. It is unfortunate that obtaining sufficiently detailed and accurate information is a challenge [2]. General information is not viewed by individuals with MS as being helpful; rather, they seek detailed, relevant information specific to their circumstances. Relevant information changes over time depending on the phase of the condition. For example, in-depth information about what to expect may be needed during the period immediately following the diagnosis. Later, such information is less useful because past experience has taught individuals with MS what to expect. During acute exacerbations, information about the costs and benefits of various drug regimes is critical. In-depth information about assistive technology may be most appropriate during the period when techniques to maintain independence are being explored. In summary, individuals with MS wish to have detailed, up-to-date, and relevant information on a just-in-time basis. Information that is too general or information that is detailed but poorly timed is not viewed as helpful. The role of the health care provider is to serve as a resource, guiding the individual with MS to the right level of information at the right time.

*Identifying the costs/benefits of activities—less is not necessarily better*

For many individuals with MS, crafting a life means taking part in valued activities despite the many barriers that may arise, including fatigue, cognitive-communication changes, limited mobility, and so on. Participants during in-depth interviews have described a process of setting priorities in the face of physical, cognitive, social, and environmental barriers along with identifying needs, resources, and strategies for accomplishing the activities [41]. They appear to develop unique and complex ways of dealing with symptoms so that they can participate in valued activities. Decisions to participate in various activities are made based on weighing the costs versus benefits of participation.

Maintaining paid employment is an excellent example of the cost-versus-benefit balance that must be achieved [16]. Employment has personal and financial benefits, and some participants view work as therapeutic. Although work is highly valued, the costs include having less time and energy for things outside work and needing to curtail other activities. Many have been given advice to "take it easy" or to do less because of MS. Such advice, although well intended, is not always consistent with the goals and preference of the individual living with MS. Making management decisions based on a careful weighing of the costs and benefits of the activity for an individual is central to health care communication in MS. For example, making decisions about whether or not to maintain employment may involve weighing many factors including the stress of the job versus the stresses of unemployment (financial considerations, lack of health care benefits, loss of professional identity, social isolations, increased focus on pain and disability). Because the costs and benefits are different for every individual, decisions are different. The role of the health care provider is to assist in reflecting on the costs and benefits of participation as a tool in decision making.

*Avoid decisions during periods of crisis*

The management of life with MS requires many decisions. These decisions are dependent on having sufficient information and weighing the balance of costs versus benefits of the various options. A partnership between the health care provider and individual with MS is clearly necessary. The final advice related to health care communication is to avoid making decisions during periods of crisis. During such periods, problem solving is less likely to be effective. For example, the timing of departure from employment is best not made during periods of exacerbation when individuals with MS may be compliant with or vulnerable to advice from experts without weighing personal factors. The best practice would be for health care providers to encourage those living with MS who are experiencing an exacerbation to wait before making important decision. Decisions should be made during periods when full resources can be devoted to reflecting on appropriate choices. Having an emergency plan in place before the crisis is an excellent way to lessen stress.

**Summary**

Health care professionals participating in rehabilitation for people with MS can play a critical role in enhancing limited outcomes such as enhanced mobility, reductions in symptoms such as pain and depression, and the metaoutcome—participation. This role will be significantly more effective if the health care professional acknowledges and validates the different perspectives of the professional and the patient and recognizes the expertise of the patient who has lived with MS in the context of his or her life. Assuming this role effectively requires that the health care professional develop a collaborative relationship with the patient and understand that the role may change depending on the stage of MS and the individual's circumstances.

## References

[1] Webster BD. All of a piece: a life with multiple sclerosis. Baltimore (MD): Johns Hopkins University Press; 1989.

[2] Thorne S, Con A, McGuinness L, et al. Health care communication issues in multiple sclerosis: an interpretative description. Qual Health Res 2004;14(1):5–22.

[3] Ironside PM, Scheckel M, Wessels C, et al. Experiencing chronic illness: cocreating new understanding. Qual Health Res 2003;13(2):171–83.

[4] Miller CM. The lived experience of relapsing multiple sclerosis: a phenomenological study. J Neurosci Nurs 1997;29(5):291–301.

[5] Finlayson M, Van Denend T. Experiencing the loss of mobility: perspectives of older adults with MS. Disabil Rehabil 2003;25(20):1168–80.

[6] Reynolds F, Prior S. Sticking jewels in your life: exploring women's strategies for negotiating an acceptable quality of life with multiple sclerosis. Qual Health Res 2003;13(9):1225–51.

[7] Courts NF, Buchanan EM, Werstlein PO. Focus groups: the lived experience of participants with multiple sclerosis. J Neurosci Nurs 2004;36(1):42–7.

[8] Stuifbergen A, Rogers S. Health promotion: an essential component of rehabilitation for persons with chronic disabling conditions. Adv Nurs Sci 1997;19(4):1–20.

[9] O'Day B. Barriers for people with multiple sclerosis who want to work: a qualitative study. J Neurol Rehabil 1998;12(3):139–46.

[10] Magnus E. Everyday occupations and the process of redefinition: a study of how meaning in occupation influences redefinition of identity in women with a disability. Scand J Occup Ther 2001;8(3):115–24.

[11] Yorkston KM, Klasner ER, Swanson KM. Communication in context: a qualitative study of the experiences of individuals with multiple sclerosis. Am J Speech-Lang Pathol 2001; 10(2):126–37.

[12] Thorne SE, Paterson BL. Two decades of insider research: what we know and don't know about chronic illness experience. Annu Rev Nurs Res 2000;18:3–25.

[13] Loveland CA. The experiences of African Americans and Euro-Americans with multiple sclerosis. Sex Disabil 1999;17(1):19–35.

[14] Somerset M, Peters TJ, Sharp DJ, et al. Factors that contribute to quality of life outcomes prioritised by people with multiple sclerosis. Qual Life Res 2003;12:21–9.

[15] Kramer AM. Rehabilitation care and outcomes from the patient's perspective. Med Care 1997;35(Suppl 6):JS48–57.

[16] Johnson K, Yorkston KM, Klasner ER, et al. The cost and benefits of employment: a qualitative study of experiences of individuals with multiple sclerosis. Arch Phys Med Rehabil 2004;85(2):201–9.

[17] Dijkers MP. Individualization in quality of life measurement: instruments and approaches. Arch Phys Med Rehabil 2003;84(4 Suppl 2):S3–15.

[18] International Classification of Function, Disability, and Health. World Health Organization. Available at: http://www3.who.int/icf/icftemplate.cfm. Accessed December 10, 2001.

[19] Desrosiers J, Noreau L, Rochette A, et al. Predictors of handicap situations following post-stroke rehabilitation. Disabil Rehabil 2002;24(15):774–85.

[20] Law M. Participation in the occupations of everyday life. Am J Occup Ther 2002;56:640–9.

[21] Bonder BR, Wagner MB. Functional performance in older adults. 2nd edition. Philadelphia: F.A. Davis; 2001.

[22] Herzog AR, Ofstedal MB, Wheeler LM. Social engagement and its relationship to health. Clin Geriatr Med 2002;18(3):593–609 [ix].

[23] Willer B, Rosenthal M, Kreutzer JS, et al. Assessment of community integration following rehabilitation for traumatic brain injury. J Head Trauma Rehabil 1993;8(2):75–87.

[24] Whiteneck GG, Charliefue SW, Gerhart KA, et al. Quantifying handicap: a new measure of long-term rehabilitation outcomes. Arch Phys Med Rehabil 1992;73:519–26.

[25] Finlayson M, Impey M, Nicolle C, et al. Self-care, productivity and leisure limitations of people with multiple sclerosis in Manitoba. Can J Occup Ther 1998;65(5):299–308.

[26] Dijkers M. Measuring the long-term outcome of traumatic brain injury: a review of the Community Integration Questionnaire. J Head Trauma Rehabil 1997;126:74–91.

[27] Johnston MV, Miklos CS. Activity-related quality of life in rehabilitation and traumatic brain injury. Arch Phys Med Rehabil 2002;83(Suppl 2):S26–38.

[28] Singh-Manoux A, Richards M, Marmot M. Leisure activities and cognitive function in middle age: evidence from the Whitehall II study. J Epidemiol 2003;57(11):907–13.

[29] Wang H, Karp A, Winblad B, et al. Late-life engagement in social and leisure activities is associated with a decreased risk of dementia: a longitudinal study for the Kungsholmen Project. Am J Epidemiol 2002;155(12):1081–7.

[30] Sorensen LV, Axelsen U, Avlund K. Social participation and functional ability from age 75 to age 80. Scand J Occup Ther 2002;92:71–8.

[31] Verghese J, Lipton RB, Katz MJ, et al. Leisure activities and the risk of dementia in the elderly. N Engl J Med 2003;348(25):2508–16.

[32] Hakim EA, Bakheit AM, Bryant TN, et al. The social impact of multiple sclerosis: a study of 305 patients and their relatives. Disabil Rehabil 2000;22(6):288–93.

[33] Rothwell PM, McDowell Z, Wong CK, et al. Doctors and patients don't agree: cross sectional study of patients' and doctors' perceptions and assessments of disability in multiple sclerosis. BMJ 1997;314:1580–3.

[34] Koopman W, Schweitzer A. The journey to multiple sclerosis: a qualitative study. J Neruosci Nurs 1999;31(1):17–25.

[35] Somerset M, Campbell R, Sharp DJ, et al. What do people with MS want and expect from health-care services? Health Expect 2001;4:29–37.

[36] Finlayson M. Concerns about the future among older adults with multiple sclerosis. Am J Occup Ther 2004;58(1):54–63.

[37] Baker LM. Sense making in multiple sclerosis: the information needs of people during an acute exacerbation. Qual Health Res 1998;8(1):106–20.

[38] Boeijue HR, Duijnstee MSH, Grypdonck MHF, et al. Encountering the downward phase: biographical work in people with multiple sclerosis living at home. Soc Sci Med 2002;55(6):881–93.

[39] Leino-Kilpi H, Luoto E, Katajisto J. Elements of empowerment and MS patients. J Neurosci Nurs 1998;30(2):116–23.

[40] Halpern SP. The etiquette of illness. New York: Bloomsbury; 2004.

[41] Yorkston KM, Johnson K, Klasner ER, et al. Getting the work done: a qualitative study of individuals with multiple sclerosis. Int J MS Care 2003;5(3):89.

ELSEVIER
SAUNDERS

Phys Med Rehabil Clin N Am
16 (2005) 595–602

PHYSICAL MEDICINE
AND REHABILITATION
CLINICS OF
NORTH AMERICA

# Index

*Note:* Page numbers of article titles are in **boldface** type.

# N

## Please Print:

Name _____

Address _____

City_____ State _____ ZIP _____

## Method of Payment

❑ Check (payable to **Elsevier**; add the applicable sales tax for your area)

❑ VISA ❑ MasterCard ❑ AmEx ❑ Bill me

Card number _____ Exp. date _____

Signature _____

Staple this to your purchase order to expedite delivery

---

**Adolescent Medicine Clinics**
- ❑ Individual $95
- ❑ Institutions $133
- ❑ *In-training $48

**Anesthesiology**
- ❑ Individual $175
- ❑ Institutions $270
- ❑ *In-training $88

**Cardiology**
- ❑ Individual $170
- ❑ Institutions $266
- ❑ *In-training $85

**Chest Medicine**
- ❑ Individual $185
- ❑ Institutions $285

**Child and Adolescent Psychiatry**
- ❑ Individual $175
- ❑ Institutions $265
- ❑ *In-training $88

**Critical Care**
- ❑ Individual $165
- ❑ Institutions $266
- ❑ *In-training $83

**Dental**
- ❑ Individual $150
- ❑ Institutions $242

**Emergency Medicine**
- ❑ Individual $170
- ❑ Institutions $263
- ❑ *In-training $85
- ❑ Send CME info

**Facial Plastic Surgery**
- ❑ Individual $199
- ❑ Institutions $300

**Foot and Ankle**
- Individual $160
- Institutions $232

**Gastroenterology**
- ❑ Individual $190
- ❑ Institutions $276

**Gastrointestinal Endoscopy**
- ❑ Individual $190
- ❑ Institutions $276

**Hand**
- ❑ Individual $205
- ❑ Institutions $319

**Heart Failure (NEW in 2005!)**
- ❑ Individual $99
- ❑ Institutions $149
- ❑ *In-training $49

**Hematology/ Oncology**
- ❑ Individual $210
- ❑ Institutions $315

**Immunology & Allergy**
- ❑ Individual $165
- ❑ Institutions $266

**Infectious Disease**
- ❑ Individual $165
- ❑ Institutions $272

**Clinics in Liver Disease**
- ❑ Individual $165
- ❑ Institutions $234

**Medical**
- ❑ Individual $140
- ❑ Institutions $244
- ❑ *In-training $70
- ❑ Send CME info

**MRI**
- ❑ Individual $190
- ❑ Institutions $290
- ❑ *In-training $95
- ❑ Send CME info

**Neuroimaging**
- ❑ Individual $190
- ❑ Institutions $290
- ❑ *In-training $95
- ❑ Send CME info

**Obstetrics & Gynecology**
- ❑ Individual $175
- ❑ Institutions $288

**Occupational and Environmental Medicine**
- ❑ Individual $120
- ❑ Institutions $166
- ❑ *In-training $60

**Ophthalmology**
- ❑ Individual $190
- ❑ Institutions $325

**Oral & Maxillofacial Surgery**
- ❑ Individual $180
- ❑ Institutions $280
- ❑ *In-training $90

**Orthopedic**
- ❑ Individual $180
- ❑ Institutions $295
- ❑ *In-training $90

**Otolaryngologic**
- ❑ Individual $199
- ❑ Institutions $350

**Pediatric**
- ❑ Individual $135
- ❑ Institutions $246
- ❑ *In-training $68
- ❑ Send CME info

**Perinatology**
- ❑ Individual $155
- ❑ Institutions $237
- ❑ *In-training $78
- ❑ Send CME info

**Plastic Surgery**
- ❑ Individual $245
- ❑ Institutions $370

**Podiatric Medicine & Surgery**
- ❑ Individual $170
- ❑ Institutions $266

**Primary Care**
- ❑ Individual $135
- ❑ Institutions $223

**Psychiatric**
- ❑ Individual $170
- ❑ Institutions $288

**Radiologic**
- ❑ Individual $220
- ❑ Institutions $331
- ❑ *In-training $110
- ❑ Send CME info

**Sports Medicine**
- ❑ Individual $180
- ❑ Institutions $277

**Surgical**
- ❑ Individual $190
- ❑ Institutions $299
- ❑ *In-training $95

**Thoracic Surgery (formerly Chest Surgery)**
- ❑ Individual $175
- ❑ Institutions $255
- ❑ *In-training $88

**Urologic**
- ❑ Individual $195
- ❑ Institutions $307
- ❑ *In-training $98
- ❑ Send CME info

---

*To receive in-training rate, orders must be accompanied by the name of affiliated institution, dates of residency and signature of coordinator on institution letterhead. Orders will be billed at the individual rate until proof of resident status is received.

*(side margin)* Order your subscription today. Simply complete and detach this card and drop it in the mail to receive the best clinical information in your field.

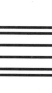

# BUSINESS REPLY MAIL

FIRST-CLASS MAIL     PERMIT NO 7135     ORLANDO FL

POSTAGE WILL BE PAID BY ADDRESSEE

PERIODICALS ORDER FULFILLMENT DEPT
ELSEVIER
6277 SEA HARBOR DR
ORLANDO FL  32821-9816